Food – biochemistry and nutritional value

Food – biochemistry and nutritional value

David S. Robinson
Procter Professor of Food Science
Procter Department of Food Science
The University of Leeds

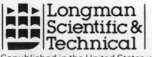
Longman
Scientific &
Technical

Copublished in the United States with
John Wiley & Sons, Inc., New York

Longman Scientific & Technical,
Longman Group UK Limited,
Longman House, Burnt Mill, Harlow,
Essex CM20 2JE, England
and Associated Companies throughout the world.

Copublished in the United States with
John Wiley & Sons, Inc., 605 Third Avenue, New York, NY 10158

First published 1987

British Library Cataloguing in Publication Data
Robinson, David S.
  Food-biochemistry and nutritional value.
  1. Food
  I. Title
  641.1   TX353
  ISBN 0-582-49506-7

Library of Congress Cataloging in Publication Data
Robinson, David S., 1935–
  Food: biochemistry and nutritional value.

  Bibliography: p.
  Includes index.
  1. Nutrition. 2. Food – Composition. I. Title.
[DNLM: 1. Biochemistry. 2. Food Analysis. 3. Nutritive
Value. QU 50 R659f]
QP141.R535 1987   641.1   86-21522
ISBN 0-470-20735-3 (Wiley, USA only)

Set in Linotron 202 10/12pt Times

Produced by Longman Group (FE) Limited
Printed in Hong Kong

Contents

Appendices   484

Preface

This text has grown out of a need by an internationally broad based industry and its graduate employees to understand the action of enzymes in foods and the variable nature and nutritive value of food ingredients. While many long, but detailed specialist texts and review articles are now available on starch, sugars, lipids, oxidative enzymes, vitamins, etc., I have attempted to condense and distil the essential information into a critical and comprehensive text devoted to the biochemistry and nutritional value of food.

A considerable proportion of food ingredients are normally available at sources distant from the consuming populations. Such foods are harvested, moved and stored wherein the quality may deteriorate due to indigenous enzyme action and infestation. The cellular control of enzymatic activity is diminished in post-harvest foods so that substrates become more readily available for hydrolysis and oxidation. The increasing production of chilled fresh foods is increasing the awareness of the ability of enzymes to discolour and taint. While many of the effects of indigenous enzymes are negative, for example the decomposition of starch catalysed by α- and β-amylases and the production of off-flavours by lipases, enzymes may also be used as processing aids. For citrus fruits, microbial nomilin acetyl lyase and limonate dehydrogenase may be used to remove bitter compounds. For fermented foods various glycolytic pathways used by microorganisms are well known, but now pre-treatment with enzymes may be used to influence the availability of substrates for subsequent microbial growth. In the future the food biochemist may be able to define desirable pathways for the production of enhanced flavour and aroma in fresh foods, chilled foods and fermented foods.

There is an increased awareness by the consumer and government that the nutritive value and composition of the diet is important for health and well-being. The relationship of diet to health is an expanding, fascinating and controversial field. The food biochemist will be able to justify to the manufacturer and consumer the optimisation of the nutrient content of foods. For example, it is now known that polyunsaturated fatty acids are required for the biosynthesis of prostaglandins, leucotrienes and thromboxanes. Linoleic and α-linolenic acids are essential dietary fatty acids, whereas the higher and more unsaturated fatty acids may all be essential metabolites. Likewise retinoic acids, which are also essential metabolites, are now known to control cell growth and cell division. The consumption of sucrose is falling and there is now dietary advice for total fat intake, cholesterol and common salt. Regulatory agencies are modifying their recommendations for the daily intake of protein, fats, mineral and vitamins by population groups and these aggregated pressures are leading the food manufacturer to re-examine his ingredients and re-evaluate his processes.

Conversely there are many misconceptions of the needs for so-called 'health foods'. However, the composition and mode of action of even dietary fibre, which is a heterogeneous mixture of polysaccharides not hydrolysed by human enzymes, is not fully understood. Furthermore, the presence of proteinase inhibitors and toxic haemagglutinins in most fresh plant foods is generally unrecognised. Digestive intolerances of substances like lactose and metabolic intolerance of galactose, as present in hydrolysed whey, are now recognisable diseases caused by deficiencies of human enzymes.

I have sought to produce a text which provides not only knowledge of the chemical structures of the main food components, but also a greater insight into the ways in which the action of enzymes change the composition, texture, nutritive values and acceptability of food. The text is suitable for B.Sc. Honours undergraduate food scientists, Mastership post-graduate taught course students who have first degrees in biological sciences, and as a reference text for research students, scientists carrying out research into the chemistry and biochemistry of food and industrialists. However, I have tried not to clutter the text with references but aimed to produce a readable but also authoritative presentation. Therefore references are given for factual data, and guidance is provided to recent review articles at the end of each chapter.

The book anticipates a basic knowledge of biochemistry. The text is wide ranging and sectionalised for carbohydrates, proteins, lipids, minor constituents and the post-harvest action of enzymes. Data for the nutritive value of foods is given where it is considered to be reliable. In the text there is no delineation into either food commodities or foods of plant and animal origin. Appendices are provided for quick reference and as an *aide-mémoire* to the well understood primary metabolic biochemical pathways; hence it has been possible to restrict the bulk of the text to the biochemistry and nutritive value of foods.

ACKNOWLEDGEMENTS

My greatest thanks go to my secretary, Mrs E. Romanec, who mastered my handwritten text and the word processor and to my wife, Audrey, for the preparation of figures and checking of proofs. I wish to thank all the following people: Dr J. W. Gramshaw, Dr P. R. Hayes, Dr J. E. McKay, Dr Kathryn M. McLellan, Mrs J. Ryley, Dr G. Stainsby and Dr B. L. Wedzicha for their evaluation and critical appraisal of the text. Also Mr J. A. Fish, Dr F. Olga Flint, Dr Patricia H. Moulding, Dr H. G. Muller and Mrs S. Salmon for providing photographic or graphic material. Dr D. H. Buss, Professor J. Edelman, Dr A. Graveland, Dr Kjell Janné, Dr B. J. Miflin and Professor W. Pilnik kindly provided useful information, often before publication. Mr A. B. Haigh and Mr D. Ohara of the University of Leeds Audio Visual Service, University Printing services and Dr M. J. W. Povey also gave valuable help. I am indebted to Mr B. Normington (Technical and Engineering Graphics, Huddersfield) for his outstanding drawings and to the authors and publishers who gave permission to copy tables and figures.

Abbreviations and Glossary of Terms

ABBREVIATIONS

Å: 1 nm = 10 ångström units
A: antigen
AB: antibody
ADP: adenosine diphosphate
ADP: glucose: adenosyl diphosphoglucose
AMP: adenosine monophosphate
ATP: adenosine triphosphate
ATPase: adenosine triphosphatase
cAMP: cyclic AMP
DE: dextrose equivalent
DGDG: diglycosyl diglyceride
DiHETE: dihydroxyeicosatetranoic acid
DHSS: Department of Health and Social Security
DMA: dimethylamine
E_0': standard oxidation reduction potential at pH 7.0
FAD: flavin adenine dinucleotide (oxidised form)
$FADH_2$: flavin adenine dinucleotide (reduced form)
FAO: Food and Agricultural Organisation
Fru$f$: fructofuranose
F-1-P: fructose-1-phosphate
F-6-P: fructose-6-phosphate
ΔG^{01}: standard free energy change at pH 7.0
Gal$p$: galactopyranose
Gal$p$A: galacturonic acid in the pyranose form
gc/ms: gas chromatography–mass spectrometry
GDP: guanosine diphosphate
Glc$p$: glucopyranose
G-6-P: glucose-6-phosphate

GMP: guanosine monophosphate
GRAS: generally recommended as safe
GSH: reduced glutathione
GSSG: oxidised glutathione
HPETE: hydroperoxyeicosatetraenoic acid
GTP: guanosine triphosphate
HPLC: high performance liquid chromatography
Ile: isoleucine
IMP: inosine monophosphate
IUB: International Union of Biochemistry
IUPAC: International Union of Pure and Applied Chemistry
JECFA: Joint Expert FAO/WHO Committee on Food Additives
K_m: Michaelis constant
MAFF: Ministry of Agriculture, Fisheries and Foods
Mb: myoglobin
MbO_2:   oxomyoglobin
MetMb: metmyoglobin
MGDG: monoglycosyl diglyceride
NAD^+:   nicotinamide adenine dinucleotide (oxidised form)
NADH: nicotinamide adenine dinucleotide (reduced form)
$NADP^+$:   nicotinamide adenine dinucleotide phosphate (oxidised
              form)
NADP: nicotinamide adenine dinucleotide phosphate (reduced form)
NAS: National Academy of Science
NOMb: nitric oxide myoglobin
NOMetMb: nitric oxide metmyoglobin
NRC: National Research Council
Pi: inorganic orthophosphate
PPi: inorganic pyrophosphate
ppm: parts per million
PQQ coenzyme: pyrroloquinoline coenzyme
RDA: recommended daily amount
Rha$p$:   rhamnopyranose
R-6-P: ribose-6-phosphate
TCA: tricarboxylic acid cycle
TMA: trimethylamine
TMAO: trimethylaminoxolate
TPP: thiamin pyrophosphate
UDP: uridine diphosphate
UDP-galactose: uridine diphosphate galactose
UDP-glucose: uridine diphosphate glucose
UMP: uridine monophosphate
UTP: uridine triphosphate
WHO: World Health Organisation
Xly$p$:   xylopyranose

GLOSSARY OF TERMS

acalins: cottonseed proteins.

actin: a globular protein (2S) which forms long linear polymers (F-actin). The globular units of F-actin interact with the myosin heads during the contraction of the muscle sarcomere.

amino acid score: ratio of the amount of amino acid in a food to that present in a reference protein.

annato: a yellow carotenoid pigment obtained from the seed pods of *Bixa orellana* used for the colouring of butter, margarine and cheese.

anomers: diastereomers differing in configuration at C-1 of the sugar pyranose and furanose rings.

carbonyl proteinase: contains carboxyl groups of Asp in the enzyme active site.

caseins: a group of phosphoproteins which interact to form suspended micelles in milk. The caseins are precipitated at acid pH values and by the action of chymosin.

cathepsins: proteinases which are contained within lysosomes.

chylomicrons: spherical droplets of emulsion with diameters $0.03\ \mu\text{m}$ to $0.06\ \mu\text{m}$.

Coberine: a palm oil product that has been interesterified to produce a solid fat with melting characteristics which resemble cocoa butter.

cocoa butter: obtained from *Theobroma cacao* as the lipid with a sharp melting point used in the manufacture of chocolate.

colipase: a protein of approximately eighty-five amino acid residues which aids the action of pancreatic lipase by absorption to emulsified oil droplets.

cyclic AMP: adenosine $3',5'$-cyclic monophosphate.

cysteine proteinases: contain a cysteine residue in the enzyme active site.

desmosine: a natural cross-link formed by the condensation of lysyl aldehydes and lysyl ε-amino groups in elastin.

dietary essential: a substance which must be present in the diet as it cannot be synthesised by living tissues.

emulsifying agents: substances that aid the suspension of either oil drops in water or water droplets in oil.

endo-enzymes: catalyse the cleavage of covalent bonds linking the residues in the central parts of polymer chains.

erucic acid: a fatty acid containing twenty-two carbon atoms with one double bond at C-13 found in some *Brassica spp*.

essential metabolite: a substance which is synthesised by living tissues and is an essential component of metabolic processes, e.g. arachidonic acid (C20 : 4).

exo-enzymes: catalyse the cleavage of covalent bonds linking the terminal residues at the ends of polymer chains.

galactosamine: 2-aminogalactose.
gelatinisation: formation of a jelly-like semi-solid material imbibing substantial amounts of water, e.g. during the swelling of starch grains.
gliadins: wheat prolamins.
glucosamine: 2-aminoglucose.
glucosinolate: thioglucoside.
glutenins: the high molecular weight prolamine polymers which are insoluble in alcohol solvents. Glutenins are cross-linked by disulphide bonds.
glycolipids: glycosyldiacylglycerols.
goitrin: 5-vinyloxazolidine-2-thione is formed from some thioglucosides present in *Brassica spp*. and may cause goitre.

hairy zones: regions of linear polymers with a number of short side chains.
hordeins: barley prolamins.

Illipe butter: naturally occurring fat obtained from *Shorea stenoptera* and resembles cocoa butter with a relatively sharp melting point.
isodesmosine: an isomeric form of desmosine.

lectins: (haemagglutinins) proteins able to cause the agglutination of red blood cells, mainly found in plant foods.
legumins: the 11S storage protein of plant seeds.
limit dextrin: the branched polysaccharide residue remaining after hydrolysis of starch or glycogen catalysed by α- and β-amylases.
lingual lipases: lipases secreted by glands at the base of the tongue.
linoleic acid: an eighteen-carbon atom n : 6 fatty acid which contains two double bonds that are methylene interrupted by one–CH_2 group.
α-linolenic acid: an eighteen-carbon atom n : 3 fatty acid which contains three double bonds that are methylene interrupted.
γ-linolenic acid: an eighteen-carbon atom n : 6 fatty acid which contains three double bonds that are methylene interrupted.
lysophospholipid: the monoacyl derivatives of sn-glycerol-3-phosphate.

menaquinones: K-vitamers synthesised by microorganisms. Prenyl derivatives of naphthaquinones.
methylene interrupted double bonds: double bonds which are not conjugated and are separated by one–CH_2 group.
monenoic acids: fatty acids which contain only one double bond.
mycoprotein: a fibrous protein food derived from *Fusarium graminearum* (Schwabe).
myofibrillar sarcomere: the basic structural unit of muscle containing

the linear actin and myosin filaments.

myosin: the main multimeric linear muscle protein containing globular heads present in the muscle sarcomere. Complexes with the protein actin to form actomyosin as the main structural element of muscle.

ovoinhibitors: inhibitors of enzymes found in the eggs of avian species.

phytic acids: phosphate esters of myoinositol.

phytoquinones: K-vitamers found in plants. Phytyl derivatives of naphthaquinones.

polymorphic: a substance which crystallises in two or more distinct forms, each of which have a different physical appearance and different melting points.

polyols: sugar alcohols such as sorbitol, mannitol, inositol, and glycerol.

polyunsaturated fatty acids: fatty acids which contain more than one double bond in the alkane chain.

prolamins: proteins which are soluble in 70 per cent (v/v) ethanol generally obtained from seeds.

resistant starch: retrograded starch which is resistant to enzymatic hydrolysis.

retinoids: chemical derivatives of vitamin A, retinal or retinoic acids.

retrogradation: re-association of amylose polymers in a starch gel. Causes loss of gel structure and solubility to form a precipitate.

rigor mortis: a stiffening of muscle which occurs after death due to the increased association of the actin and myosin filaments.

secalins: rye prolamins.

serine proteinases: contain a serine residue in the enzyme active site.

sialic acid: N-acetylneuraminic acid, an aldol addition product formed from mannosamine and pyruvic acid.

smooth zones: regions of linear polymers without side chains.

stabiliser: substances which stabilise suspensions of colloidal particles and emulsions of oil-in-aqueous phases often by a thickening of the aqueous phase.

starch blockers: substances which inhibit the hydrolysis of starch by digestive enzymes, generally inhibitors of α-amylase.

syneresis: contraction of a gel due to the exudation of fluid and association of the polymer material from within a gel.

tropomyosin: a cable-like protein which lies within the grooves or between coiled linear actin polymers.

vicilins: the 7S storage protein of plant seeds.
viscoelastic: a material which can flow like a liquid but recover its shape like a solid.
vitamers: different chemical derivatives of similar chemical composition that can substitute for a given vitamin.

water activity, a_w: the ratio between the vapour pressure of water in a solution or food and that of pure water at the same temperature.
whey: the liquid filtrate remaining after the removal of coagulated caseins during the manufacture of cheese.

zymogen: the inactive precursor of enzymes. Generally contains an extension peptide which blocks the active site of the enzyme.

Standard single letter notations and abbreviations for amino acids

A	Ala	Alanine
C	Cys	Cysteine
D	Asp	Aspartic acid
E	Glu	Glutamic acid
F	Phe	Phenylalanine
G	Gly	Glycine
H	His	Histidine
I	Ile	Isoleucine
K	Lys	Lysine
L	Leu	Leucine
M	Met	Methionine
N	Asn	Asparagine
P	Pro	Proline
Q	Gln	Glutamine
R	Arg	Arginine
S	Ser	Serine
T	Thr	Threonine
V	Val	Valine
W	Trp	Tryptophan
Y	Tyr	Tyrosine
Z	Glx	Glutamate or Glutamine
X		Undetermined

Part I
Food carbohydrates

INTRODUCTION

Historically the term 'carbohydrate' has been used to classify those substances with the empirical formula $C_n(H_2O)_n$, as the hydrates of carbon. This simple definition has been extended so that the class generally includes sugar alcohols, amino sugars, anhydro sugars and deoxy sugars. There are a substantial number of introductory texts in biochemistry, organic chemistry or food science, which list fully the very large number of structural isomers for carbohydrates that theoretically can be proposed and synthesised. However, the synthesis, properties and the chemical reactions of unusual monosaccharides are not of concern to the food scientist, the food industry, the public analyst or the consumer.

The number of naturally occurring free monosaccharides in foods is few, and is limited mainly to D-glucose, D-fructose and L-ascorbic acid. Only small amounts of D-galactose, sugar alcohols and myoinositol have been detected in foods. However, the sugar alcohols xylitol, sorbitol and mannitol, which strictly are not carbohydrates, are of increasing interest to the food scientist because of their use as humectants in intermediate moisture foods. Seeds and root crops contain a restricted number of di- and trisaccharides. The term 'oligosaccharide' is used for polymers containing less than ten monosaccharide units; polysaccharides are higher polymers and are complex gums, seaweed and bacterial mucilages, plant seed arabinans, mannans, starch, cellulose, pectins and animal glycogen. Glycoproteins which occur in plant cells and in animal foods such as milk and egg contain a small number of monosaccharide units including galactose, mannose, glucosamine and galactosomine as short oligosaccharide units. The best-known disaccharide is sucrose obtained from sugar-beet (*Beta vulgaris, var. rapa*), or from sugar-cane (*Saccharum officinarum*). The disaccharide lactose, found in animal milk, is synthesised in the mammary gland. Small amounts of maltose (the repeating disaccharide unit of starch) and cellobiose (the repeating unit of cellulose) arise from enzymatic hydrolysis of the higher polymers and are found in fruits and vegetables.

The food processor, who uses isolates of soybean or other legume seeds, is likely to be concerned with the presence of raffinose, stachyose and small amounts of other oligosaccharides in such products. D-Raffinose is found in sugar-beet – but not in sugar-cane – cereals, root crops and molasses prepared from sugar-beet. Stachyose is the only frequently occurring tetrasaccharide found in root crops and legumes. Both raffinose and stachyose are described as members of the raffinose family of sugars and are thought to cause flatulence in humans due to fermentation by intestinal microorganisms. For this reason, and also because of the availability of improved chromatographic techniques for the resolution of carbohydrates, the occurrence of the raffinose family of oligosaccharides is being increasingly investigated.

In the human diet, the main food sources of monosaccharides are honey, jam and marmalade preserves, syrups, and confectionery products. Confectionery products are characterised by the inclusion of a sweetening carbohydrate to produce products which range from boiled sweets and Turkish delight gels to cakes. Fruits and vegetables, such as bananas and potatoes, cereals and legume seeds are prime sources of starch. Canned fruits contain added syrup which may contain added glucose or glucose–fructose syrups, but in the United Kingdom the sugar content of the added syrup must consist of at least 75 per cent of sucrose. Manufactured fruit pie fillings contain fruit, sugars and, often, chemically modified starches. The total invert sugar content of tomato paste and purée represents from 50 to 65 per cent of the dry solids and for tomato ketchup from 10 to 25 per cent of the dry solids. Other dietary sources of carbohydrate, and in particular of added sucrose, include citrus and blackcurrant fruit juices, squashes and cordials, and comminuted drinks prepared from whole citrus fruits rather than from the juice itself. Minor sources of dietary carbohydrate include marzipan, with not less than 75 per cent of solid carbohydrate which is generally present as invert sugar, glucose syrup, pickles, sauces and nuts.

For polysaccharides, traditional common names are used, but the terms glucan, mannan or galactan arise from Recommendations (IUPAC–IUB 1982a, see Reference list, Ch. 1, p. 57) for the name to provide information on chemical structure. Homoglycans yield one type of monosaccharide only on hydrolysis, whereas heteroglycans yield more than one type of monosaccharide.

CHAPTER 1

Mono- and oligosaccharides in foods

MONOSACCHARIDES

Only D-glucose and D-fructose occur substantially in animal and plants as free monosaccharides. Other monosaccharides sometimes detected in plants in small amounts, such as D-galactose, D-mannose, D-xylose and D-rhamnose, may represent products from either chemical or enzymatic hydrolysis of oligosaccharides of the raffinose series of sugars or from polysaccharides such the hemicelluloses.

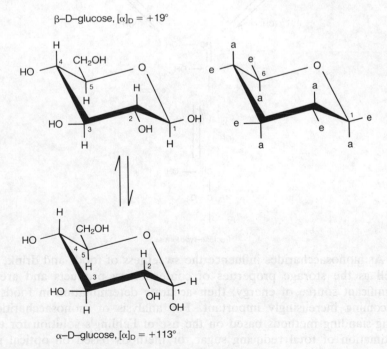

Fig. 1.1   The $^4C_1$ chair conformation of D-glucose

D-Glucose, $C_6H_{12}O_6$

At equilibrium in distilled water glucose is mainly present as a mixture of α- (36 %) and β-pyranoses (64 %) in the $^4C_1$ conformation (Fig. 1.1). X-ray and nuclear magnetic resonance studies have established for mono-, di- and polysaccharides that the pyranose rings exist in the chain conformations. The chain forms are slightly flexible and variations up to 3° in bond angles seem possible. The β-diasteromer is obtained on crystallisation from pyridine and the α-diasteromer on crystallisation from water as a monohydrate. Mutarotation is catalysed by either H^+ or OH^- ions or mutarotases. All hexose sugars, including di- and trisaccharides where the hydroxyl group on the C-1 atom remains unsubstituted, can undergo ring opening to the open chain carbonyl form and hence reduce Fehling's solution. The mechanism of the Fehling's reaction for sugars with a potentially free carbonyl group on either C-2 or C-3 involves first a base-catalysed transformation to an enediol, which is then easily oxidised to an aldonic acid.

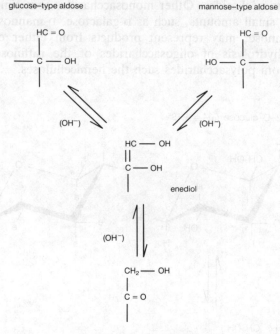

As monosaccharides influence the sweetness of foods and drink, as well as the storage properties of confectionery products and are a significant source of energy, their accurate determination in foods is becoming increasingly important. For analysis of monosaccharides, long-standing methods based on the use of Fehling's solution for the estimation of total reducing sugar, or methods based on optical rotation are still used, but owing to the presence of other unknown reducing sugars, errors may be incurred. Increasingly, instrumental techniques such as gas–liquid chromatography and high performance liquid chromatography and enzymatic assays are being introduced, particularly for quality control in the food-manufacturing industries.

Gas–liquid chromatography for the analysis of monosaccharides has proved useful, but there is a need to prepare volatile derivatives which may then require a long chromatographic time to resolve large numbers of derived anomers. Alternatively monosaccharides can be analysed after reduction and acetylation as the alditol acetates. High performance liquid chromatography (HPLC) of underivatised mono- and oligosaccharides affords a more rapid assay (15 min. per sample), but for HPLC the methods available for detection of carbohydrates are restricted to unspecific changes in refractive index. For carbohydrates there is poor absorption in the ultraviolet region. For HPLC analysis it is also necessary to prepare a clear solution which will not damage the expensive bonded phase solid supports. Nevertheless, these newer methods are more reliable than paper chromatographic procedures previously used. The results of such analyses have been published for citrus fruits, juices and other fruit products. The precise amounts of the sugars found in fruits varies considerably between cultivars and the values given in Table 1.1 are merely representative of the average amounts found. Generally, a very considerable range of values for the amounts of sugars present in different varieties of fruits at various stages of ripeness have been found. As shown in Table 1.1, while sucrose is readily hydrolysed by invertase to glucose and fructose there is no obvious arithmetic relationship for the glucose and fructose contents of the different fruits. However, generally oranges and peaches contain greater amounts of sucrose.

Table 1.1 Monosaccharides of some fruits

Fruit or fruit product	Fructose	Glucose (g/100 g)[†]	Sucrose
Pear (ripe Bartlett)	8.9	1.2	1.1
Plum, purple	3.5	3.4	2.0
Prune, Californian	16.0	23.4	—
Sweet Cherry, English	7.2	4.7	—
Blackberry, English	2.9	3.2	0.2
Peach, English	1.5	0.9	6.7
		(g/100 ml)[‡]	
Apple juice	6.4	3.1	1.1
Orange juice	3.0	2.2	5.2
Tomato juice	1.7	1.2	—

([†] Wrolstad and Schallenberger 1981; [‡] Li and Schuhmann 1983).

Although the increased interest of nutritionists in the amounts of sugars present in many products is resulting in an increased need for more accurate analyses, it is worth noting that the composition of many food materials is extremely complex and therefore the application of analytical methods to foods is far from simple. In fruit juices, preserves, soups and comminuted meat products the cellular structure of either the fruit or animal tissue has often been destroyed by pressing or homogenisation. Enzymes, previously present in discrete organelles are released, which catalyse changes in the composition of the food during storage and processing unless proper precautions are taken. Homogenisation can be carried out under refrigeration and followed quickly by pasteurisation to minimise the action of hydrolytic and even oxidative enzymes. Alternatively, for fresh juices the enzymatic catalysed changes can only be restrained by careful refrigeration.

Many of the enzymatic assays for analysis of sugars have been developed by biochemists for use with solutions of pure substrates or purified extracts. However, the application of such assay techniques to complex unfractionated foods must be treated more cautiously, with great care taken to verify the reliability of the enzymatic assays for different complex food homogenates or extracts. Fortunately such verification can often be achieved by sequential omission of individual enzymes from a multi-enzyme system for assay of sugars. Often the activity of unwanted enzymes in the food can be diminished through a short time–high temperature heat-treatment of the food homogenate before assay. Overall the main and most important advantage of enzymatic assay arises from the large number of specific analyses which can be completed quickly, but only when the validity of the method has been established for a particular food extract. Furthermore, enzymatic assays are particularly useful for estimating amounts of minor constituents as, for example, lactose in butter. Enzymatic assays are also particularly valuable for estimating in mixtures the amounts of the individual sugars – glucose (obtained from corn syrups) and sucrose and lactose which are often present in products like ice-cream. The isolation of microbial cytoplasmic membrane-bound dehydrogenases now permits more specific assays for a number of carbohydrates including lactose and cellobiose. Some of these enzymes are listed in Table 1.2 and many of the experimental details for these methods are given by Ameyama (1982). In the future hydrolases are likely to become increasingly available in very pure states, which can then be used to sequence monosaccharide residues in polysaccharide chains. Also purer glycosidases for binding to solid supports, with a high degree of substrate specificity, may become increasingly available through advances in genetic engineering.

Table 1.2 Cytoplasmic enzymes for assay of some carbohydrates †

Substrate	Enzyme/organism	Products	Electron acceptor
D-Glucose	Glucose dehydrogenase *Pseudomonas fluorescens*	δ-Lactone	Ferricyanide or 2,6-dichlorophenolindophenol‡
D-Glucose	Glucose dehydrogenase *Gluconobacter oxydans* subsp. *suboxydans*	δ-Lactone	NADP
D-Fructose	Fructose dehydrogenase *Gluconobacter oxydans* subsp. *industrius*	5-Keto-D-fructose	Ferricyanide or 2,6-dichlorophenolindophenol‡
D-Galactose	Galactose oxidase *Dactylium dendroides*	Galactose dialdehyde + H_2O_2	Oxygen
D-Galactose	Commercial galactose oxidases	Galactose dialdehyde + H_2O_2	Oxygen
D-Galactose	Galactose dehydrogenase *Pseudomonas fluorescens*	δ-1,5-Lactone, γ-1,4-Lactone or D-Galactonic acid	NAD
Hexoses Glucose Galactose Maltose Cellobiose Lactose	Hexose oxidase *Chondrus crispus* (red alga)	δ-Lactone + H_2O_2 γ-Lactone + H_2O_2	Oxygen Oxygen
D-Gluconic acid	Gluconate dehydrogenase *Pseudomonas, Klebsiella, Serratia* and *Acetobacter* spp.	2-keto-D-gluconate	Ferricyanide or 2,6-dichlorophenolindophenol‡
Cellobiose	Cellobiose dehydrogenase	Cellobionic acid	NAD, FAD
Lactose	Cellobiose dehydrogenase	Lactobionic acid	NAD, FAD

(†After Ameyama 1982).
‡ The use of 2,6-dichlorophenolindophenol is mediated by phenazine methosulphate.

Glucose oxidase (EC 1.1.3.4) β-D-glucose:oxygen-oxidoreductase

Glucose oxidase is a fungal enzyme which requires flavin adenine dinucleotide (App. I) as a hydrogen acceptor. In the absence of oxygen, reduced flavin adenine dinucleotide accumulates (Fig. 1.2) with a loss of absorbance at 377 and 455 nm. The glucose oxidase is very specific for β-D-glucose (K_m 3 × 10^{-2} M) and therefore is suitable for assay of extracts which contain in addition to glucose other reducing sugars. Generally there is sufficient mutarotation of α-D-glucose probably catalysed by contaminating aldose-1-epimerase (EC 5.1.3.3; mutarotase), for the oxidation of all the glucose to occur quickly at room temperature. The lactone product is rapidly hydrolysed to gluconic acid in aqueous solution. The amount of hydrogen peroxide formed in the presence of oxygen, can be determined through the peroxidase (EC 1.11.1.7) coupled oxidation of either o-dianisidine or 4-aminophenzone and phenol to form a dye which is measured at 460 nm, or 505 nm, respectively. Interference may be caused by the presence of other reducing agents such as ascorbic acid and glutathione or catalase which can decompose hydrogen peroxide. Other possible sources of error can arise from the presence of other FAD-dependent enzymes present in the food extract, such as D-amino acid oxidases and succinate dehydrogenase which also catalyse the reduction of oxygen to hydrogen peroxide.

$$Enz - FADH_2 + O_2 \rightleftharpoons Enz - FAD + H_2O_2$$

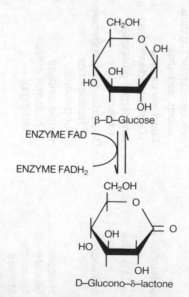

β–D–Glucose

ENZYME FAD

ENZYME FADH₂

D–Glucono–δ–lactone

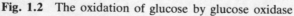

Fig. 1.2   The oxidation of glucose by glucose oxidase

However, interference by such enzymes can be detected by omission of the glucose oxidase enzyme from the assay mixture. Furthermore, such interfering enzymes as well as hydrolases and any catalase present can often be denatured by a short heat-treatment of the food extract before assay. Assays with glucose oxidase, can be used to determine the glucose content of a large number of samples and are therefore useful as screening methods to detect adulteration of foods by glucose syrups. For example, honey contains a mixture of D-glucose (approximately 32 %) and D-fructose (approximately 38 %). The presence of glucose in excess of 32 per cent on a wet weight basis for a large number of samples is readily determined with the enzymatic assay. Similarly, excess glucose for a large number of fruit juices may also be detected by enzymatic assay. Industrial use of the glucose oxidase enzyme has included both the removal of glucose from egg white before drying, in order to reduce non-enzymic browning reactions, and the removal of oxygen from packaged foods.

Glucose-6-phosphate dehydrogenase (EC 1.1.1.49)
D-glucose-6-phosphate : NADP⁺-oxidoreductase

After conversion of glucose to glucose-6-phosphate (G-6-P) by hexokinase (EC 2.7.1.1) the amount of glucose present in a food extract can be determined accurately by use of a coupled enzymatic assay using glucose-6-phosphate dehydrogenase. First, D-glucose is phosphorylated by hexokinase in the presence of adenosine-5'-triphosphate (ATP) – App. II – to form G-6-P and adenosine-5'-diphosphate (ADP).

$$\text{D–glucose + ATP} \underset{}{\overset{\text{hexokinase}}{\rightleftharpoons}} \text{G–6–P + ADP}$$

Secondly, the yeast glucose-6-phosphate dehydrogenase specifically catalyses the oxidation of G-6-P and requires nicotinamide adenine dinucleotide phosphate (NADP) – App. I – as hydrogen acceptor.

$$\text{G–6–P + NADP}^+ \underset{\text{dehydrogenase}}{\overset{\text{glucose–6–P}}{\rightleftharpoons}} \text{6–phosphogluconate + NADPH + H}^+$$

With a sufficient amount of the glucose-6-phosphate dehydrogenase present in the assay mixture, the rate of NADPH production, measured at 340 nm, is equivalent to the rate of phosphorylation of glucose and therefore the concentration of free glucose. The intermediate lactone formed is hydrolysed rapidly to 6-phosphogluconate. Possible errors can arise in a number of ways to which attention is infrequently directed: consider the sequence of the enzymic reactions in the order given above, first, product inhibition by G-6-P can reduce the activity of hexokinase and secondly, the reduction catalysed by the dehydrogenase does not easily go to completion due to inhibition by NADPH. However, both these effects can be minimised through the use of sufficient glucose-6-phosphate dehydrogenase, so that the rate of removal of G-6-P is increased. However, the presence of glucose-6-phosphatase, which may be present in foods, can also deplete the yield of G-6-P. Contamination of the assay solutions with either G-6-P, or alternative sources of G-6-P can be removed by prior incubation with glucose-6-phosphate dehydrogenase and NADP in the absence of ATP until no further absorbance increase occurs: then free glucose can be assayed by the direct addition of ATP into the test solution. Additionally, other enzymatic sources of NADPH or NADH can be detected by the omission of the glucose substrate, ATP and hexokinase. Alternatively, an observed continual decrease in absorbance at 340 nm is likely to be due to the reduction of other metabolites, such as pyruvate, oxidised glutathione. These effects can be minimised by prior heat-treatment of the extracts.

Sample calculation for the glucose content of honey

Honey (0.5 g) was diluted in water (1 litre) to give solution A. Buffer solution (pH 7.6, 2.50 ml) was placed in a dry spectrophotometer cell (1 cm path length) followed by an NADP solution (100 μl), an ATP solution (100 μl), solution A (200 μl) and 10 μl of a glucose-6-phosphate dehydrogenase preparation. The absorbance at 340 nm was then 0.040 when read against water in the reference cell. A solution of hexokinase (10 μl) was added to the cell and 15 min. later the absorbance was 0.435. When the procedure was repeated using water in place of solution A, the absorbance values were 0.030 and 0.040, respectively.

Calculate the weight of glucose present in 100 g of the honey.

The molar extinction coefficient ϵ_{340} is 6.3×10^3 mole^{-1} cm^{-1} for NADPH.

$$\text{glucose} \xrightleftharpoons[]{\text{ATP}} \text{G-6-P} \xrightleftharpoons[]{\text{NADP}^+} \text{6-phosphogluconate} + \text{NADPH} + \text{H}^+$$

The change in absorbance ($\triangle A_{340}$) for NADPH produced
= (0.435 − 0.04) minus change for water blank (0.04 − 0.03)
= 0.385
Therefore the cuvette solution contained

$\dfrac{0.385}{6.3 \times 10^3}$ moles of NADPH per litre

Therefore 1 litre of solution A (0.5 g of honey) contained

$$\frac{0.385}{6.3 \times 10^3} \times \frac{2.92}{0.2} \text{ moles of glucose}$$

(1 mole of G-6-P reduces 1 mole of NADP to NADPH)
Therefore 100 g of honey contained

$$\frac{0.385}{6.3 \times 10^3} \times \frac{2.92}{0.2} \times \frac{100}{0.5} \text{ moles of glucose}$$

= 0.178 moles of glucose
= 32.04 g of glucose

For a number of hexoses, as referred to above, alternative enzymatic assays have been developed which are based on the oxidation of free unphosphorylated hexoses. The assays can be linked to the electron transport chain in microbial cytoplasmic membranes constituting an oxidase system, where either potassium ferricyanide or 2,6-dichlorophenolindophenol can be used as terminal electron acceptors. Potassium ferricyanide is frequently employed, because of its simplicity for routine estimations, and the velocity of oxidation is determined from the rate of reduction of ferricyanide to ferrocyanide. For determination of D-glucose, the microbial enzyme β-D-glucose dehydrogenase (EC 1.1.1.47) is obtained from *Gluconobacter* or *Pseudomanas spp.* (Table 1.2).

The microbial glucose dehydrogenase does not catalyse the oxidation of fructose and only shows oxidation rates of 13, 6.5, 3.2 per cent towards D-xylose, D-galactose and maltose, respectivaly. Mutarotases (aldose-1-epimerase, EC 5.1.3.3) may be required continuously to convert all the glucose to the β-anomer. The reaction is initiated by the separate addition of the ferricyanide reagent and the reaction rate can be measured by following the reduction of ferricyanide at 420 nm. Trace amounts of glucose (2 nmole) are best determined after termination of the enzyme-catalysed oxidation. The ferrocyanide formed is determined by the addition of a ferric sulphate–Dupenol reagent and measurement of the Prussian blue colour at 660 nm.

$$\text{D-glucose} + 2 \text{ Fe(CN)}_6^{3-} \underset{\text{dehydrogenase}}{\overset{\text{glucose}}{\rightleftarrows}} \text{D-glucono-δ-lactone} + 2 \text{ Fe(CN)}_6^{4-} + 2\text{H}$$

D-fructose, D-gluconic acid and aliphatic aldehydes (Table 1.2) can also be assayed with microbial cytoplasmic membrane dehydrogenases. When oxygen is the electron acceptor, as for hexose and galactose oxidases, the peroxidase-coupled assay with *o*-dianisidine can be utilised. When NAD$^+$ is electron acceptor it is important to establish the absence of NADH oxidases in the food extracts and the samples of enzymes used, by means of separate test additions of NADH.

D-fructose, $C_6H_{12}O_6$

Fructose is a 2-ketohexose, which in the crystalline state and at equilibrium in distilled water exists mainly in the more stable β-pyranose form which is responsible for sweetness. Fructose is the sweetest natural sugar (Table 1.5). Therefore mixtures of the ketohexose with synthetic sweeteners may permit a reduction in energy intake of the order of 70 per cent in beverages, while still maintaining a high soluble solids content and a low water activity. Fructose reduces Fehling's solution via the enediol rearrangement which results in the formation CuI and D-gluconic acid. It is more easily degraded than glucose with acids, but can be a better non-enzymic browning agent than other reducing sugars with amino acids. Fructose is metabolised independently of insulin in the liver and hence is useful for diabetic foods. It is absorbed slowly from the intestine into the blood supply and has little effect on insulin release in man.

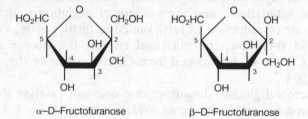

α–D–Fructofuranose   β–D–Fructofuranose

Fig. 1.3 The chemical structure of fructose

Free fructose, together with glucose and sucrose, is found in fruits and honey and can exist in solution in the furanose conformation. Fructose is a component of short chain oligosaccharides and in particular of the raffinose family of sugars. Fructose is also the main constituent of some polysaccharides (fructans) such as inulin found in many plant tubers. In foods, fructose is always found in the presence of other optically active and Fehling's-reducing carbohydrates and therefore the traditional chemical methods for the specific analysis of fructose are cumbersome. Alternatively, enzymatic assays make use of the action of hexokinase, which catalyses the phosphorylation of the 2-ketohexose to D-fructose-6-phosphate (F-6-P).

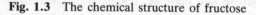

$$\text{D–fructose} + \text{ATP} \xrightleftharpoons[\quad]{\text{hexokinase}} \text{F–6–P} + \text{ADP}$$

Then through the use of glucose-6-phosphate isomerase (EC 5.3.1.9) as a second enzyme, F-6-P is isomerised to G-6-P which is then determined by the glucose-6-phosphate dehydrogenase – NADP assay. Any glucose initially present can be estimated separately with glucose-6-phosphate dehydrogenase prior to the isomerisation step. However,

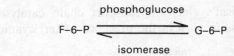

$$\text{F-6-P} \underset{\text{isomerase}}{\overset{\text{phosphoglucose}}{\rightleftharpoons}} \text{G-6-P}$$

to date the enzymic assay of fructose is unfortunately dependent on the use of the non-specific hexokinase which is able to catalyse the phosphorylation of D-glucose, D-mannose and D-glucosamine. Nevertheless, the use of more specific fructokinases, or those hexokinases with lower K_m values for fructose, could improve the specificity of the enzymic assay for fructose. Various enzymatic reactions which lead to G-6-P are shown in Fig. 1.4. Additionally, the presence of other enzymes in the food extract, such as invertase or phosphatases and other kinases, together with phosphorylated sugars can give false results for the assay of fructose. However, appropriate procedures can be carried out to check for false results: the presence of F-6-P can be detected in the absence of either hexokinase or ATP (reaction E-1); interference by glucose can be detected in the absence of phosphoglucose isomerase (reaction E-4); other sources of NADPH or NADH which will increase the absorbance at 340 nm can be detected by addition to the food extract of only NADP or only NAD (reaction E-2); the activity of contaminating enzymes in the extract may be reduced by heat-treatment.

A more specific and separate assay for fructose uses a microbial cytoplasmic membrane, fructose dehydrogenase obtained from *Gluconobacter spp*. This microbial cytoplasmic enzyme which is linked

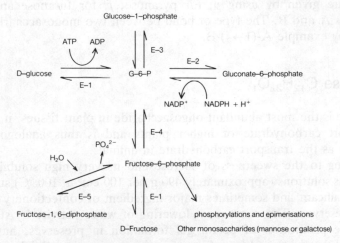

Fig. 1.4 Enzymic reactions leading to D-glucose-6-phosphate
E-1 hexokinase (EC 2.7.1.1)
E-2 glucose-6-phosphate dehydrogenase (EC 1.1.1.49)
E-3 phosphoglucomutase (EC 2.7.5.5)
E-4 glucose-6-phosphate isomerase (EC 5.3.1.9)
E-5 fructose-1, 6-diphosphatase (EC 3.1.3.11)

to the microorganism's electron transport chain catalyses only the oxidation of fructose *in vitro* in the presence of ferricyanide.

$$\text{D-fructose} + 2\,[\text{Fe(CN)}_6]^{3-} \underset{\text{dehydrogenase}}{\overset{\text{fructose}}{\rightleftharpoons}} \text{5-ketofructose} + 2\,[\text{Fe(CN)}_6]^{4-} + 2\text{H}^+$$

The concentration of fructose can be measured by either the initial reaction rate or end-point methods (App. VII). The reaction is unaffected by the presence of other sugars such as glucose, F-6-P, G-1-P, D-gluconate or mannose. Therefore the enzyme is particularly valuable for the direct assay of samples of foods containing fructose in the presence of other sugars. However, again, overestimates may be obtained in the presence of invertase which catalyses the hydrolysis of sucrose and some other fructan oligosaccharides.

DISACCHARIDES

Nomenclature

The chemical structures of disaccharides, and small oligosaccharides, are frequently written in an abbreviated form using a series of symbols. Common sugars are designated by the first three letters. These are based on the IUPAC–IUB (1982b). Ring size and anomeric configuration are given by using *p*, for pyranose; *f*, for furanose and the symbols A and B. The type of bond between two monosaccharides is given by example A-(1→4)-B.

Sucrose $C_{12}H_{22}O_{11}$

Sucrose is the most abundant oligosaccharide in plant tissues, it is the transport carbohydrate of higher plants and is thus analogous to glucose as the transport carbohydrate in animals.

Owing to the sweetness of sucrose and its very high solubility in aqueous solutions (approximately 490 g per 100 cm^3 at 100 °C) sucrose is a significant and sometimes major ingredient of confectionery foods and preserves. The consequent lowering of water activity by sucrose and the promotion of pectin gel formation in preserves, have all ensured the continued use of sucrose as a preservative. Fondants with a low moisture content of from 10 to 12 per cent are sucrose syrups containing added glucose to reduce the crystallisation of sucrose. Sucrose is an added substrate for microorganisms in fermented sausages. Commercially sucrose is readily available in a crystalline state (crystallite size 300 μm) and a separate microcrystalline powder

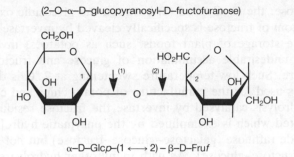

Fig. 1.5 The chemical structure of sucrose

which has a larger surface area for adsorption of colours and flavours which can be dissolved very quickly is available. Caramel is obtained by heating concentrated solutions of sucrose.

In the disaccharide molecule (Fig. 1.5) the anomeric hydroxyl groups of each monosaccharide unit are involved in the 1→2 glycosidic bond and thus the disaccharide is non-reducing. Sucrose is easily hydrolysed by dilute acids, and thus by the relatively small quantities of acid present in citrus and soft fruit preserves. The ease of hydrolysis is due to the planar structure of the furanose ring, and is characteristic of furanoid oligosaccharides and the fructan polysaccharide inulin. The mixture of glucose and fructose produced by hydrolysis of sucrose is known as invert sugar. Invert sugar can be manufactured by the invertase-catalysed process which requires 0.15 per cent (w/v) invertase at 60 °C for 8 hours. Alternatively, the acid process requires a pH value of 2.15 obtained by the addition of 0.1 per cent HCl for 2 hours at 71 °C. For the manufacture of soft-centred chocolates, added invertase catalyses the degradation of the solid sucrose paste after solidification of an outer chocolate coating. The ease of hydrolysis in dilute acids is used to advantage by the food industry during the manufacture of desserts, preserves and boiled sweets, where the presence of from 10 to 15 per cent of invert sugar prevents the crystallisation of sucrose.

Isomaltulose (6-O-α-D-glucopyranosyl-D-fructofuranose), produced by isomerisation of sucrose by a number of microorganisms, and its reduced derivatives have been suggested as alternatives to sucrose. These derivatives of sucrose are non-cariogenic.

Invertase (EC 3.2.1.26) β-D-fructofuranoside fructohydrolase

Yeast invertase was one of the first enzymes discovered and is responsible, together with sucrose synthetase in living plants, for the hydrolysis of sucrose: the O–C bond (2) between the glycosidic oxygen atom and C-2 atom of fructose is specifically cleaved by invertase (Fig. 1.5). During the storage of plant foods, such as potatoes, invertase can cause the undesirable accumulation of glucose and fructose at low temperature. Such low-temperature sweetening at 2 °C is detrimental in potatoes used for the manufacture of potato chips and crisps.

For hydrolysis catalysed by invertase the fructose residue must be unsubstituted which is exemplified by the enzymatic hydrolysis of the trisaccharide raffinose (galactose–glucose–fructose) but not melezitose (glucose–fructose–glucose). As with many other hydrolyase enzymes, in the presence of high concentrations of substrate, a transferase-catalysed reaction may be observed – where fructose residues are transferred to other molecules of either sucrose or the hydrolysis products, glucose and fructose. Such transferase activity may be significant during the commercial manufacture of concentrated glucose–fructose syrups, but is less important in enzymatic assays where the concentration of the sugars is much lower. The extracellular yeast invertases are glycoproteins of high molecular weight containing up to 50 per cent of carbohydrate and are relatively resistant to heat denaturation. Also, further increased thermostability can be achieved by coupling to solid dextran supports, although for the latter modification the K_m values are generally increased due to the restricted access of substrate to the enzyme.

Some invertases are claimed to be activated by inorganic phosphate or Group I metals. Also a proteinaceous invertase inhibitor is claimed to be active in potatoes at 10 °C, but not at 5 °C where cold sweetening can take place. High concentrations of sucrose required in confectionery products also inhibit yeast invertase.

Other sources of invertase include bacteria such as *Streptococcus mutans*, which can be responsible for tooth decay, and *Bacillus subtilis*. Acid and alkaline invertases are present in higher plants such as sugar-cane where the action of the enzymes reduce the yield of sucrose.

α-Glucosidase (EC 3.2.1.20), α-D-glucoside glucohydrolase

α-Glucosidase is present in all plant tissues and was originally called maltase because of its use in the brewing industry. Unlike invertase, α-glucosidase catalyses cleavage of the C_1–O bond (1) of the glucose moiety of the α,1→2 glycosidic bond in sucrose (Fig. 1.5). The site of action of either α-glucosidase or β-fructofuranosidase can be established by the use of isotopically labelled ^{18}O water. α-Glucosidase catalyses the hydrolysis of maltose or other small oligosaccharides containing D-glucose α,1→4 linked residues at the non-reducing end of the molecule. Consequently, for specific hydrolysis of sucrose invertase is preferred, as the enzyme only acts on oligosaccharides which contain the fructose residue in the β-furanose form.

Numerous α-glucosidases have been described for fungi, bacteria, animals and plants. The most extensively studied enzyme is from malted barley, which also shows transglycosylase activity that can result in the synthesis of maltotriose from maltose. Galactose and xylose can also act as acceptor molecules. Thus the transglycosylation reaction, which results from competition between water and sugar molecules, is likely to restrict the commercial use of the soluble enzyme for production of glucose syrups where the concentration of reactants and products is high in static solutions; however, the use of the more expensive α-glucosidases bound to solid supports may minimise transglycosylation reactions. Erythritol and D-glucono-δ-lactone are inhibitors of barley invertase.

Sucrose cannot be assayed directly as an appropriate oxidising enzyme has not been found. Consequently, estimation of the amount of sucrose present in foods such as fruit juices, sweetened milks, chocolate or preserves depends on prior enzymatic-catalysed hydrolysis to form glucose. Such glucose, produced by inversion catalysed by β-fructofuranosidase, can be determined through either the use of the coupled hexokinase and glucose-6-phosphate dehydrogenase or glucose oxidase-catalysed reactions. The amount of free glucose originally present in the food extract is estimated prior to the enzyme-catalysed hydrolysis with β-fructofuranosidase. Alternatively, large amounts of free glucose can be removed by prior oxidation with glucose oxidase; the liberated hydrogen peroxide is easily removed by the action of catalase. Both glucose oxidase and catalase used for such pre-treatment of the food extract can be deactivated by heat-treatment before estimation of sucrose. The fructose produced by the action of invertase can also be assayed directly using the cytoplasmic membrane-bound fructose dehydrogenase from *Gluconobacter oxydans* subsp. *industrius*, although this enzyme has not been widely used in the food industry or associated analytical laboratories.

The analysis of mixtures of glucose, fructose and sucrose has been of paramount importance for establishing the authenticity and quality of natural honey, where the amount of fructose always exceeds the glucose content (Table 1.3). It is essential to maintain a need for authentic honey as pollination of important crops is dependent on the honey-bee. One of the main changes that occurs during the conversion of nectar to honey is evaporation of water to less than 20 per cent. During this period, and later, a number of different enzyme-catalysed reactions that require nectar invertase and honey-bee α-glucosidase, take place and result in the production of substantially glucose and fructose together with small amounts of a large number of di- and trisaccharides (Table 1.11). The deliberate addition to honey of extra

Table 1.3 The average composition of
honey

Substrate	Composition (%)
Water	17.2
Fructose	38.2
Glucose	31.3
Sucrose	1.3
Maltose	7.3
Oligosaccharides	1.5

(Doner 1977).

glucose or sucrose to achieve the required sugar solids content is indicated by a positive optical rotation. However, the adulteration of honey with high fructose–glucose syrups prepared commercially by the action of glucose isomerase on glucose syrup is more difficult to ascertain. Resort to pollen counts or chromatographic analysis of adventitious oligosaccharides is then necessary to test the authenticity of honey. Also a more complicated definitive test based on $^{13}C/^{12}C$ isotope ratios has been proposed (White and Doner 1978), as the carbon isotopes in carbon dioxide are separated less during photosynthesis in corn and sugar-cane (C-4 plants). Thus starch and sucrose obtained from these C-4 plants contain a greater abundance of the ^{13}C isotope. The use of glucose syrup in jams is indicated when the

Table 1.4 The sugar content of selected food materials

Food	Sucrose (%)	Invert sugar (%)
Golden syrups[†]	32	48
Golden syrups[‡]		
acid converted (DE 55)[§¶]	—	
acid/enzyme (DE 70)	—	
enzyme converted (DE 65)	—	
Honey	1.3	—
Jam	25–30	20–40
Diabetic jam (containing 60–65 % sorbitol)	—	2–4
Maple syrup[‡]	83	—

([†] Egan *et al*. 1981; [‡] Howling 1979; [§] Doner and Hicks 1982).
[¶] Dextrose equivalent (DE): The DE value of a solution is the equivalent concentration of D-glucose measured by the reduction of Cu^{2+} to Cu^+ expressed as a percentage on a dry weight basis. A DE 45 syrup contains 45 per cent of reducing sugars expressed as equivalents of glucose on a dry weight basis. Therefore, the DE value for anhydrous glucose is 100 and for unhydrolysed starch is zero.

optical rotation is positive, but here the use of such syrups is beneficial to the manufacturers of jam at lower temperatures in vacuum pans where inversion of added sucrose is much reduced. The sugar content of some sucrose-derived products is given in Table 1.4.

Maple syrup, manufactured from the sap of *Acer saccharum* or *A. nigram*, contains mainly sucrose (Table 1.4). The smaller amounts of glucose and fructose found in maple syrups are believed to be formed during evaporation of the sap which is originally mainly free of hexoses, although small amounts of galactose, pentoses and oligosaccharides are present in maple syrup. Adulteration with cane sugar can be detected by the isotope ratio method as the sugars in pure maple syrup contain approximately 24 per cent of ^{13}C (Carro *et al.* 1980).

For commercial purposes sucrose is extracted from sugar-cane (*Saccharum officinarum*), and sugar-beet (*Beta* var. *rapa*). Sugar-cane, a C-4 plant grown in subtropical countries, yields a juice which contains up to 23 per cent of sucrose, whereas sugar-beet grown in temperate climates such as Northern Europe gives a juice which contains up to only 15 per cent sucrose. Crude extracts of sugar-beet can be readily distinguished from sugar-cane due to the occurrence of the trisaccharide, raffinose, only in *Beta vulgaris*, var. *rapa*. Purification of the juice requires the removal of gums and waxes which are adsorbed to a calcium carbonate precipitate obtained by bubbling of carbon dioxide. Subsequent filtration and decolorisation are with charcoal, and after evaporation at reduced pressure granulated sugar is obtained by crystallisation. Golden syrup is manufactured from the

Glucose (%)	Fructose (%)	Other oligosaccharides (%)
—	—	
31	—	59
43	—	57
34	—	66
31	38	9
4	3	—

Table 1.5 The relative sweetness of sugars[†]

Sugar	Relative sweetness
Sucrose	100
Fructose	180
Glucose	70
Galactose	32
Maltose	32
Lactose	32
Lactulose[‡]	55

(Mäkinen and Söderling 1980).

[†] The relative sweetness of various sugars is a function of concentration. Consequently the literature values vary slightly.

[‡] Lactulose is prepared by the alkaline isomerisation of D-lactose.

remaining supernatant liquor, after partial hydrolysis with dilute sulphuric acid and neutralisation with calcium carbonate. The syrup containing sucrose (30 %) and invert sugar (45 %) is obtained by concentrating under reduced pressure.

The relative sweetness of sucrose and other common sugars is given in Table 1.5. As fructose is almost twice as sweet as sucrose a considerable amount of development work has been directed towards the economic production of fructose as a substitute sweetener for sucrose. The preference for sweet substances is not restricted to man, nor is the sweet reaction restricted to mono- and oligosaccharides. Other sweeteners are cyclamates, aspartame and the protein thaumatin. The recognition of sweetness in mammals resides in the structure of the taste buds. For sweet molecules, including the dipeptide ester aspartame, it has been postulated, based on the shapes of a series of 'sweet' molecules, that bonding of the molecule to the taste bud receptor site is due to two hydrogen bonds and a third hydrophobic site. Molecular models for the sweet receptor site have to take into account the recognition of many different substances such as leucine, aspartame and saccharin in addition to carbohydrates. The biochemistry of the interaction of the sweet molecule with a taste bud receptor site, presumably on a taste bud membrane protein, is probably the initial step for recognition of sweetness. The further physiological mechanism by which different molecules are distinguished and provide the nervous stimulus is unknown.

It is likely that sucrose is formed during the low-temperature sweetening of potatoes which is then hydrolysed by invertase to produce fructose and glucose. It is suggested by Ap Rees *et al.* (1981) that the primary biochemical pathway of the synthesis of sucrose during the cold sweetening of potatoes requires the enzyme-catalysed hydrolysis of starch to form hexose phosphates which are then converted to sucrose phosphate through the action of sucrose phosphate synthase (EC 2.4.1.14). Sucrose phosphatase (EC 3.1.3.24) would then be responsible for the liberation of free sucrose.

$$\text{UDP--glucose} + \text{F--6--P} \underset{}{\overset{\text{sucrose phosphate}}{\underset{\text{synthase}}{\rightleftharpoons}}} \text{sucrose--6--phosphate} + \text{UDP}$$

$$\text{H}_2\text{O} + \text{Sucrose--6--phosphate} \underset{\text{phosphatase}}{\overset{\text{sucrose}}{\rightleftharpoons}} \text{sucrose} + \text{phosphate}$$

$$\text{H}_2\text{O} + \text{Sucrose} \overset{\text{invertase}}{\rightleftharpoons} \text{glucose} + \text{fructose}$$

However, the removal of fructose as the 'cold-sweetening' agent can be induced by raising the environmental temperature from 2 to 10 °C which causes sucrose and starch synthesis.

Lactose $C_{12}H_{22}O_{11}$

The structural formula for lactose shows the presence of a β-glycosidic link between the anomeric carbon atom of galactose and the C-4 atom of the glucose residue (Fig. 1.6). The hydroxyl group on the C-1 atom of the glucose residue remains unsubstituted: thus mutarotation can occur and lactose reduces Fehling's solution. Lactose is not as readily hydrolysed by acid as sucrose, due to the absence of a furanose ring. Lactose is less sweet than the two constituent monosaccharides and affords a means of supplying a significant source of energy-yielding carbohydrate to the suckling animal without imparting excessive sweetness. In humans, lactose acts as a mild laxative where its digestion is lower than that of sucrose. Lactose is synthesised, in the mammary

4–O–β–D–galactopyranosyl–D–glucopyranose

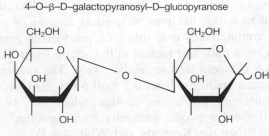

β–D–Gal*p*–(1 → 4)–D–Glc*p*

Fig. 1.6 The chemical structure of lactose

Table 1.6 Lactose content of some
mammalian milks

Mammal	Carbohydrate (%)
Cow	4.8
Human	7.0
Sheep	4.5
Goat	4.7
Reindeer	2.4
Buffalo, Indian	4.8
Camel	5.0
Horse	6.6
Llama	5.3

(With permission from T. H. Nickerson 1974).

Table 1.7 Lactose content of some milk products

Milk product	Lactose (%)	Water (%)
Skimmed milk	5.1	90.5
Cream (18 % fat)	4.1	74.5
(36 % fat)	3.3	58.0
Dried whole milk	38	2
Dried skimmed milk	53	2
Sweetened condensed milk		
(c. 43 % sucrose)	11.4	26.5
Yoghurt	4.6	86
Butter	0.18–0.4	16

(Bell and Whittier 1965).

glands of mammals from UDP-galactose and N-acetylglucosamine, by
the enzyme N-acetyllactosamine synthase (EC 2.4.1.90). In the presence of the milk protein, lactalbumin, the synthase is modified to
produce lactose instead of N-acetyllactosamine. The lactose content of
some mammalian milks, likely to be used as sources of human food,
and for some commercially available milk products is given in Tables
1.6 and 1.7. Cow's milk and human milk contain from 4.5 to 5.5 and
from 5.5 to 8.0 per cent lactose, respectively. The mammalian milks
also contain small amounts, from 0.3 to 0.6 per cent of tri- to hexa-
saccharides containing the lactose residue, which may be responsible
for passing on species-specific immunity to some infectious diseases
from parent to offspring (Kennedy and White 1983).

Commercially lactose is isolated from whey, which contains approximately 4.7 per cent lactose and up to 5 million tons of this disaccharide

are available annually. For the manufacture of 1 kg of cheese, 10 litres of milk are required leaving approximately 9 litres of whey. Unfortunately dried whey contains approximately 70 per cent lactose and thus has a high dietary energy value. Lactose crystallises in two forms, namely the stable α-hydrate and the β-anhydride. The solubility of lactose at 0 °C is very low (<5 g per 100 g of water) and large crystals of α-hydrate (approximately 10 μm) cause sandiness in products such as ice-cream and sweetened condensed milk. To prevent the formation of large α-crystals due to slow nucleation, such products can be seeded with very small crystals of lactose. At low-moisture values (<8 %) lactose exists as a viscous concentrate in spray-dried milk. However, if the moisture content is allowed to increase α-lactose crystals may form. Alternatively, lactose can be hydrolysed to the constituent monosaccharides by β-galactosidase, but the dietary energy value of the food product remains high.

(β-Galactosidase) (EC 3.2.1.23) β-D-galactoside galactohydrolase

The enzyme, sometimes known as lactase, catalyses the hydrolysis of lactose for yeasts, bacteria and fungi and is found in the intestines of young mammals. The most widely used industrial enzyme is obtained from *Kluyveromyces lactis*. The enzyme is also synthesised by *Streptococcus lactis* and *Lactobacillus bulgaricus* which are used in cheese and yoghurt manufacture, respectively. The yeast and bacterial enzymes show maximal activity at neutral pH values, whereas the fungal enzymes from *Aspergillus niger*, described as acid lactases, show optimal enzymatic activity over the range pH 3.5 to 5.5. Owing to its low pH optimum the fungal lactase is preferred for removal of lactose from acid whey where the lower pH value restricts the growth of unwanted microorganisms. Therefore the acid lactases are the most suitable for immobilisation and the enzyme is stable up to 65 °C. The neutral lactases are more suitable for the hydrolysis of lactose in whole milk at a pH value of 6.8, but then greater care is needed to restrict the growth of microorganisms. Alternatively, the enzyme can be added aseptically to pasteurised milk during packaging. Galactosidases, like other glycosidases, can exhibit glycosyl transferase activity at high substrate concentrations, which results in the formation of new oligosaccharides, like allolactose (6-O-β-D-galactopyranosyl-D-glucopyranose). The advantages gained by the hydrolysis of lactose in milk products include increased sweetness, with a consequent reduced requirement for additional carbohydrate, and the absence of crystallisation of lactose in frozen products. In ice-cream at least 20 per cent of the sucrose can be replaced by hydrolysed lactose syrups. Lactase can also be used to remove lactose from milk concentrates, where the disaccharide may cause aggregation of caseins during freezing. For fermented products the monosaccharides produced through the action of lactase are readily available carbon sources for a number of micro-organisms and therefore use of the enzyme will permit the use of lactase-deficient microorganisms for the manufacture of new products. The cheese-ripening process is also accelerated through the use of lactase and if hydrolysed whey syrup is added to yoghurt, pre-evaporation in order to concentrate the raw milk may no longer be necessary. Neutral lactase-treated milk is available for populations where lactose intolerance may frequently occur.

Galactose dehydrogenase (EC 1.1.1.48)

The most common enzymatic method for the estimation of lactose first requires hydrolysis of the disaccharide by β-galactosidase to the constituent monosaccharides followed by the estimation of the released galactose. The liberated galactose is assayed with galactose dehydro-genase and the increase in absorbance due to the formation of NADH is measured at 340 nm. Alternatively, the liberated glucose can be assayed using hexokinase and glucose-6-phosphate dehydrogenase.

$$\text{D–galactose} + \text{NAD}^+ \xrightleftharpoons[\text{dehydrogenase}]{\text{galactose}} \text{D–galactono–δ–lactone} + \text{NADH}$$

The D-galactono-1,5-lactone can rearrange to the 1,4-1actone and both are readily hydrolysed to D-galactonic acid. During the analysis obvious sources of error may arise from the presence of other NAD-dependent enzymes such as lactate dehydrogenase. Also β-galactosidases with high glycosyl transferase activity will reduce the yield of galactose and therefore the apparent lactose content of the analyte. Alternatively, other sources of galactose may arise from naturally occurring galactose-containing oligosaccharides, such as raffinose and stachyose through the action of any contaminating α-galactosidase. As with other NAD-linked enzymatic assays NADH oxidases should be absent from the test solutions. It is claimed that L-arabinose is also oxidised by galactose dehydrogenase, which there-fore indicates that the configuration of the hydroxyl group on the C-4 atom of D-galactose is important for recognition of the substrate by the dehydrogenase enzyme.

Galactose oxidase (EC 1.1.3.9)

This copper-dependent enzyme can be extracted from the fungus

Dactylium dendroides. Galactose oxidase is quite specific for the oxidation of the primary hydroxyl group at the C-6 atom of α-D-galactose. Oxygen acts as the electron acceptor.

$$\text{D-galactose} + O_2 \underset{\text{oxidase}}{\overset{\text{galactose}}{\rightleftharpoons}} \text{D-galactohexodialdo-1,5-pyranose} + H_2O_2$$

Through racemisation an equimolar mixture of the two enantiomers (D- and L-forms) of the oxidised galactose is produced. For measurements of the rate of reaction with either an oxygen electrode or by spectrophotometry, the test solutions and enzyme preparations used must be free of catalase. The hydrogen peroxide liberated can be determined by use of a coupled peroxidase assay. As with the assay of glucose which uses the corresponding glucose oxidase, deleterious effects may arise due to the destructive action of hydrogen peroxide on the assaying enzyme. Further, some of the chromogens or their oxidised products may inhibit galactose oxidase or peroxidase.

Cellobiose dehydrogenase (EC 1.1.5.1)

Lactose is oxidised through the action of cellobiose dehydrogenase (Ayers and Eriksson 1982) to lactobionic acid (Fig. 1.7). Potentially this is a most useful enzyme, as the amount of lactose in a food extract might be assayed directly without interference from glucose, which may be naturally present in samples. The enzymatic reaction is terminated by the addition of periodate in sulphuric acid which then oxidises lactobionic acid to glyoxylic acid and excess periodic acid can be destroyed by ethylene glycol. Addition of L-lactate dehydrogenase (EC 1.1.1.27) and NADH reduces glyoxylate to glycolate and therefore the amount of lactose originally present in the test solution can be related to a decrease in absorbance at 340 nm.

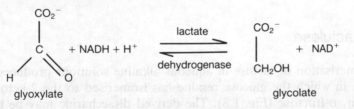

Possible errors might arise from either the oxidation by periodate of α-hydroxy acids, such as aldonic acids, present in foods to produce glyoxylic acid, or through the action of other NADH-dependent dehydrogenases to form NAD^+. Cellobiose is also oxidised by the enzyme, but is unlikely to be present in milk-based products. For this enzyme there may be other potential uses for removing lactose from milk powders and whey products with a resultant nutritional benefit,

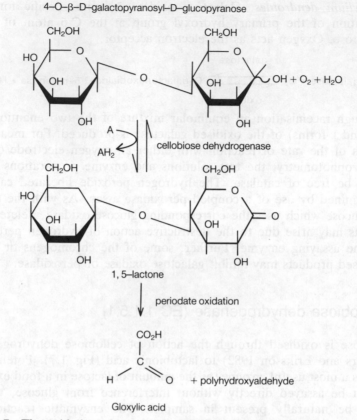

Fig. 1.7 The oxidation of lactose by cellobiose dehydrogenase

but the mode of action of the enzyme is not fully understood and the reactive superoxide anion (O_2^-) may be one of the products (Ayers and Eriksson 1982).

D-Lactulose

Isomerisation of lactose in aqueous alkaline solutions produces lactulose in which the glucose residue has isomerised to the 2-ketohexose form, D-fructose (Fig. 1.8). The derived disaccharide may be present in heat-processed milk products and is claimed to be beneficial for infant foods due to enhancement of a *Lactobacillus bifidus* flora in the intestine. Hicks *et al.* (1984) have described a process for conversion of up to 80 per cent of whey lactose to lactulose. However, lactulose is not hydrolysed by the mammalian enzymes, β-galactoxidase and invertase, but is hydrolysed by the enzymes of *E. coli* and therefore is possibly fermented in the large intestine. Consequently, as for other

(4–O–β–D–galactopyranosyl–D–fructofuranose)

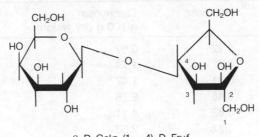

β–D–Gal*p*–(1 → 4)–D–Fru*f*

Fig. 1.8 The chemical structure of lactulose

such non-digestible carbohydrates which can later be fermented by gut microorganisms, flatulence may be enhanced.

HIGHER OLIGOSACCHARIDES

Raffinose series of sugars

Whereas only two disacchaarides are known for animals, namely lactose for mammals and α, α-trehalose for insects (Fig. 1.9), plants contain significant amounts of various tri- and tetrasaccharides. Many of these are stored in individual organs and separate organelles. In plants, the oligosaccharides are stored in the vacuoles, whereas starch is accumulated in the chloroplasts and soluble glucan polymers in the plastids. It has been claimed that greater amounts of the di- and trisaccharides accumulate in these organelles during cold stress, where they may serve as cryoprotectants. However, only small quantities of some of the oligosaccharides have been found.

α, α–Trehalose

(1–O–α–D–glucopyranosyl–D–glucopyranose)

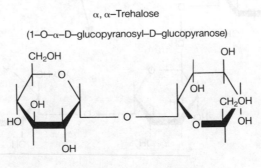

α–D–Glc*p*–(1 ⟷ 1)–α–D–Glc*p*

Fig. 1.9   The chemical structure of trehalose

Table 1.8 The raffinose series of sugars in legume flours

Legume	Raffinose	Stachyose g/100 g dry weight	Verbascose
Fababean	0.22	0.67	1.45
Field pea	0.6	1.71	2.30
Lentil	0.31	1.47	0.47
Lima bean	0.46	2.76	0.31
Lupin	0.82	4.11	0.48
Navy bean	0.37	2.36	0.05
Soybean	1.15	2.85	—

(Soluski, *et al.* 1982).

To date no significant commercial use has been made of the raffinose series of sugars, although substantial quantities of the trisaccharide raffinose and related oligosaccharides are available as by-products, after both the isolation of sucrose from sugar-beet and gluten from wheat flour. As raffinose and the tetrasaccharide stachyose are claimed to be responsible for digestive abnormalities such as flatulence, which is often associated with the ingestion of plant foods like soybean flour and soybean concentrates, knowledge of the origin and occurrence of the trisaccharides and other closely related substances belonging to the so-called raffinose family is important. For soybean the amounts of raffinose and stachyose (Table 1.8), can represent 16 per cent of the total soluble carbohydrate.

The trisaccharide raffinose is composed of a sucrose moiety and an additional residue of α-D-galactose (Fig. 1.10). Stachyose which is

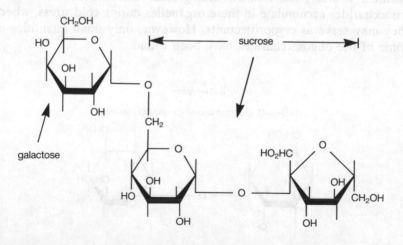

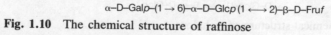

α–D–Gal*p*–(1 → 6)–α–D–Glc*p* (1 ⟷ 2)–β–D–Fru*f*

Fig. 1.10 The chemical structure of raffinose

Table 1.9 The ratio of galactose and fructose residues in the raffinose ascending series of sugars

Oligosaccharide	Galactose : fructose
Sucrose	0
Raffinose	1 : 1
Stachyose	2 : 1
Verbascose	3 : 1
Ajugose	4 : 1

often the most significant oligosaccharide present in storage organs is almost as widely found as raffinose in plants. The tetrasaccharide molecule contains another additional D-galactose residue which is linked through an α-1,6-glycosidic bond to the C-6 atom of the galactose residue of raffinose (Table 1.9): the terminal galactose residue in stachyose as in raffinose, is also therefore non-reducing. Stachyose has the structure of α-D-Galp-(1→6)-α-D-Galp-(1→6)-α-D-Glcp-(1→2)-β-D-Fruf. When raffinose is found in high concentrations it is nearly always, and certainly should be assumed, to be accompanied by stachyose. Also there may be traces of the higher homologues, verbascose and ajugose, which contain an additional one and two residues of α-(1→6) linked α-D-galactose, respectively.

Treatment of any of the oligosaccharides with α-D-galactosidase (EC 3.2.1.22) causes the release of galactose:

a–galactosidase

$$\text{raffinose} + \text{H}_2\text{O} \rightleftharpoons \text{sucrose} + \text{galactose}$$

In germinating beans, naturally occurring α-galactosidases catalyse the hydrolysis of stachyose to raffinose, sucrose and galactose, so that a mixture of α-D-galactose oligosaccharides, sucrose and free galactose is found in germinating beans. Commercially, α-D-galactosidase, free of invertase, has been used for increasing the yield of crystalline sucrose from sugar-beet. Raffinose also reduces the crystallisation of sucrose and may accumulate in molasses to concentrations of from 7 to 8 per cent. Raffinose is also hydrolysed by β-fructofuranosidase as the fructose residue of the trisaccharide occupies a terminal position in the molecule. Hence the presence of sucrose and other fructosides will interfere with any assay for raffinose based on the use of invertase. However, the galactose : fructose ratio should provide a guide to the amounts of raffinose-type oligosaccharides present in a plant food product. The theoretical molar ratio for galactose to fructose for the different α-galactosyl oligosaccharides derived from sucrose is given in Table 1.9.

The enzyme α-D-galactosidase is not synthesised by man and it is widely accepted that such oligosaccharides are fermented in the colon by colonic microorganisms such as *Clostridium perfringens*. However, the oligosaccharides which are water soluble can be removed from food ingredients by washing, aided by enzymatic treatment with either α-D-galactosidase or invertase. In the traditional preparation of oriental foods such as tempeh and soy sauce, the oligosaccharides seem to be hydrolysed during the fermentation process.

Umbelliferose (α-D-Gal*p*-(1→2)-α-D-Glc*p*-(1→2)-β-D-Fru*f*) which is a galactosyl derivative of sucrose linked glycosidically to the C-2 of the glucose moiety has been identified in Umbellifers but not in the closely related order Cornales. Other oligosaccharides of minor importance to food but generally of unknown toxicity are found in a number of diverse plants. However, most of these naturally occurring oligosaccharides also possess a chemical structure based on sucrose. Moreover, where an additional residue of glucose is attached to the fructose residue of sucrose, the trisaccharide, for example, melezitose (Fig. 1.11) cannot be hydrolysed by β-D-fructofuranosidase.

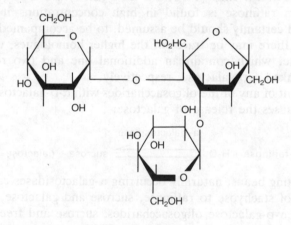

α–D–Glc*p*–(1 ⟷ 2)–β–D–Fru*f*–(3 → 1)–α–D–Glc*p*

Fig. 1.11 The chemical structure of melezitose

Maltose and melibiose (Fig. 1.12) present in fruits and vegetables may arise from enzymatic hydrolysis of either the higher polymers, such as starch and galactans, or from raffinose and stachyose. In ripening fruits where the cellular structure and compartmentalisation of enzymes is disrupted, such autolytic reactions may predominate. Furthermore, during the preservation of fruits by drying, or during the manufacture of juices and concentrates from citrus fruits or stone fruits, the release and ready mixing of various enzymes with susceptible substrates is likely to result in depolymerisation of polysaccharides and transglycosidase-catalysed reactions. The action of

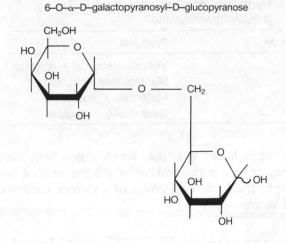

6–O–α–D–galactopyranosyl–D–glucopyranose

α–D–Gal*p*–(1 → 6)–D–Glc*p*

Fig. 1.12 The chemical structure of melibiose

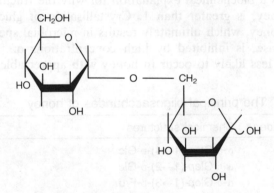

6–O–α–D–glucopyranosyl–D–glucopyranose

β–D–Glc*p*–(1 → 6)–D–Glc*p*

Fig. 1.13 The chemical structure of gentobiose

β-fructofuranosidase on the raffinose series of oligosaccharides which are regarded as primary products in plants is shown in Table 1.10. Both melebiose and gentobiose (Fig. 1.13) are derived from raffinose and gentianose, respectively.

During storage and processing of plant foods such as honey the complexity of the oligosaccharides increases. The nectar oligosaccharides collected by honey-bees are subjected to enzymatic hydrolysis by naturally occurring plant enzymes and other hydrolytic and transferase enzymes present in the digestive tract of the bee. A major trisac-

Table 1.10   Hydrolysis of plant oligosaccharides by
β-fructofuranosidase

Oligosaccharide	Products
Verbascose	Verbascotetraose + fructose
Stachyose	Manniotriose + fructose
Raffinose	Melibiose + fructose
Gentianose	Gentobiose + fructose

charide present in honey is erlose, which arises from the transglucosidase activity of bee α-glucosidase: a glucose residue is transferred
from sucrose to the 4-hydroxyl group of a glucose residue of a second
molecule of sucrose.

$$\text{sucrose} + \text{sucrose} \underset{\text{a–glucosidase}}{\overset{\text{bee}}{\rightleftharpoons}} \text{erlose} + \text{fructose}$$

The other trisaccharides and disaccharides (Table 1.11) present in
honey are expected to similarly arise by the action of transglycosidases.
Indeed the preferential transfer of glucose residues to disaccharides in
honey offers a biochemical explanation for why the fructose : glucose
ratio of honey, is greater than 1. Crystallisation of glucose (granu-
lation) in honey, which ultimately results in microbial spoilage of the
aqueous phase, is inhibited by high concentrations of fructose and
therefore is less likely to occur in honey with appreciable transgluco-

Table 1.11   The principal oligosaccharides of honey

Oligosaccharide	Chemical structures
Maltose	α-D-Glcp-(1→4)-D-Glc
Kojibiose	α-D-Glcp-(1→2)-D-Glc
Turanose	α-D-Glcp-(1→3)-D-Fru
Isomaltose	α-D-Glcp-(1→6)-D-Glc
Sucrose	α-D-Glcp-(1→2)-β-D-Fruf
Maltulose	α-D-Glcp-(1→4)-D-Fru
Nigerose	α-D-Glcp-(1→3)-D-Glc
α,β-trehalose	α-D-Glcp-(1→2)-β-D-Glc
Gentiobiose	β-D-Glcp-(1→6)-D-Glc
Erlose	α-D-Glcp-(1→4)-α-D-Glcp-(1→2)-β-D-Fruf
Panose	α-D-Glcp-(1→6)-α-D-Glcp-(1→4)-D-Glc
Maltotriose	α-D-Glcp-(1→4)-α-D-Glcp-(1→4)-D-Glc
Isokestose	α-D-Glcp-(1→2)-β-D-Fruf-(1→2)-β-D-Fruf
Melezitose	α-D-Glcp-(1→3)-β-D-Fruf-(2→1)-α-D-Glcp
Isomaltotetrose	α-D-Glcp-(1→4)-α-D-Glcp-(1→4)-α-D-Glcp-(1→4)-D-Glc

(After Doner 1977).

sides activity. Other insects, such as aphids, are also able to cause the hydrolysis, and possibly synthesis, of small oligosaccharides, for example honeydew is obtained from the syrups secreted by insects feeding on plant phloem sap. The trisaccharide melezitose present in many plants, and particularly in honeydew, may arise through glycosyl transfer reactions which require a transglucosidase from aphids and other insects. Many of the oligosaccharides and particularly those derived from fructose or sucrose, which contain additional residues of glucose may be of insect rather than plant origin as a glucosyl transferase is present in insect saliva. The complex mixtures of oligosaccharides found in honey have not been fractionated due to the limited resolution of available chromatographic techniques.

PLANT GLYCOSIDES

Anthocyanins

Monosaccharides and oligosaccharides are important substituent groups of anthocyanins. Anthocyanins are glycosides of anthocyanidins. The colour is determined by the hydroxylation of the B-ring (App. XI). Chemical hydrolysis of the glycosidic bond during heat processing of fruit products causes loss of colour. The β-glycosyl substituent at C-3 of the aglycones stabilises the natural colour of the anthocyanins; enzymatic decoloration can occur as a result of specific hydrolysis of the O-glycosidic bond by anthocyanin-β-glycosidases. A K_m value of 123 μM has been reported for such an enzyme obtained from *Aspergillus niger* and gluconolactone has been shown to be a very

Table 1.12 Some carbohydrates of flavonoids

Monosaccharide	Disaccharide	Trisaccharide
D-Glucose	Gentiobiose (Glc-β1→6-Glc)	Gentiotriose (Glc-β1→6-Glc-β2→6-Glc)
D-Galactose	Sophorose (Glc-β2→2-Glc)	Xylosylrutinose (L-Rha α1→6-Glc-β1→2-Xyl)
D- and L-Arabinose	Rutinose (L-Rha α1→6-Glc)	Glucosylrutinose (L-Rha α1→6-Glc-β1→2-Glc)
D-Xylose	Neohesperidose (L-Rha α1→2-Glc)	
L-Rhamnose	Apiosylglucose (Api β1→6-Glc)	

(Harborne 1973).

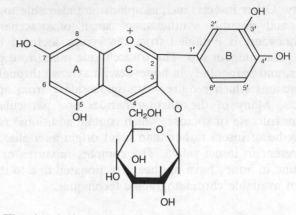

Fig. 1.14   The chemical structure of cyanidin-3-glucoside

potent competitive inhibitor (K_i, 2.3 μM) (Blom and Thomassen 1985). The range of sugars glycosidically linked in flavonoids is substantial and includes mono-, di- and trisaccharides and acylated sugars (Table 1.12). The 3-glucoside (Fig. 1.14) of cyanidin occurs widely in plants and is the principal component of blackberries, whereas the 3-arabinoside is the main purple component of cocoa seeds. The 3-rutinoside is also widely found in many plants. In anthocyanins, the hydroxyl group at position 5 is also frequently glycosylated. The flavylium cation being electron deficient is highly reactive and exists as a resonant structure. Anthocyanins are unstable in alkaline solution and are degraded by peroxides and sulphur dioxide. Decoloration with

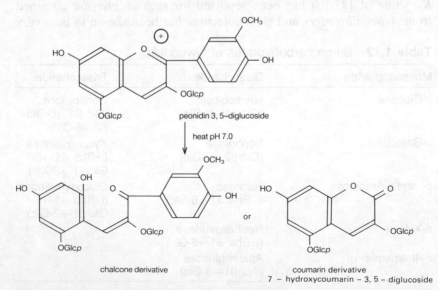

Fig. 1.15   The thermal degradation of anthocyanins

sulphur dioxide involves the reversible formation of an adduct with the carbonium ion to the c-ring at position 4. Such decolorisation may be prevented by substitution at position 4. On thermal decomposition the anthocyanins and anthocyanidin bases are decomposed by opening of the pyrone ring or loss of the B-ring (Jurd 1972) (Fig. 1.15).

The colour intensity and stability of anthocyanins are increased by intermolecular association (generally known as copigmentation), metal ion chelation and probable interaction with substituents in the oligo-saccharide moieties. Intramolecular interactions between acylating caffeic acid and the phenolic groups of the B-ring have been suggested for anthocyanins in decorative plants. Copolymerisation between anthocyanins and other flavonoids occurs to produce more stable polymerised colours. The dimer and larger units are linked by an intermolecular carbon–carbon bond between the 4- and 8-positions of the monomers. A typical reaction between cyanidin-3-glucoside and catechin is shown in Fig. 1.16. The higher polymers are termed generally proanthocyanidins.

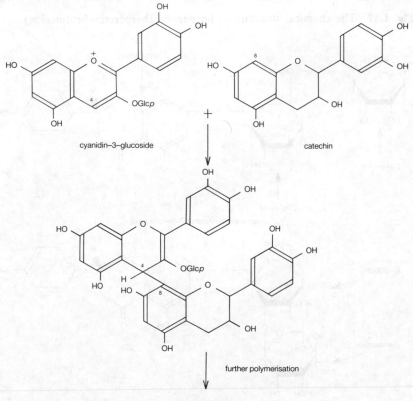

Fig. 1.16 Copolymerisation of flavonoids

Other flavonoid compounds, namely the flavonols, chalcones and aurones, make a significant contribution to yellow colours where the sugar may be present in the 3-,3'-,7- or 4'-positions. Substituents on the 7- and 4-positions can often be removed by β-glucosidase. Up to 60 mg per kg of the flavonols, quercetin and kaempherol, have been found in some varieties of onions and leaf vegetables (Bilyk and Sapers 1985). Glycosidically substituted flavanones are colourless compounds, of which the most significant economically are narginin and hesperidin. These substances can be measured in citrus juices by a direct ultra-violet spectrophotometric method. Hesperidin, although tasteless,

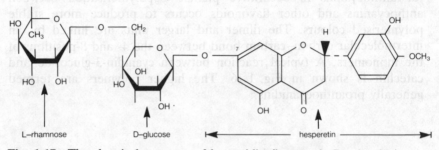

Fig. 1.17 The chemical structure of hesperidin (hesperetin-7-rutinoside)

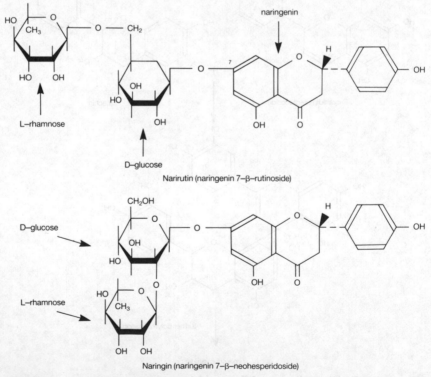

Fig. 1.18 Rutinosides of naringenin

crystallises in damaged fruit, orange juice products and on the surfaces of evaporators used for the manufacture of citrus juice concentrates. Hesperidin is the glycoside of hesperetin (3′,5,7-trihydroxy-4′-methoxyflavanone (Fig. 1.17). Naringin may also crystallise but is mainly responsible for bitterness in grapefruit products. The disaccharide unit (neohesperidose) consists of α-D-rhamnosyl(1→2)-β-D-glucopyranose and is linked glycosidically to the 7-hydroxyl group of naringenin (4′,5,7-trihydroxylflavanone). All citrus flavanone neohesperidosides are bitter. This disaccharide moiety differs only in the glycosidic linkage from the corresponding naringenin 7-β-rutinoside which is tasteless. Thus bitterness is due to the presence of the β 1→2 glycosidic link in naringin (Fig. 1.18): minor changes in the chemical structure of the flavanone moiety destroy bitterness and the corresponding flavone hesperidosides are tasteless. Also enzymatic debittering is possible with narginase from *Asperqillus niger* which contains α-rhamnosidase (EC 3.2.1.40) and β-glucosidase.

$$\text{H}_2\text{O} + \text{naringin} \xrightleftharpoons{\text{a–rhamnosidase}} \text{prunin} + \text{rhamnose}$$

$$\text{H}_2\text{O} + \text{prunin} \xrightleftharpoons{\text{β–glucosidase}} \text{naringenin} + \text{glucose}$$

Owing to product inhibition by glucose, and the presence of substantial amounts of this sugar in citrus juices, the reaction does not generally go to completion, but prunin (nargingenin-7-β-glucopyranoside) has approximately one-third of the bitterness of naringin.

In the presence of alkali the flavanone ring is opened to form a chalcone. These are very sweet compounds, have been proposed as intermediates in flavonoid biosynthesis, and can be stabilised by reduction to the extremely sweet dihydrochalcones (Fig. 1.19).

Betalaines

In place of anthocyanins as colouring substances, betalaines are glycosides which are found in yellow (betaxanthins) and red pigments (betacyanins) in one plant order the Centrospermae. Betanin is the main red pigment of beetroot (*Beta vulgaris*) which contains a β-glucosyl moiety (Fig. 1.20). The pigment is relatively stable within the pH range from 3.0 to 7.0 although excess heat can change the red beetroot type colour to pale brown (Harmer 1980). The betalaines are water-soluble nitrogen-containing pigments; they are immonium derivatives of betalamic acid which is synthesised from 3′,4′-dihydroxyphenylalanine (DOPA). The red betacyanin pigment of beetroot, betanin, is produced by addition of a second molecule of DOPA as cyclic DOPA to the open chain aldehyde group of betalamic

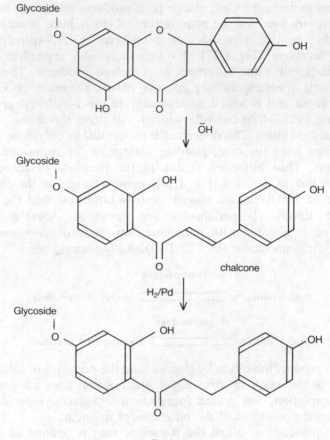

Fig. 1.19   The ring opening of flavones to form chains

acid to form a Schiff base compound (betanidin). Betanin is the 3′,O-substituted glucoside. In other plant species, disaccharide and trisaccharide substituents on either of the hydroxyl groups have been found. The yellow betaxanthins which are not glycosylated are synthesised from the betalamic acid intermediate by an addition reaction with the α-amino groups of simple amino acids such as proline, methionine or aspartate to form a Schiff base type product.

An unrelated glycoside is cycasin, which is a carcinogen and is found in the palm-like cycad trees of the Cycadaceae. Hydrolysis catalysed by β-glucosidase liberates the aglycone, methylazomethanol $CH_3-N=N-CH_2OH$ that decomposes to methylate nucleic acids – a reaction which accounts for the carcinogenic character of cycasin.

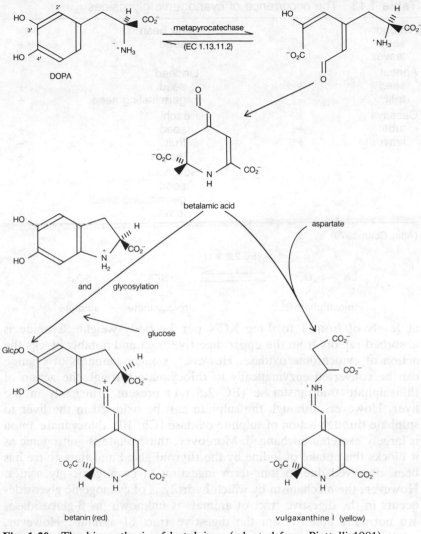

betalamic acid

aspartate

and   glycosylation

glucose

betanin (red)

vulgaxanthine I (yellow)

Fig. 1.20 The biosynthesis of betalaines (adapted from Piattelli 1981)

Cyanogenic glycosides

Cyanide anion is produced in plant materials through the enzymatic-catalysed hydrolysis of O-β-glycosides of α-hydroxynitriles (cyanogenic glycosides). For some plants, the occurrence of cyanogenic glycosides is restricted to the leaves (e.g. sorghum), whereas in others such as peach, the stone seeds but not the fruits are cyanogenic (Table 1.13). The cyanide liberated by enzymatic action is acutely toxic to animals

Table 1.13 The occurrence of cyanogenic glycosides

Almond		Lima bean	
seed	+	seed	+
leaves	+		
Apricot		Linseed	
seed	+	seed	+
fruit	−	germinating seed	+
Cassava		Peach	
tuber	+	seed	+
leaves	+	fruit	−
		leaves	+
		Sorghum	
		seed	−
		germinating seed	+
		leaves	+

(After Conn 1979).

$$\text{CN}^- + \text{S}_2\text{O}_3^{2-} \underset{}{\overset{\text{(EC 2.8.1.1)}}{\rightleftharpoons}} \text{SCN}^- + \text{SO}_3^{2-}$$

thiosulphate   thiocyanate   sulphite

at levels of from 1 to 7 mg KCN per kg body weight. Cyanide is absorbed rapidly from the upper digestive tract and notably blocks the action of cytochrome oxidase. However, smaller amounts of cyanide can be converted enzymatically to thiocyanate through the action of thiosulphate thiotransferase (EC 2.8.1.1) present principally in the liver. However, although the sulphite can be oxidised in the liver to sulphate through action of sulphite oxidase (Ch. 10), thiocyanate anion is largely excreted unchanged. Moreover, thiocyanate is goitrogenic as it blocks the uptake of iodine by the thyroid gland and thus goitre has been observed due to long-term ingestion of cyanogenic glycosides. However, the mechanism by which hydrolysis of cyanogenic glycosides occurs in the digestive tract of animals is unknown, as β-glucosidases are normally absent from the digestive tract of animals. However, small quantities of cyanide may arise from the hydrolysis of cyanogenic glycosides by intestinal and rumen microorganisms, or from the action of microbial contaminants prior to ingestion of cyanogenic foods.

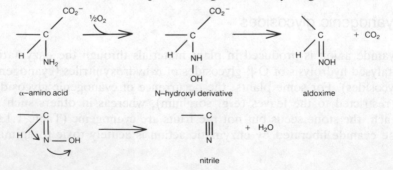

The cyanogenic glycosides are synthesised by glycosylation of the α-hydroxynitriles which are derived from oxidation of the amino group of common α-amino acids. The final step requires hydroxylation of the nitrile in the α-position to produce the hydroxynitrile for glycosylation:

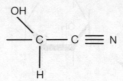

the hydroxynitrile group itself being unstable. The most common cyanogenic glycosides are linamarin and dhurrin (Fig. 1.21) found in the Leguminosae and Euphorbiacae which includes cassava (*Manihot spp.*). Amygdalin (Fig. 1.22) which contains a disaccharide is found in the Rosaceae family.

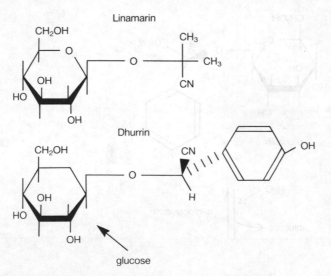

Fig. 1.21 The chemical structure of cyanogenic glycosides

The liberation of cyanide anion from the glycosides is catalysed by β-glucosidase. For amygdalin, found in bitter almonds, where the glycosyl substituent is a disaccharide unit, three enzymes act sequentially. There are three enzymes present in almond emulsion and the catalytic action of the third, a lyase usually present in all cyanogenic plants, results in the formation of cyanide and benzaldehyde.

mandelonitrile

mandelonitrile $\rightleftharpoons$ $C_6H_5CHO + HCN$

lyase
(EC 4.1.2.10)

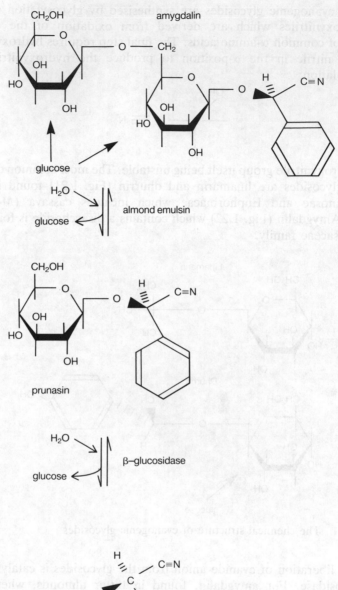

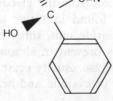

(R)–mandelonitrile

Fig. 1.22   The action of glycosidases on cyanogenic glycosides

Thus two or sometimes three enzymes are required to liberate cyanide from glycosides, and there is reason to believe that at least some of the plant species contain very specific enzymes for the hydrolysis of the different cyanogenic glycosides. To enable further utilisation of the plant species, such as sorghum leaves or cassava, it should be possible to select cultivars which are low in either the cyanogenic glycosides or the relevant hydrolytic enzymes. Alternatively, controlled fermentation might be encouraged in harvested foods in order to release hydrogen cyanide, which then may be trapped as a useful raw material for the chemical industry.

Steroidal glycosides

Saponins are glycosides of commonly triterpenoids (App. X) and also more specifically the steroids. Generally the steroidal hydroxyl group at C-3 forms the glycosidic link to the oligosaccharide moiety which may contain glucose, galactose, rhamnose or xylose. The steroidal glycosides also include the cardiac glycosides of which the *Digitalis* group have been the most widely investigated. During food processing, the saponins produce unwanted foams as the molecule consists of hydrophilic carbohydrate and hydrophobic steroidal moieties. The soybean might contain up to 0.6 per cent of saponin which may be responsible for astringency in soya products.

Solanine, present in green potatoes, and tomatine, in the leaves and unripe fruit of the tomato plant, are glycosidic steroidal alkaloids (glycoalkaloids, Fig. 1.23) found in members of the Solanaceae. Tomatine is deglycosylated in ripe tomato extracts to the steroidal alkaloid, 3-β-hydroxy-5α-pregn-16-en-20-one. The steroidal glycoalkaloids in the potato are claimed to be toxic and teratogenic but levels below 20 mg per 100 g are thought to be acceptable. In commercially available tubers, 95 per cent of the steroidal glycosides consists of α-chaconine and α-solanine. These compound differ only by the residues linked through the 3β-hydroxy group of solanidine, the parent aglycone. Other potato glycoalkaloids have been reported. However, for the sugar moiety, only four monosaccharides, glucose, galactose, xylose and L-rhamnose, have been found in the form of di-, tri- and tetrasaccharides. Recently a method of fast atom bombardment mass spectrometry has been described for identification of the intact glycoalkaloids (Price *et al.* 1985).

Thus, in conclusion, many secondary metabolites of plants are glycosylated and an overwhelming number are found naturally. Glycosidic linkages between carbon, nitrogen, oxygen or sulphur can occur to form C-glycosides and N-glycosides. Some are known to affect the digestion of foods by animals and exert toxic properties. Overall,

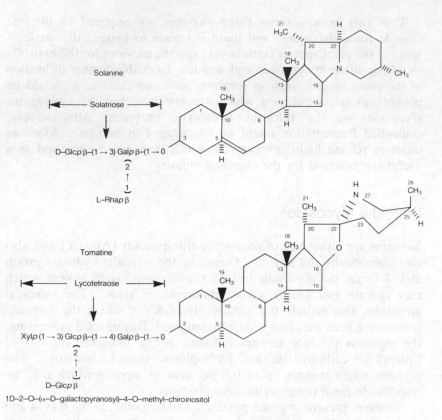

Fig. 1.23 The chemical structure of the glycoalkaloids solanine and
tomatine

glycosylated secondary products in plants increase the solubility of the
aglycones in water and decrease their chemical reactivity, which is
particularly apparent for the phenolic derivatives.

INOSITOLS

There are nine possible stereoisomers of inositol (hexahydroxycyclo-
hexane). Seven of the isomers have been found to occur naturally.
Myoinositol (Fig. 1.24) together with its various derivatives, is the
most frequently occurring inositol. Asymmetry is created by substitution of the hydroxyl groups. In dried tea leaves, myoinositol represents
up to 10 per cent of the total weight. The most common derivatives
of myoinositol found in all plants are monomethyl ethers, glycosides
and phosphate esters, and to a smaller extent dimethyl ethers. The
phosphate ester is synthesised through the enzymatic transformation
of glucose-6-phosphate to 1L-myoinositol-1-phosphate by the action of
myoinositol-1-phosphate synthase (EC 5.5.1.4).

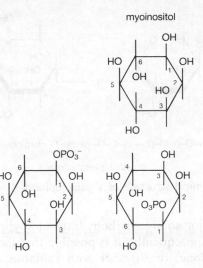

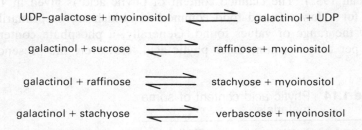

1L–myoinositol–1–phosphate   1D–myoinositol–1–phosphate

Fig. 1.24 The chemical structure of myoinositol

During the synthesis of galactose-containing oligosaccharides, such as raffinose and stachyose, the glycoside galactosyl-myoinositol has been shown to act as a donor substrate for galactose residues. Myoinositol first acts as a galactosyl acceptor from UDP-galactose to form galactinol (the α-D-galactopyranoside of myoinositol), which then acts as a galactosyl donor to either sucrose, raffinose or other precursors of the galactose-containing oligosaccharides.

UDP–galactose + myoinositol   ⇌   galactinol + UDP

galactinol + sucrose   ⇌   raffinose + myoinositol

galactinol + raffinose   ⇌   stachyose + myoinositol

galactinol + stachyose   ⇌   verbascose + myoinositol

It is probable that in some plants one enzyme is capable of catalysing two or more of the above reactions. UDP-galactose is an activated form of galactose where the hydroxyl group of the C-1 atom. of galactose is esterified to a diphosphate (App. II).

Other α-D-galactopyranosylcyclitols (the galactopinitols, Fig. 1.25) have been detected in soybean and chick peas. The galactopinitols, which are glycosides of O-methyl-D-chiroinositols may also act as transfer intermediates for the biosynthesis of galactose-containing oligosaccharides. They are likely to coexist with raffinose and stachyose in legumes and other plant materials and cyclitols have been claimed to

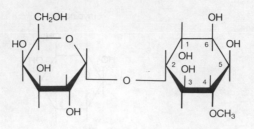

α–D–Gal*p*–(1 → 2)–4,–O–methyl–D–chiroinositol

(a galactopinitol isomer)

Fig. 1.25 The chemical structure of a galactopinitol

represent the major soluble carbohydrate of soybean (Schweizer and Horman 1981). Consequently, it is possible that these substances may be responsible alone, or together with raffinose and stachyose, for flatulence often associated with the consumption of legumes such as the soybean. Furthermore, the presence of α-D-galactosylcyclitols may lead to false values for amounts of raffinose if based on assays for galactose alone.

The term phytate is generally assumed to include the hexaphosphate esters of not only myoinositol but also the hexaphosphate esters of all the other stereoisomeric inositols. Phytates are biologically important as they represent a store for phosphorus (Table 1.14). The content of phytate in foods is normally based on analysis of precipitated ferric–phytate complexes. A ratio of 4Fe : 6P is assumed for the molecular structure of a ferric–phytate complex (Thompson and Erdman 1982). The claimed content of phytic acid is given in Table 1.14 for a few selected food commodities which serves primarily to show the range of values found. Generally, a phosphate content of 28.2 per cent is assumed for phytic acid. However, the presence of

Table 1.14 Phytic acid content of some materials

Food commodity	Phytic acid (%)
Cereals	0.5–1.8
Legumes	0.4–2.10
Rapeseed	2.0–4.0
Cottonseed	2.6–4.8
Plant products	
Wheat gluten	2.1
Rapeseed meal	3–5
Soybean meal	1.4–1.6

(Reddy *et al.*1982).

lower phosphate esters in foods which gives rise to the chemical heterogeneity of inositol phosphates limits the application of such a simple procedure. However, mixtures of inositol phosphates can now be resolved at low pH values, where the net charge per molecule is small, by ion exchange chromatography. The affinity of the phosphate esters to the anion exchanger is proportional to both the total number of phosphate groups and the number of adjacent equatorial phosphate groups (Cosgrove 1978).

The term 'phytic acid' can have a more restricted use for the hexakis-O-phosphate ester of myoinositol (IP_6) but generally the term has encompassed the hexaphosphate esters of the other inositol isomers. IP_6 is synthesised from myoinositol-1-phosphate through the action of phosphoinositol kinase and phosphotransferases. The structural formula for phytic acid (Fig. 1.26) is not absolutely certain, but it is possible that the uncertainty may be due to the formation of anhydrides between the individual phosphate groups – a reaction which could easily occur during the isolation, purification and drying of phytic acids. Phytate and probably lower esters complex through ionic bonding to the essential dietary metals such as calcium, magnesium and zinc. The lower phosphate–inositol esters are formed during sequential dephosphorylation of phytic acid through the action of a phytase enzyme (myoinositol hexakis, dihydrogen phosphate phosphohydrolase). Numerous studies have indicated that phytates reduce the bio-availability of Mg, Ca, Zn and Fe in monogastric animals, which means that the presence of substantial amounts of phytate in the diet could give rise to mineral deficiencies. Complexes may be formed between the anionic side chains of proteins, metal cations and the phosphate groups of phytates (Fig. 1.26). Thus the increased availability and use of many new plant products, such as soybean isolates, bran products or other plant proteins, which all may contain substantial amounts of phytates may give rise to mineral deficiencies, unless phytate-free products are developed. Thus the use of phytases available from plants and microorganisms to degrade phytate is likely to increase.

In the undamaged plant cell phytases seem to have little effect on

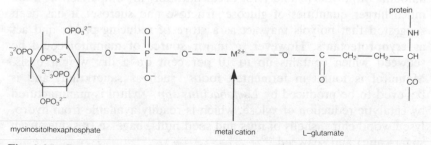

myoinositolhexaphosphate   metal cation   L–glutamate

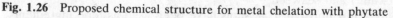

Fig. 1.26 Proposed chemical structure for metal chelation with phytate

phytic acid until disruption of the material takes place through either autolysis or mechanical damage. The pH optima for phytases is generally between 4.0 to 5.5 pH units, and the optimum temperature ranges from 40 to 60 °C. Mammalian phytases have not been identified, although phytases might be synthesised by intestinal microorganisms. The hydrolysis catalysed by phytases in plants seems to be closely regulated, probably through the action of inhibitors and control mechanisms for the biosynthesis of the enzyme. Such control may help to explain why the action of phytases is claimed to be rapid in fermented bread prepared from a 75–90 per cent extraction wheat, but slow for the 95–100 per cent extraction products. Similarly up to 75 per cent of phytate may be hydrolysed during the manufacture of soya-fortified bread, whereas the separate soya preparations possess little or no phytase activity. The amount of phytate in soybean can also be reduced through the enzymatic action of fungal phytases, although where the phytate is located in the seed coat or germ part, the phytate content of derived products can be reduced by mechanical milling processes. Also phytates are water soluble and provided the phytate–protein complexes can be broken, by the judicious use of salts and control of pH values, it is possible to obtain protein concentrates free of phytates through the use of isoelectric precipitation. Ultrafiltration also offers a means for reducing the phytate content of manufactured plant seed protein concentrates.

POLYHYDRIC ALCOHOLS

Pentitols, hexitols and shorter chain polyols are strictly not carbohydrates, but due to a similar polyhydroxyl structure and hence because of similar chemical properties the polyols are generally considered together with carbohydrates. Furthermore, from the nutritional point of view, polyols when metabolised enter the metabolic pathways for monosaccharides and also yield approximately the same order of energy per mole on complete oxidation. In plants, only small amounts of polyols (Table 1.15) occur naturally in comparison with the much larger quantities of glucose, fructose and sucrose. It has been suggested that polyols may act as a store of reducing power and act as cryoprotectants. However, a major source of mannitol could be seaweed which contains up to 10 per cent on a dry weight basis. Mannitol is found in fermented foods, such as sauerkraut, and is believed to be produced by *Lactobacillus spp*. Xylitol is manufactured by catalytic reduction of xylose, which is readily available from hydrolysed wood chips, shells of nuts and seed hulls, bagasse (residues from sugar-cane) and seaweed.

Only a few polyhydric alcohols have been used as food ingredients.

Table 1.15 The amounts of polyols in some fruits

Fruit	Xylitol[†] (mg/100 g)
Blackcurrant	7.0
Cranberry	2.1
Raspberry	2.6
Rowanberry	8.1
	Glucitol (sorbitol) (g/100 g)
Apple[‡]	0.2–1.0
Pear[‡]	1.2–2.8
Plum[‡]	0.6–2.01
Peach[‡]	0.5–1.29

([†] Makinen and Söderling 1980; [‡] Wrolstad and Shallenberger 1981).

These have included glycerol, propylene glycol and maltitol, glucitol, mannitol and xylitol (Fig. 1.27). Lycasin (R) is a glucose–maltose syrup with a high content of maltitol manufactured by hydrogenation of β-amylase digests of corn or potato starch. The process and application of the products are covered by patents. Lycasin 80/55, has a solids content of 80 per cent and a dextrose equivalent of 55 before hydrogenation. The commercial product contains monosaccharide alcohols (8 %), disaccharide alcohols (50–55 %), trisaccharide alcohols (20–25 %) and higher alcohols (15–20 %); the sweetness is

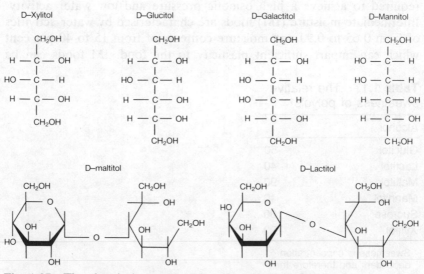

Fig. 1.27 The chemical structure of some polyols used in foods

Table 1.16   Solubility in water of polyhydric
              alcohols

Alcohol	Solubility at 25 °C (g/100 g of water)
Glucitol[†]	251
Glycerol[†]	∞
Lactitol	206
Mannitol[†]	22
Propylene glycol[†]	∞
Xylitol[‡]	68

([†] From Griffin and Lynch 1975; [‡] from Hyvönen *et al.* 1982).

from 75 to 80 per cent that of sucrose (Rockstrom 1980). Lactitol (4-
O-β-D-galactopyranosyl-D-glucitol) prepared by hydrogenation of
lactose has been suggested for use in instant soups, beverages, ice-
cream and dietetic foods where sucrose can be replaced. The alcohols
used are readily soluble in water (Table 1.16), exhibit variable viscosities and possess sweetness, so that they may be used in non-glucose
and sucrose products. Mixtures of polyols, which are more stable than
reducing sugars, are used to change the viscosity of foods and are
particularly important for imparting sweetness (Table 1.17). Also
bactericidal activity has been reported for a range of polyols. When
used in confectionery products crystallisation can be reduced by the
inclusion of from 5 to 10 per cent of sorbitol to increase the shelf life
of fondants and fruit fillings in biscuits. To prevent microbiological
deterioration and hence increase the storage time at ambient temperature, large amounts of polyols, up to 75 per cent by weight, may be
required to achieve a high osmotic pressure and low water activity.
Intermediate moisture (IM) foods are characterised by water activities
of from 0.65 to 0.90 and moisture contents of from 15 to 40 per cent
which can impart sufficient plasticity to the food. IM foods can be

Table 1.17   The relative
sweetness of polyols[†]

Alcohol	
Glucitol	50
Lactitol	40
Maltitol	90
Mannitol	40
Sucrose	100
Xylitol	90

[†] Sweetness is concentration
 dependent and therefore the
 values given are not absolute.

manufactured by soaking particulate foods in an infusion solution which may contain sucrose (11 %), NaCl (12 %), glucitol (19 %) and glycerol (9 %) as humectants, which permit relatively high moisture levels providing food ready to consume. Cheese and jam are older and more familiar examples of IM foods. For dietary confectionery products polyhydric-alcohols may account for up to 90 per cent of the product.

Absorption from the intestine of glucitol and xylitol is slow so that the intake of large amounts (more than 50 g) may result in a high osmotic pressure in the colon and flatulence. Both glucitol and xylitol are metabolised by conversion first to fructose and then to triose phosphates. The regulatory factor is polyol dehydrogenase (EC 1.1.1.21) – now aldehyde reductase.

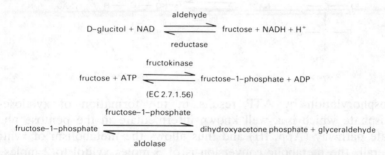

$$\text{D-glucitol} + \text{NAD} \underset{\text{reductase}}{\overset{\text{aldehyde}}{\rightleftharpoons}} \text{fructose} + \text{NADH} + \text{H}^+$$

$$\text{fructose} + \text{ATP} \underset{\text{(EC 2.7.1.56)}}{\overset{\text{fructokinase}}{\rightleftharpoons}} \text{fructose-1-phosphate} + \text{ADP}$$

$$\text{fructose-1-phosphate} \underset{\text{aldolase}}{\overset{\text{fructose-1-phosphate}}{\rightleftharpoons}} \text{dihydroxyacetone phosphate} + \text{glyceraldehyde}$$

Therefore for foods which contain these polyols there is no reduction in the available metabolic energy content of the food, although for mannitol there seems to be little metabolic conversion. However, the polyols are not metabolised quickly by oral bacteria and thus are useful for reducing dental decay. Also, with the exception of maltitol, they do not cause rapid changes in the levels of blood glucose and are therefore useful in diabetic foods. However, both glucitol and xylitol are converted to α-glycerophosphate via fructose and therefore both polyols could theoretically increase the synthesis of triglycerides for which α-glycerophosphate may be a regulatory factor.

Maltitol is thought to be hydrolysed by α-glucosidase to glucose and glucitol, thus eventually providing the same metabolic energy value as molar quantities of sucrose. Consequently, maltitol may be assimilated more rapidly than the simpler alcohols. On the other hand lactitol is claimed to be only slowly hydrolysed to galactose and glucitol by human β-galactosidase, although the intestinal microorganism, E. Coli, may be able to adapt to utilise the reduced disaccharide. Also it is thought possible that lactitol, like lactulose, may encourage the development of a *Lactobacillus bifidus* flora in the intestine. For xylitol the rate of intestinal transport is no more than 60 per cent of that for glucose, but the polyol is substantially metabolised in the liver. Xylitol which is a normal metabolite of the liver is converted through the pentose-phosphate cycle (App. III) to fructose-6-phosphate (F-6-P), which is then oxidised to carbon dioxide and water to yield an almost identical amount of energy to that obtained from oxidation of glucose. Alternatively, fructose-6-phosphate can be converted to glucose and ultimately glycogen in the liver. Xylitol is oxidised to xylulose by the non-specific cytoplasmic aldehyde reductase in the liver, where the rate of oxidation is controlled by the concentration of xylitol and the activity of the enzyme. The enzyme is not allosterically controlled. However, the hydrogen acceptor is NAD and therefore there may occasionally be competitive inhibition of xylitol oxidation by ethanol or glucitol.

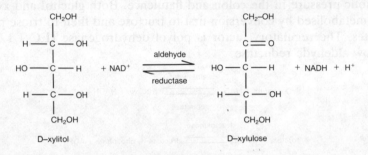

Phosphorylation by ATP results in the formation of xylulose-5-phosphate which is a well known intermediate in the pentose phosphate pathway (App. III) and thus allows the metabolism of xylitol. Overall, the metabolic conversion is of 3 moles xylitol to 2 moles of F-6-P and 1 mole of glyceraldehyde-3-phosphate. R-5-P is obtained after oxidation of G-6-P by glucose-6-phosphate dehydrogenase. Thus the main regulatory factors are likely to be aldehyde reductase, ATP and glucose-6-phosphate dehydrogenase. Transketolase, a key enzyme in the metabolism of xylitol, is a thiamin-dependent enzyme and thus an adequate amount of thiamin pyrophosphate is required to saturate the enzyme. Xylitol is fortunately assimilated through the above metabolic reactions, because it is a normal intermediate in the uronic acid cycle. A tolerable dose may be of the order of from 20 to 40 g per day of xylitol without causing osmotic diarrhoea, but adaptation to increasing amounts of xylitol has been claimed. Many of the polyols possess laxative properties and may be prescribed separately for this purpose.

ASSIMILATION OF CARBOHYDRATES

In man, the principal digestible carbohydrates consumed in the diet are starch, glycogen, lactose and sucrose. The hydrolysed products of α-glycosidically-linked polysaccharides, such as starch, are small oligosaccharides. The sources of secreted enzymes are saliva, pancreatic juice and the intestinal mucosa. The secretions represent a considerable fluid volume and so reduce the viscosity of food and facilitate its

solution. Final hydrolysis of lactose, sucrose and the small oligosaccharides occurs in the lumen of the intestine, and is catalysed by intestinal brush border disaccharidases located close to the cellular specific
active transport mechanisms for translocation of the resultant monosaccharides. In the intestine, the mucosal surface area is increased by
villi, the extent of which varies in man according to age and disease.
The brush border disaccharidases are β-galactosidase (lactase) and the
α-glucosidases sucrase, isomaltase, maltase and trehalase. Disaccharides are not absorbed from the small intestine. Glucose is also released
by glucoamylase-catalysed hydrolysis of small oligosaccharides arising
from starch and dextrins. Glucose which may be transported against
a blood-to-intestinal lumen concentration gradient shares a sodium-
coupled active transport system with galactose. Therefore, although
there may be other transport systems for glucose, it is possible that the
presence of significant amounts of dietary galactose may competitively
reduce the uptake of glucose. After assimilation glucose can either be
used directly for the production of energy, or stored in the liver and
muscles in the form of glycogen or in fatty tissue as triglycerides. The
interrelated physiological processes are controlled by insulin and other
hormones. In the case of fructose, any carrier system merely aids the
simple diffusion of fructose into the blood, as there is not an opposing
blood-to-intestinal concentration gradient for fructose. Therefore,
normally fructose never reaches the colon where it would be rapidly
fermented by microorganisms.

Digestive intolerance of carbohydrates

A failure to assimilate dietary monosaccharides is due to deficiences
of either hydrolytic enzymes, or the energy-dependent transport
system, which in either case results in carbohydrate intolerance.
However, lactose deficiency, and the consequent malabsorption of
lactose, is now considered to be the normal state for a large proportion
of the world's adult population: approximately 90 per cent of Chinese
and Arab populations suffer from an inability to assimilate lactose. A
sucrase deficiency has been found in the North American Eskimo
population. In most mammals the enzymatic activity of lactase declines
with age and congenital deficiency of lactase is rare. Many of the
disaccharidase deficiencies can result from intestinal mucosal damage
which may be induced by infections, diseases and physical defects of
intestinal function. Although enteric microorganisms are normally
confined to the colon, the establishment of a flora in the upper small
bowel may result in proteolysis of the disaccharidases and transport
systems that will bring about malabsorption of carbohydrates. An
inherited malabsorption of glucose or galactose due to a failure of
energy-dependent Na-coupled transport system is rare. Deficiencies of
the disaccharidase as well as deficiencies in the transport capacity for

the monosaccharides, will give rise to specific intolerances of, for example, lactose or sucrose, or a more general carbohydrate intolerance.

The presence of unabsorbed carbohydrates in the intestinal lumen creates a high osmotic pressure which reduces the diffusion of water and minerals into the blood plasma, so that excessive carbohydrate is fermented separately by microorganisms in the colon. Consequently, overgrowth of faecal microorganisms may occur coupled to the production of carbon dioxide and hydrogen to cause abdominal distention and probable further mucosal damage. The symptoms of carbohydrate intolerance are flatulence, abdominal distention, diarrhoea and acid stools. Fermentation in the colon can result in an increased concentration of hydrogen in the breath of mammals that may provide a simple sensitive and non-invasive diagnostic test for intolerance of food carbohydrates.

Metabolic intolerance of carbohydrates

Although it is well known that diabetics are unable to control the levels of glucose in the blood, it is not generally known that other hexoses such as galactose and fructose cannot be metabolised by some individuals. For D-galactose, accumulation of this sugar is normally prevented by rapid enzyme-catalysed epimerisation to D-glucose in the liver. The epimerisation at the C-4 of galactose requires the sequential action of three enzymes and the overall expenditure of energy in the form of ATP. The galactose residue is phosphorylated by galactokinase, UDP-galactose is formed and then epimerised to UDP-glucose.

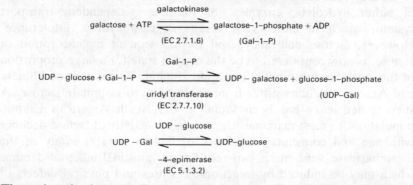

The epimerisation reaction incorporates an oxidation at the C-4 atom of galactose to form an intermediate keto group which is then reduced to form the new hydroxyl group of D-glucose which lies below the plane of the pyranose ring. The epimerase requires NAD/NADH as co-factor, which is believed to act in a cyclic manner as hydrogen acceptor during the oxidative step and hydrogen donor during the final reductive step. The reversible epimerase reaction is also important for the synthesis of galactose-containing polysaccharides where dietary galactose is insufficient. The deficiency disease, galactosemia, is due to absence of the enzyme galactose-1-phosphate uridyltransferase (EC 2.7.7.10); galactose and D-galactinol are two of the toxic products which accumulate although other toxic products may be formed from galactose-1-phosphate. Enlargement of the liver and jaundice are symptoms. Also galactose is excreted in the urine and may accumulate in the eye where there is no epimerase.

From fruits, vegetables and dietary sucrose, up to 100 g per day of fructose may be taken as food for normal individuals. There are two different mechanisms in the liver and adipose tissues for the phosphorylation of D-fructose. The assimilated fructose enters the liver easily and is phosphorylated rapidly through the action of fructokinase (EC 2.7.1.4) to fructose-1-phosphate (F-1-P). Without further phosphorylation F-1-P is cleaved directly by fructose-1-phosphate aldolase to glyceraldehyde and dehydroxyacetonephosphate in normal individuals. Thus in liver, fructose is converted to the trioses and metabolised through the glycolytic pathway (App. III) or utilised for the synthesis of glucose and ultimately glycogen. Normally the activity of fructokinase is high in the liver without allosteric control by ATP or AMP. Therefore the initial steps in the metabolism of fructose through F-1-P – unlike fructose-6-phosphate (F-6-P) – are poorly controlled and can quickly affect the levels of ATP, inorganic phosphate and nucleotides. However, slow absorption from the digestive tract, coupled with such a direct metabolism of fructose by the liver, does mean that fructose has very little affect on blood glucose levels, and is therefore useful as a sweetener and energy source in diabetic foods. Hereditary intolerance of fructose is rare and is due to the absence of the specific aldolase or fructokinase. Alternatively, and particularly in adipose tissue, where the concentration of glucose is low, F-6-P can be formed by the action of hexokinase. In the placenta and eye lens, fructose can be metabolised by first reduction to sorbitol and then oxidation to glucose.

KEY FACTS

1.   Of the low molecular weight monosaccharides only substantial amounts of glucose, fructose, sucrose and lactose occur in foods.
2.   Enzymatic methods of analysis afford rapid highly sensitive and specific methods for assay in admixture. Microbial cytoplasmic membrane dehydrogenases have been identified for the direct analysis of glucose, fructose and galactose using ferricyanide as the electron acceptor.
3.   The greater abundance of ^{13}C in corn starch can be used as a

basis for detection of adulteration of honey in 'maize' high-fructose syrups.

4.   Cold sweetening of potatoes is due to the accumulation of sucrose and fructose. At higher temperatures they are metabolised by oxidation or indirect conversion to starch.

5.   Dried milk products contain substantial amounts of lactose. The disaccharide is a readily available source of energy. Large crystals (10 μm) cause sandiness in condensed milks and ice-cream. A high proportion of the world's population is lactose intolerant.

6.   Seeds contain a restricted number of di- and trisaccharides of which those of the raffinose family are the most dominant. Such α-galactosides and their inositol derivatives may cause flatulence in humans.

7.   Deficiencies in humans of intestinal disaccharidases cause digestive intolerance of carbohydrates. Metabolic intolerance of galactose and fructose may be due to deficiencies of galactose-4-epimerase and fructokinases in the liver.

8.   Some glycosides of flavonoids (anthocyanins) are responsible for water-soluble, but heat-labile colours in fruits. Other glycosides may be responsible for bitterness in citrus products. Cyanogenic glycosides and some steroidal glycosides are potentially toxic.

REFERENCES

Ameyama, M. (1982) 'Enzymic microdetermination of D-glucose, D-fructose, D-gluconate, 2-keto-D-gluconate, aldehyde and alcohol with membrane-bound dehydrogenases', in *Methods in Enzymology*, vol. 89 *Carbohydrate Metabolism*, part D (ed. Wood, W. A.). Academic Press, London.

Ap Rees, T., Dixon, W. L., Pollock, C. J. and Franks, F. (1981) 'Low temperature sweetening of higher plants', in *Recent Advances in the Biochemistry of Fruits and Vegetables* (eds Friend, J. and Rhodes, M. J. C.). Academic Press, London.

Ayers, A. R. and Eriksson, K. E. (1982) 'Cellobiose oxidase from *Sporotrichum pulverulentum*', in *Methods in Enzymology*, vol. 89 *Carbohydrate Metabolism*, part D (ed. Wood, W. A.). Academic Press, London.

Bell, R. W. and Whittier, E. O. (1965) in *Fundamentals of Dairy Chemistry* (eds. Webb, B. H. and Johnson, A. H.). AVI Publishing Co., Westport, Connecticut.

Bilyk, A. and Sapers, G. M. (1985) 'Distribution of quercetin and kaempferol in lettuce, kale, chive, garlic chive, leek, horseradish, red radish and red cabbage tissues', *J. Agric. Food Chem.*, **33**, 226–8.

Blom, H. and Thomassen, M. S. (1985) 'Kinetic studies of strawberry anthocyanin hydrolysis by a thermostable anthocyanin-β-glycosidase from *Aspergillus niger*', *Food Chem.*, **17**, 157–8.

Carro, O., Hillaire-Marcel, C. and Cagnon, M. (1980) 'Detection of adulterated maple products by stable carbon isotope ratio', *J. Assoc. Off. Anal. Chem.*, **63**, 840–4.

Conn, E. E. (1979) 'Cyanogenic glycosides', in *Biochemistry of Nutrition* 1, *International Revue of Biochemistry*, vol. 27 (eds. Neuberger, A. and Jukes, J. H.). University Park Press, Baltimore.

Cosgrove, D. J. (1978) 'The isolation and identification of inositol phosphate intermediates by ion exchange chromatography', in *Cyclitols and Phosphoinositides* (eds. Wells, W. A. and Eisenberg, F. jun.). Academic Press, New York.

Doner, L. W. (1977) 'The sugars of honey – a review', *J. Sci. Food Agric.*, **28**, 443–6.

Doner, L. W. and Hicks, K. B. (1982) 'Lactose and the sugars of honey and maple: Reactions, properties, and analysis', in *Food Carbohydrates* (eds. Lineback, D. R. and Inglett, G. E.). AVI Publishing Company, Westport, Connecticut.

Egan, H., Kirk, R. S. and Sawyer, R. (1981) *Pearson's Chemical Analysis of Foods*, 8th edn. Churchill Livingstone, Longman, London.

Griffin, W. C., Lynch, M. J. (1975) 'Polyhydric alcohols', in *Handbook of Food Additives*, vol. 1, 2nd edn. (ed. Furia, T. E.). CRC Press, Cleveland, Ohio.

Harborne, J. B. (1973) 'Flavonoids', in *Phytochemistry Organic Metabolites*, vol. II (ed. Miller, L. P.). Van Nostrand Reinhold Company, New York.

Harmer, R. A. (1980) 'Occurrence, chemistry and application of betanin', *Food Chem.*, **5**, 81–90.

Hicks, K. B., Raupp, D. L. and Smith, P. W. (1984) 'Preparation and purification of lactulose from sweet cheese whey ultra-filtrate', *J. Agric. Food Chem.*, **32**, 288–92.

Howling, D. (1979) 'The general science and technology of glucose syrups', in *Sugar, Science and Technology* (eds. Birch, G. G. and Parker, K. J.). Applied Science Publishers, London.

Hyvönen, L., Koivistoinen, P. and Volrol, F. (1982) 'Food technological evaluation of xylitol', *Adv. in Food Res.*, **28**, 373–403.

IUPAC–IUB, (1982a) Joint Commission on Biochemical Nomenclature (JCBN) 'Polysaccharide nomenclature. Recommendations 1980', *Eur. J. Biochem.*, **126**, 439–41.

IUPAC–IUB, (1982b) Joint Commission on Biochemical Nomenclature (JCBN) 'Abbreviated terminology of oligosaccharide chains. Recommendations 1980', *Eur. J. Biochem.*, **126**, 433–7.

Jurd, L. (1972) 'Some advances in the chemistry of anthocyanin-type plant pigments', in *The Chemistry of Plant Pigments, Advances in Food Research*, supplement 3 (ed. Chichester, C. O.). Academic Press, London.

Kennedy, J. F. and White, C. A. (1983) *Bioactive carbohydrates in Chemistry, Biochemistry and Biology*. Ellis Horwood, Chichester.

Li, B. W. and Schuhmann, P. J. (1983) 'Sugar analysis of fruit juices: content and method', *J. Food Sci.*, **48**, 633–53.

Mäkinen, K. K. and Söderling, E. (1980) 'A quantitative study of mannitol, sorbitol, xylitol and xylose in wild berries and commercial fruits', *J. Food Sci.*, **45**, 367–71.

Nickerson, T. H. (1974) in *Fundamentals of Dairy Chemistry* 2nd edn. (eds. Webb, B. H., Johnson, A. H. and Alford, J. A.). AVI Publishing Co, Westport, Connecticut.

Piattelli, M. (1981) 'The betalains: Structure, biosynthesis and chemical taxonomy', in *The Biochemistry of Plants. A Comprehensive Treatise*, vol. 7 *Secondary Plant Products* (ed. Conn, E. E.). Academic Press, New York.

Price, K. R., Mellon, F. A., Self, R., Fenwick, G. R. and Osman, S. F. (1985) 'Fast atom bombardment mass spectrometry of *Solanum* glycoalkaloids and its potential for mixture analysis', *Biomed. Mass Spectrom.* **12**, 79–85.

Reddy, N. R., Sathe, S. K. and Salunkhe, D. K. (1982) 'Phytates in legumes and cereals', *Adv. in Food Res.*, **28**, 1–92.

Rockström, E. (1980) 'Lycasin hydrogenated hydrolysates', in *Carbohydrate Sweeteners in Foods and Nutrition* (eds. Koivistoinen, P. and Hyvönen, L.). Academic Press, London.

Schweizer, T. F. and Horman, I. (1981) 'Purification and structure determination of three α-D-galactopyranosylcyclitols from soya bean', *Carbohydr. Res.*, **95**, 61–71.

Soluski, F. W., Elkowicz, L. and Reichert, R. D. (1982) 'Oligosaccharides in eleven legumes and their air-classified protein and starch fractions', *J. Food Sci.*, **47**, 498–502.

Thompson, D. B. and Erdman, J. W. (1982) 'Structural model for ferric phytate: Implications for phytic acid analysis', *Cereal Chem.*, **59**, 525–8.

White, J. W. and Doner L. W. (1978) 'Sugars and sugar products. Mass spectrometric detection of high-fructose corn syrup in honey by use of $^{13}C/^{12}C$ ratio : collaborative study', *J. Assoc. Off. Anal. Chem.*, **61**, 746–50.

Wrolstad, R. E. and Shallenberger, R. S. (1981) 'Free sugars and sorbitol in fruits – A compilation from the literature', *J. Assoc. Off. Anal. Chem.*, **64**, 91–102.

ADDITIONAL READING

Chandra, R. K. (1984) *Food Intolerance*. Elsevier Science Publishing Co., New York.

Cheryan, M. (1980) 'Phytic acid interactions in food systems', *CRC* in *Crit. Rev. Food Sci. Nutr.* **13**, 297–335.

Holub, B. J. (1986) 'Metabolism and function of myoinositol and inositol phospholipids', *Ann. Revs. Nutr.*, **6**, 563–97.

Kennedy, J. F. and White, C. A. (1983) *Bioactive carbohydrates in Chemistry, Biochemistry and Biology*. Ellis Horwood, Chichester.

Koivistoinen, P. and Hyvönen, L. (1980) *Carbohydrate Sweeteners in Foods and Nutrition*. Academic Press, London.

Lifshitz, F. (1982) *Carbohydrate Intolerance in Infancy*. Marcel Dekker, New York.

Lineback, D. R. and Inglett, G. E. (1982) *Food Carbohydrates*. AVI Publishing Co., Westport, Connecticut.

Preiss, J. (1980) *The Biochemistry of Plants. A Comprehensive Treatise*, vol. 3

Carbohydrates: Structure and Formation (eds. in chief, Stumpf, P. K. and Conn, E. E.). Academic Press, New York.

Reddy, N. R., Sathe, S. K. and Salunke D. K. (1982) 'Phytates in legumes and cereals', *Adv. in Food Res.*, **28**, 1–92.

Wells, W. W. and Eisenberg, F. Jun. (1978) *Cyclitols and Phosphoinositides*. Academic Press, New York.

Ylikahra, R. (1979) 'Metabolic and nutritional aspects of xylitol', *Adv. in Food Res.*, **25**, 159–80.

CHAPTER 2

Food polysaccharides

Polysaccharides are high polymers in which many monosaccharides of various types are covalently linked by glycosidic bonds. For polysaccharides, traditional common names are used but the terms glucan, mannan or galactan arise from recommendations to provide information on chemical structure. Homoglycans yield one type of monosaccharide only on hydrolysis, whereas heteroglycans yield more than one type of monosaccharide. The polysaccharides may also be classified on the basis of both their physical properties and on the presence of the various types of monosaccharides. Starch and cellulose (glucans) are homopolymers consisting of repeating glucose units but are readily distinguished by their different physical properties, starch being granular and cellulose being fibrous. To the food scientist these differences are important, for starch forms useful gels and pastes, whereas cellulose forms insoluble micelles and crystalline products. Other polysaccharide molecules which contain polymers of different monosaccharides are heteropolymers. Frequently these are used by the food industry as gelling agents, thickeners and stabilisers. The overall shape of the polymer chains is determined mainly by the bond angles between the monosaccharide units. The conformational formula, comprising an equatorial–equatorial β-(1→4) glycosidic bond, for the cellobiose unit of cellulose is given in Fig. 2.1. It can be readily deduced that such a polymer will exist mainly as an extended drawn out linear chain. The disaccharide unit of cellobiose is stabilised by a hydrogen bond between the hemiacetal ring oxygen and the oxygen at O-3. In cellulose the linear chains may be packed in parallel or antiparallel arrangements to form fibres. Other examples of 'ribbon-like' structures are the β-(1→4) mannans and β(1→4) xylans. Whereas in starch, the axial–equatorial glycosidic bond of the maltose unit subtends at an acute angle and allows the α-glucan chain to fold and coil. A consequence of the difference in configuration of the hydroxyl group at the C-1 atom between cellobiose and maltose is the stabilising hydrogen bond between O-3 of one residue and O-2 of its near neighbour for the

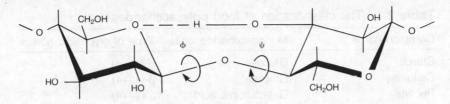

cellobiose

maltose unit

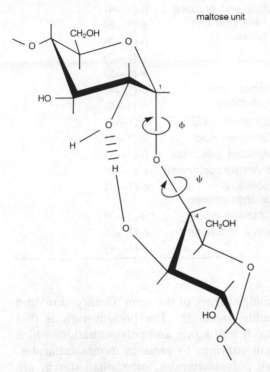

Fig. 2.1 Hydrogen bonded conformation of disaccharide units. For cellobiose, the hydrogen bond is between the ring oxygen and the C-3 hydroxyl groups of adjacent glucose residues. For maltose, the hydrogen bond is between the C-2 and the C-3 hydroxyl groups of adjacent glucose residues

maltose disaccharide unit. In the solid state, as stored in plants, amylose chains are compressed into coiled springs with an average six residues per turn. Other coiled polysaccharides are formed with β(1→3) glycosidic linkages where the O-2 atoms of the monosaccharide units project into the centre of the helix to form interchain hydrogen bonds.

Since 1975 a new dimension has been added to food polysacchar-

Table 2.1 The classification of food polysaccharides

Common name	Monosaccharide units	Type of glycosidic bonds
Starch	Glucose	α-(1→4)
Cellulose	Glucose	β-(1→4)
Pectins	Galacturonic acid	α-(1→4)
	L-Rhamnose, arabinose	β-(1→2)
	Xylose	α-(1→2)
Glucans	Glucose	β-(1→3)
Hemicelluloses containing xyloglucans and arabinoxylans	Xylose and glucose arabinose and xylose	β-(1→4)
		α-(1→6)
		β-(1→2)
		α-(1→2)
		α-(1→3)
Galactomannan	Mannose and galactose	β-(1→4)
		α-(1→6)
Alginic acid	Mannuronic acid	β-(1→4)
	L-Guluronic acid	α-(1→4)
Carrageenan	Sulphated galactose	β-(1→4)
	3,6-Anhydrogalactose	α-(1→3)
Xanthan gum	Glucose, 6-acetylmannose	β-(1→4)
	Glucuronic acid	α-(1→3)
	Pyruvyl mannose	β-(1→2)
		β-(1→4)

ides, as the consumer increasingly hears of the term 'dietary fibre' and the associated claimed benefits to health. The present view is that dietary fibre is mainly plant cell wall lignin and polysaccharides which are not hydrolysed by human enzymes to produce monosaccharides. In reality this means that all polysaccharides, other than starch, are part of the dietary fibre. Among the plant polysaccharides only starch contains the amylase susceptible α-(1→4) glucosidic bond which links the monosaccharide units. The β-(1→4) glucosidic bond of cellulose, the α-(1→4) galacturonate bonds of pectins, and the β-glycosidic bonds of galactomannans, pentosans and many other plant polysaccharides (Table 2.1) are not hydrolysed by human enzymes.

STARCH

Starch is the main storage carbohydrate of higher plants. It is found in cereal grains, leguminous seeds and fruits and is a long term reserve

Table 2.2 Sources of starch

Food commodity	Starch (%)	Food commodity	Starch (%)
Arrowroot	94	Butter bean	46
Potatoes	20.3	Haricot bean	43
Barley, pearl	84	Mung bean	34
Rice, polished	87	Red kidney bean	42
Maize	63	Lentils	51
Wheat	63	Chick pea	40
Pea	66	Red pigeon pea	45
Soya flour	12	Plantain	27
Tapioca (cassava)	25	Sweet potato	12
Oatmeal, raw	73	Yam	31

(Paul and Southgate 1978).

for later germination and growth in sprouting seeds. Starch is also the main constituent of rhizomes and tubers, for example the potato (Table 2.2). The cereal grains (the *Graminacea*), which contain different amounts of starch, have been of special importance as they have supplied during the last 3000 years, some of the basic nutritional needs of man.

The carbohydrates are the major constituent of the wheat grain, forming approximately 82 per cent of the total dry matter; they include starch (63 %), cellulose, hemicelluloses, and small amounts of the raffinose series of oligosaccharides. Starch is important, first, as a dietary source of energy and secondly because its physical properties influence the texture and acceptability of foods. In the wheat grain, starch is found in the endosperm that forms approximately 80 per cent of the total grain weight (Fig. 2.2). The selective proportions by weight of the different anatomical parts of the grain and their contribution to the food value is given in Table 2.3. All the wheat starch is contained within the endosperm, whereas the other smaller anatomical parts contain most of the lipid.

The importance of the endosperm constituents to the bread industry

Table 2.3 The chemical constituents of the wheat grain

Anatomical part	(% w/w)	Constituents			
		Starch	Protein	Fibre	Lipid
		(% of total)			
Endosperm	82	100	72	4	20
Germ	3	0	8	3	50
Bran	15	0	20	93	30

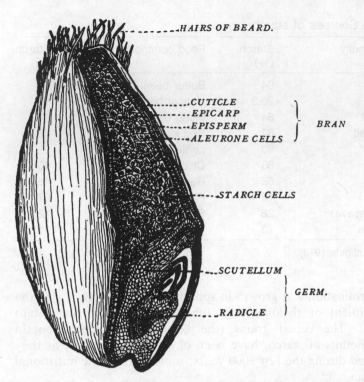

Fig. 2.2 The cereal grain. Cereal grains differ greatly in size and shape. T'eff, a grain from Ethiopia, is round and as small as a pin-head. Wheat, rye and rice are larger and elongated. Maize is the largest grain known (by courtesy of H. G. Muller, from Jago and Jago 1911)

has led to an increasing need to understand the mechanical properties of cereal grains and starch. The main aim of the wheat milling process is to separate the endosperm from the bran and germ and thus to produce flour. The bran and germ are rejected by the flour miller mainly because of their undesirable colour and the high oil content, respectively. For the separation process the wheat grain is first broken by fluted 'break rolls' to open the grain and scraped to remove the endosperm. Secondly the endosperm is reduced in size by crushing to a fine flour composed of small particles of approximately 140 μm in diameter. The aleurone layer of the wheat grain is associated with the bran fraction and contains up to 60 per cent of the total minerals of the seed as well as substantial amounts of lipid, nicotinic acid, phosphorus and dietary-important arbinoxylans. In white flour only approximately 72 per cent of the wheat grain is present, whereas the composition of wholemeal flour represents all the constituents of the original grain. During the milling of wheat the mechanical processes fragment and impinge the starch granules, which inflicts on the starch component varying degrees of mechanical damage. The physical difference between hard and soft endosperm depends on the adhesive forces between the starch granules and endosperm proteins which may be correlated with the occurrence of specific surface starch granule proteins. For hard wheats (grown in Canada, the United States and Australia), the endosperm fractures along the cell boundaries to yield a coarse gritty flour which on grinding increases starch damage. The greater degree of starch damage in the hard wheat flours enhances the absorption of water which is one of the requirements for the production of a satisfactory dough for the manufacture of bread. For bread-making, moderate amounts of mechanical damage to starch are desirable and this factor can be controlled by adjusting milling procedures. The production of satisfactory bread requires a complex balance between the amount of water used, the protein content of the flour, its damaged starch and the level of α-amylase. Damaged starch supplies the substrate for the enzymatic action of α- and β-amylases which acting in turn are important for the production by hydrolysis of fermentable glucose. Intact starch granules are resistant to enzyme attack. However, excessive starch damage or high α-amylase activity, results in an uneven loaf with large gas pockets. In wet seasons, sprouting of wheat grains is high and the biosynthesis of hydrolytic enzymes is triggered by the release of natural gibberellins. The aleurone layer of cells is the main site of biosynthesis for the endosperm-degrading enzymes. Alternatively, flours low in α-amylase activity can be supplemented with fungal α-amylase. Further grinding followed by air classification can be used to separate the wheat starch from the less dense protein in which the starch granules are embedded.

For potato starch the isolation is relatively easy, where first, milling is affected by a rotary saw to destroy the parenchyma cells in order to release the starch granules and secondly, purification is achieved by washing and settling of the granules. Likewise, for cassava starch (grown in Brazil and other countries within 30 ° latitude of the equator), owing to the low content of protein the isolation of starch is relatively simple and requires washing and peeling of roots, cell disintegration and settling of the cassava starch. For the separation of maize starch steeping in water for up to 40 hours is required to loosen the starch in the endosperm by solubilisation of the maize proteins before milling. The maize germ, which contains approximately 50 per cent of oil is first removed by flotation, and the starch is separated from the corn gluten by a cyclone system.

All starches occur as semicrystalline insoluble granules which vary in size, shape and mechanical strength. During plant growth the average size, shape and chemical composition of starch granules may change; for potato starch the average granule diameter has been claimed to increase from <10 to 50 μm as the tuber develops. In the starches of barley and wheat there are two distinct size populations of granules; the large (10–35 μm) A-granules and the smaller (1–10 μm)

B-granules. However, reported results for the proportional amounts of each type of granule can be misleading, because the smaller granules may be retained in the gluten and the larger granules may be modified further through the action of amylases during their isolation. The physically imperfect granules are referred to as damaged starch. For wheat starch, when special attention is given to the preparative methods, B-granules represent up to 30 per cent by weight of the starch.

For other food starches the granules are equally small and values which range from 8 to 50 μm have been reported. For oats the starch granules are compounded and contain a large number of separate starch particles. Such differences in size and shape can be used to identify the origin of most of the commercial starches (Fig. 2.3). Pea starch granules are often found cracked and fragmented; polyhedral granules are found in rice and maize.

Morphology of the starch grain

Storage starch is synthesised in plastids known as amyloplasts which contain, located on the inner surfaces of the membrane, the enzymes for starch synthesis. In starch grains, concentric growth rings can generally be observed which probably represent previous daily fluctuations in the biosynthesis of the starch polymers, determined by the availability of glucose arising from photosynthesis. The distances (120–400 nm) between growth rings probably represent the length of the starch molecule with the enzymes accumulating at the growth ring interfaces. The molecular axis of the starch polymer chains is perpendicular to the interfaces of the concentric growth rings and the overall growth of the starch from the centre (the hilum) of the starch grain is radial. Crystalline starch between the growth rings is birefringent.

Fig. 2.3   Bright field and polarised light photomicrographs of various
starches (bar = 50 μm)
(a) **Wheat starch**: two distinct granule types, i.e. large round
granules (Lens-shaped) and small spherical granules. Note
bright polarisation cross when lens-shaped granule is viewed
edgewise. Milling damage results in a more diffuse polarisation
cross.
(b) **Corn starch**: rounded granules from floury endosperm and
angular granules (many five-sided) from waxy endosperm.
Prominent central hilum.
(c) **Banana starch**: irregularly shaped ovoid granules, hila
extremely eccentric (see polarised light image).
(d) **Lentil starch**: ovoid or kidney-shaped granules, some
compound granules, central hila deeply fissured.
(Kindly prepared by Dr F. O. Flint.)

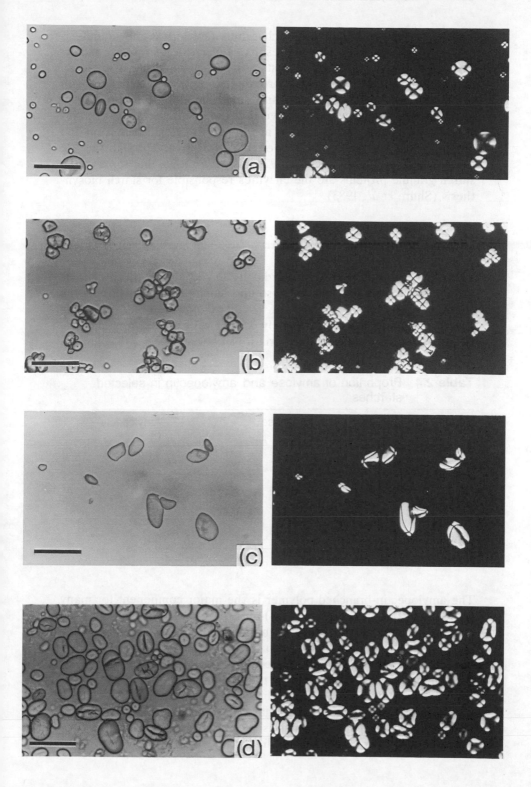

The characteristic shapes of starch grains develop as the granule is extended radially. Based on the results of electron microscopy and X-ray diffraction, it has been suggested that each molecule is made up of crystallites with lengths of approximately 7 nm. Interspersed with the starch granules are proteins and small amounts (0.5 %) of lyso-lecithins. Electrophoresis has shown that these starch granule proteins comprise a distinct group which are readily distinguished from the albumins and storage proteins (Gough *et al.* 1985). Through the use of immunofluorescence microscopy it has been shown that some of the starch granule proteins are the enzymes responsible for starch biosynthesis (Shure *et al.* 1983)

Chemical structure of starch

The polysaccharide is an α-glycosidically linked glucan which consists of two distinct components: amylose and amylopectin. Amylose is the simple mainly linear polymer of α-glucose residues and in many starches accounts for approximately 25 per cent of the total starch – although there are considerable variations between species (Table 2.4).

Table 2.4 Proportion of amylose and amylopectin in selected starches

Starch	Amylose (%)	Amylopectin (%)
Maize	26	74
Wheat	25	75
Potato	24	76
Waxy maize	1	99
Tapioca	17	83
Amylo maize	75	25

(With permission from Howling 1980).

The amylopectin-branched polymer is the major component for many well known starches. Both α-(1→4)-and α-(1→6)-glycosidic bonds are present in amylopectin, which is thought to represent the crystalline starch molecule interposed between the growth rings. The starch granules grow by gradual addition of residues of glucose to the surface of the starch granules, rather than by the addition of new material within the centre of the granules. The biosynthesis of starch involves the biosynthesis from glucose-1-phosphate and ATP, of adenosyl diphosphoglucose (ADP-glucose) which is then used as a glucose donor for the extension of α-(1→4)-glucan chains:

$$\text{glucose-1-phosphate} + \text{ATP} \xrightleftharpoons{\text{E-1}} \text{ADP-glucose} + \text{pyrophosphate}$$

$$\text{ADP-glucose} + \alpha\text{-glucan} \xrightleftharpoons{\text{E-2}} \text{glu-}\alpha\text{-glucan} + \text{ADP}$$

E-1, ADP glucose pyrophosphorylase, (EC 2.7.7.27)
E-2, starch synthase (EC 2.4.1.21)

For the synthesis of amylopectin, the α-1,6-linkages are formed by transfer of a small end part of a linear α-glucan chain to the hydroxyl group of the C-6 atom of a non-reducing terminal glucose residue.

Amylose

Amylose is a linear polymer of α-D-glucose residues, thought to be in the $^4C_1$ conformation, linked mainly by (1→4)-glycosidic bonds. The molecular weight of amylose is variable and the molecule may contain between 7500 and 50,000 residues of glucose. Solid amylose exists in three separate crystalline states A, B and C, and it has been suggested that B-amylose contains a helical structure of six α-D-glucopyransoyl residues per turn of the helix. It has been suggested that long helical structures in amylose are stabilised by hydrogen bonding between the C-2 hydroxyl group of one α-glucopyranosyl residue and a hydroxyl group of the adjacent 4-O-substituted α-glucopyranosyl unit (Fig. 2.1). However, the configuration for amylose in solution is unknown and may be substantially changed in different solvents. The types of structure in solution may vary from random to helical coils and probably includes a mixture of both types. The inclusion of iodine atoms within the helix of amylose is believed to be responsible for the blue colour of the starch–iodine complex. Other insoluble amylose complexes are also formed with both 1-butanol and thymol.

Amylopectin

2,3-Di-O-methyl-D-glucose is obtained after methylation and subsequent hydrolysis of starch or amylopectin. The number of residues of 2,3,4,6-tetra-O-methyl-D-glucose obtained from amylopectin which represents the non-reducing ends of α-glucan chains corresponds closely with the number of residues of 2,3-dimethylglucose obtained. This indicates for the amylopectin molecule that for every branch point containing an α-(1→6)-glycosidic bond, there is also one end chain which contains a non-reducing residue. The average chain length is approximately twenty-five residues of glucose which translates to approximately 4 to 5 per cent of the glycosidic bonds of the α-(1→6)-

type for amylopectin. Whereas the average chain length for glycogen, which is more ramified and water soluble than amylopectin, is from ten to fourteen residues. The molecular weight of amylopectin molecule is of the order 10^7 to 10^8. Proof of the chemical structure of the branch point has been obtained by the isolation of both isomaltose (6-O-α-D-glucopyranosyl-D-glucose) and trisaccharides which contain the α-1,6-linkage from waxy maize starch and glycogen. Other types of linkages, such as α-(1→2)-glycosidic bonds are not thought to occur in starch, although a complete understanding of the chemical structure of the amylopectin molecule has not been achieved. The use of the specific enzyme, pullulanase, for hydrolysis of the α-1,6-linkage together with β-amylase has indicated that amylopectin may exist as a cluster molecule (Manners and Matheson 1981). Based on the proposed arrangement of α-glucan chains (Fig. 2.4) in the cluster molecule different types of linear α-glucan chains (A and B) have been designated. The A and B chains, after hydrolysis catalysed by pullulanase, can be separated by molecular sieve chromatography, although the interpretation of the results is dependent on the strict use of highly purified enzymes. The chains, as shown in Fig. 2.4 are believed to be short with approximately fifteen residues of glucose, one non-reducing terminal glucose residue and only one α-1,6-linkage. The occurrence of two or more α-1,6-linkages and an average chain length of forty-five residues characterises the B chains. In the model the A chains are clustered together and are believed to represent the crystalline regions within the granules. As for amylose, helical structures for the A chains may exist in the solid state.

Technological uses of starch

The food industry has used isolated starches for three purposes. First, for the preparation of starch pastes, secondly, in the form of starch gels, and thirdly, for the manufacture of glucose, maltose or fructose syrups by hydrolysis.

STARCH PASTES AND GELS

Granular starch is mainly insoluble in cold water due to hydrogen bonding between the hydroxyl groups of the glucose residues, although very slow leaching of amylose chains can occur particularly from damaged starch granules. Such leached linear amylose chains can re-associate to produce a congealed rubbery material. This process is known as retrogradation and the product is known as retrograded starch. Solubilisation of starch granules commences at higher temperatures (approximately 55 °C) when the hydrogen bonds between glucose residues are broken. The compact starch grain then absorbs water. The

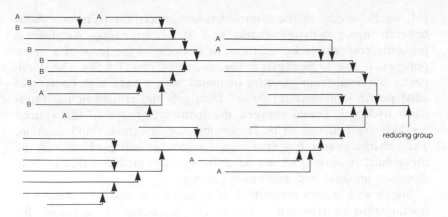

Fig. 2.4 Diagrammatic representation of a part of a molecule of
amylopectin (with permission from Manners and Matheson 1981)

Table 2.5 Initial gelatinisation temperatures for various starches

Starch	Temperature (° C)	Starch	Temperature (° C)
Barley	51.5	Sorghum	68
Potato	50	Tapioca (Brazilian)	49
Pea	57	Wheat	58
Rice	68	Waxy maize	63
Rye	57	High amylose corn	67

(Snyder 1984).

precise gelatinisation temperature is different for various starches
(Table 2.5). During gelatinisation, the crystal structure and consequently birefringence is lost permanently whereby the starch grains
swell to absorb up to 100 times their own volume of water. The
viscoelastic hot starch paste is a composite of dispersed aggregated
starch molecules, swollen starch granules and fragments and solubilised amylose. The process of gelatinisation can be followed by
viscosity measurements which show a maximum peak at the gelatinisation temperature. Later, at higher temperatures, a more gradual
increase of viscosity of hot starch paste is probably due to continuing
slow release of small amounts of exuded amylose networks. The technologist frequently observes major variations in pasting behaviour for
starches, which may be due to differences in the size of granules,
proportions of amylose, or the enzymatic action of naturally occurring
and contaminating amylases. In addition, starch always contains a
small amount of protein which can also interfere with the pasting properties and the proportion of physically damaged starch increases the
absorption of water. On cooling, starch suspensions form an elastic

gel, which is due to the intermolecular association (retrogradation) between linear amylose chains and starch granules. Amylose is primarily responsible for gelation, as it alone in the form of a linear polymer, is able to form gels at low concentrations (1.5 %). The starch pastes obtained from varieties of maize with a very high content of amylopectin (amylomaize) do not form gels and remain liquid. Inter-chain hydrogen bonds between the hydroxyl groups of the glucose residues are believed to be responsible for association and gelation. The amylose chains may exist in gels as double helices. However, the rheological behaviour of normal starch gels is probably due to both dissolved amylose and gelatinised granules.

Starch with a high proportion of amylose can also be obtained by fractionation of common starches. The fractionation technique for obtaining high amylose–starch requires the addition of 1-butanol to a hot dispersion of starch granules in order to separate on cooling an amylose–butanol complex by centrifugation or filtration. Alternatively, starch can be dissolved completely in dimethylsulphoxide – which breaks the hydrogen bonds that are responsible for the insolubility of α-amylose – prior to precipitation with butanol. Pure amylose is obtained by redissolving the butanol complex and the subsequent removal of the alcohol by distillation. However, only where there is an abundance of energy at low cost is such a fractionation process economically viable at present. For commercial use high-amylose starches require high temperatures for dispersion and gelatinisation, in order to break the hydrogen bonds between the polymer chains. High-amylose starch preparations are used where rapid setting is required for the manufacture of gums and impervious films. For other starches which contain small amounts of amylose, soft gels are formed on cooling which can be beneficial, as contraction of the gel (syneresis) and retrogradation are decreased. Chemically modified amyloses can be used to decrease the temperature required for dispersion of the amylose starch.

For starch pastes the physical properties may be modified by other substances present as either impurities or as deliberate extenders. Sodium chloride reduces the swelling and breakdown of starch gran-ules, whereas sodium hydroxide accelerates swelling; sugars compete for the molecules of water and thus limit swelling; fats inhibit swelling. For the manufacture of pre-gelatinised starch, which is obtained by drying of a hydrated starch solution before gelation, extensively physi-cally damaged starch is required. Pre-gelatinised starches are used as cold pasting products and should not require additional heating if all the starch granules have been gelatinised before drying. In order to modify the functional properties of starch, the structure of the starch granule can be strengthened by the incorporation of either substituent chemical groups or artificial cross-links. Such chemically substituted starches have been used for 25 years or more by the food industry as thickeners, stabilisers and ingredients of frozen desserts. The cross-linked starches are used to provide resistance to both heat-treatment and the disintegration of starch gels during mechanical processing. For cross-linking, bifunctional reagents, such as phosphorus oxychloride and carboxylic acid anhydrides, are used to form a bridge between the hydroxyl groups of different α-glucan chains. The chemical structure of the phosphate and adipate cross-linked starch is shown below:

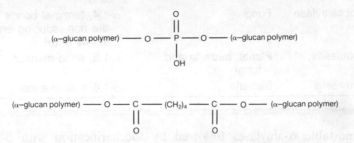

For phosphorylated starch, the maximum value for the amount of permitted phosphorus is 0.04 per cent, which corresponds to one phosphate cross-link for 500 residues of anhydroglucose, or two chains of α-glucan each containing on average 250 residues of glucose per atom of phosphorus. For adipate-derived starch, the maximum value for adipic acid is 0.12 per cent, which corresponds to one adipic acid cross-link for 750 residues of anhydroglucose. Monosubstituted derivatives are used to reduce the shrinkage of starch gels by reducing hydrogen bonding between the separate α-glucan chains of amylose. Minor substitutions of acetylated, hydroxypropylated or phosphorylated starches have generally been accepted for use in foods, although extensive toxicological studies are now in hand. The previous use of epichlorohydrin to form cross-linked starches has been withdrawn due to concern over the possible toxicity of the modifying reagent.

STARCH HYDROLYSATES

Historically, saccharide syrups, as required by the pharmaceutical and food industries, were obtained by acid hydrolysis of starch. However, the composition of such products varied considerably with some containing as little as 10 per cent of glucose and up to 72 per cent of higher oligosaccharides. For higher conversions to glucose, which required more severe acid hydrolysis conditions, undesirable by-products that affect flavour and colour are often present. Today, through the use of a range of specific enzymes, various mixtures of glucose with maltose or other higher saccharides can be obtained. The raw material has normally been corn starch obtained by the wet milling of maize although alternative sources of starch from cassava, potato and wheat are available. The processes have involved dispersion and liquefaction at approximately 105 °C of the starch in the presence of

Table 2.6 Starch hydrolysis by commercially available enzymes

Enzyme	Source	Glycosidic bonds hydrolysed
α-Amylase	Plants, bacteria and fungi	α-1,4, random endo-manner
β-Amylase	Plants and bacteria	α-1,4, penultimate bond from the non-reducing end
β-Glucoamylase	Fungi	α-1,4, terminal bonds from the non-reducing end, and slowly α-1,6
Pullulanases	Plants, bacteria and fungi	α-1,6, endo-manner
Isoamylases	Bacteria	α-1,6 endo-manner

thermostable α-amylases followed by saccharification with β-gluco-amylase of the partially hydrolysed starch which consists of mainly oligosaccharides and α-limit dextrins. An increasing number of enzymes are now available (Table 2.6) for the degradation of both amylose and amylopectin and new processes should be able to make use of enzymes active towards the α-(1→6)-bonds of amylopectin.

STARCH-DEGRADING ENZYMES

α-Amylases (EC 3.2.1.1)

The α-amylases are endo-enzymes which catalyse the hydrolysis in a random manner of the α-(1→4)-glycosidic bonds in the central regions of amylose chains and amylopectin except in the vicinity of branch

points. The activity of the enzymes is assayed by measuring the reduced ability of test solutions of starch to form the characteristic blue colour with iodine, or alternatively by measuring the decrease in viscosity of starch suspensions. Thermostable enzymes, which permit the saccharification to be carried out at high temperatures, where the process is accelerated and bacterial action is minimised, have been obtained from *Bacillus subtilis* and *Bacillus licheniformis*. Although the fungal α-amylases from *Aspergillus oryzae* are heat-labile they are described as maltogenic. The syrup produced by the action of fungal α-amylase contains maltose (50 %), maltotriose (30 %) and glucose (5 %). Commercial fungal α-amylase has also use as a bread improver by addition to wheat dough; both gas retention and loaf volume

(Couvain 1987) are increased by commercial fungal α-amylases.

α-Amylases are calcium-dependent enzymes. Although the cation is not an integral part of the active site of the enzyme, Ca^{2+} is believed to stabilise the overall conformation of the enzymes. Up to ten atoms of Ca^{2+} may be bound per mole of enzyme. The molecular weights of most α-amylase enzymes are of the order of 50,000. The optimum activity of the enzymes is observed at pH 6 to 8. α-Amylases are inactivated in acidic foods and frequently exist as different isoenzymes. The porcine α-amylase isoenzymes seem to contain two similar structural parts, both with a molecular weight of approximately 25,000 held together by a disulphide bond and possessing enzymic activity. The porcine and *Aspergillus oryzae* enzymes are glycoproteins (Robyt 1984).

β-Amylases (EC 3.2.1.2)

The β-amylases are exo-enzymes which hydrolyse the penultimate glycosidic bond from the non-reducing end of an α-glucan chain.

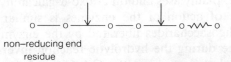

non–reducing end
residue

Like α-amylase, the β-amylases do not act on the α-(1→6)-glycosidic bonds and consequently the main product formed during the β-amylase-catalysed hydrolysis of both starch and amylopectin is a β-limit dextrin of high molecular weight. β-Amylases have been obtained from barley, wheat, rye, sweet potatoes and more recently from *Bacillus polymyxa* and *Bacillus cereus*. As the β-amylases catalyse the hydrolysis of the penultimate glycosidic bond, the low molecular weight product is mainly the disaccharide maltose. Because of the specific and limited action of β-amylases only small amounts of maltotriose and glucose are formed. The enzymes can be assayed by colorimetric methods which measure either the amounts of reducing sugar liberated from starch, or the amount of *p*-nitrophenol released after treatment with α-glucosidase of hydrolysed *p*-nitrophenol oligosaccharides. The specificity of β-amylase for the disaccharide unit at the non-reducing terminal can be explained by the presence of a pocket within the three-dimensional structure of the enzyme into which the disaccharide unit just fits. β-Amylases contain sulphydryl groups which are essential for enzymatic activity, although the optimal activity for the enzyme is usually observed in the pH range of from 4 to 5. Cereal β-amylases act in tandem with α-amylases during bread-making to produce maltose. As baking proceeds β-amylase is first inactivated. In wheat flours with high α-amylase activity, dextrins continue to be produced in the central parts of the loaf which are not then hydrolysed further by β-amylase, such that centrally a 'sticky' crumb is produced which adversely affects automatic slicing.

β-Glucoamylase (EC 3.2.1.3)

The β-glucoamylase enzymes differ from β-amylase mainly in so far as the enzyme catalyses the release of single glucose residues from the non-terminal ends of α-glucan chains. β-Glucoamylases can be assayed by either measurements of reducing sugar liberated, or now very specifically with the enzymes available for the determination of small quantities of glucose in aqueous solutions. Glucoamylase also catalyses the hydrolysis, albeit slowly, of α-(1→6)-glycosidic bonds. Thus theoretically starch can be completely hydrolysed to glucose by β-glucoamylase, but in practice resynthesis of maltose and isomaltose takes place probably through transferase-catalysed reactions. The β-glucoamylase from *Aspergillus niger* is a glycoprotein (MW 97,000) and optimum enzymic activity is observed at pH 5.0 (Robyt 1984). For β-glucoamylase, β-amylases and other exo-α-glucan hydrolyases (Table 2.7) the mode of action of the enzymes is similar as the glucose, maltose and oligosaccharides liberated by the enzymes are always β-anomers. Hence during the hydrolytic reaction inversion of configuration of the hydroxyl group at the C-1 atom of the glucose residues takes place. This type of inversion can be explained through the direct addition of a molecule of water from above the plane of the sugar ring towards the carboxyl groups of postulated acetal–ester intermediates (Fig. 2.5).

For α-amylase-catalysed hydrolysis inversion at the C-1 atom of the glucose residues does not occur. This type of hydrolytic reaction, where the configuration is retained, can be explained by addition of a molecule of water directed from below the plane of the sugar ring towards the anomeric carbon atom of an acetal–ester intermediate (Fig. 2.5).

Table 2.7 The occurrence of microbial exo-glucanhydrolases

Source	Products formed
Streptomyces griseus	Maltotriose + limit dextrin
Enterobacter aerogenes	Maltohexaose + limit dextrin
Bacillus licheniformis	Maltopentaose + limit dextrin
Pseudomonas stutzeri	Maltohexaose + limit dextrin
Aspergillus niger	Glucose + limit dextrin
Rhizopus species	Glucose + limit dextrin
	Maltose + limit dextrin

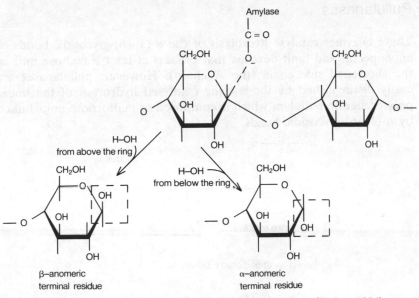

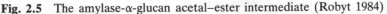

Fig. 2.5 The amylase-α-glucan acetal–ester intermediate (Robyt 1984)

Debranching enzymes

Isoamylases (EC 3.2.1.68) and pullulanases (EC 3.2.1.41) have been termed 'debranching enzymes' which are likely to be extremely valuable for improving the saccharification of starch, as even most purified high-amylose starches normally contain at least 7 per cent of amylopectin. Increased yields for glucose, a reduced requirement for glucoamylase and a shorter period of time for the reaction have all been claimed (Norman 1982). The debranching enzymes have also proved useful for structural studies on amylopectin.

Isoamylases

These enzymes which catalyse the hydrolysis of the α-(1→6)-glycosidic bonds of amylopectin, glycogen and oligosaccharides have been obtained from a number of different microorganisms (*Pseudomonas amyloderamose* and *Flavabacteria spp.*). The minimum structural requirements for the substrates are separate maltose and maltotriose units linked by an α-(1,6)-glycosidic bond:

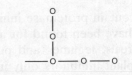

maltosyl–(1 → 6)–α–D–maltotriose unit

Pullulanases

These enzymes catalyse hydrolysis of the α-(1→6)-glycosidic bonds of amylopectin and limit dextrins that possess at least a maltose unit in the shortened side chain (the A chain). However, pullulanases are easily distinguished by the specific catalysed hydrolysis of the linear polysaccharide pullulan, which is composed of maltotriose units linked by α-(1→6)-glycosidic bonds.

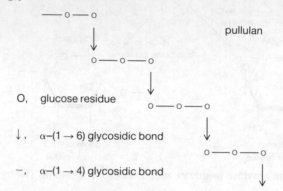

Pullulanases catalyse the hydrolysis of the α-(1→6)-linkages in a random manner to liberate maltotriose. Norman (1982) has claimed that a pullulanase from a *Bacillus sp.* is more heat stable than the isoamylases. Thus its use is preferred in conjunction with β-glucoamylase in order to increase the yield of D-glucose from starches and amylopectin.

The manufacture of glucose syrups from starch has been expanded further by the development of an enzymatic isomerisation process for the conversion of D-glucose to D-fructose. Immobilised glucose isomerase from *Bacillus coagulans* and other soluble inexpensive microbial and fungal isomerases are now available for the manufacture of a wide range of products containing different glucose : fructose ratios of varying sweetness. High-fructose syrups (42 % fructose) produced using immobilised enzymes can be used in beverages, flavour concentrates, jams and preserves, although there are some limitations due to the hygroscopic and crystalline properties of fructose.

AMYLASE INHIBITORS

Just as plant materials contain proteinase inhibitors, inhibitors also of a proteinaceous nature have been found for amylases. Such inhibitors have been found in cereals, legumes and potato tubers (Table 2.8) although generally the plant inhibitors only inhibit higher animal and insect α-amylases. Small non-protein molecules inhibit β-amylase and

Table 2.8 Amylase Inhibitors

Source	Enzyme inhibited	Type
Kidney beans[†]	α-Amylase	Protein
Oats[†]	α- and β-Amylases	Protein
Potato[†]	α-Amylase	Non-protein
Rye[†]	α-Amylases	Protein
Wheat[†]	α- Amylase	Protein
Streptomyces griseosporeus[‡] YM-25	α-Amylase	Thermostable proteins
Streptomyces N280[§]	α-Amylase	N-containing oligosaccharides
Streptomyces diastaticus and amylostaticus[¶]	α-Amylase and β-Glucoamylase	Oligosaccharides – amylostatins
Schardinger dextrins[†]	β-Amylase	Cyclic oligosaccharides
Chemical reagents[†]	α- and β-Amylases and β-glucoamylase	D-Glucono-1,5-lactone
Chemical reagents[†]	α- and β-Amylases	Maltobionolactone
Chemical reagents[†]	α- and β-Amylase and β-glucoamylase	5-Amino-5-deoxy-D-glucopyranose
Chemical reagents[†]	β-Amylase and β-glucoamylase	Maltosylamine

([†] Robyt 1984; [‡] Goto *et al.* 1983; [§] Takeshi *et al.* 1983; [¶] Fukuhara *et al.* 1982).

glucoamylases. The occurrence and action of amylase inhibitors have been reviewed by Whitaker (1983) and Robyt (1984). The activity of the inhibitors in extracts can be assayed by their interference with the hydrolysis of starch catalysed by amylases. One unit of inhibitor activity has been defined as that which produces an inhibition of 50 per cent of enzymatic activity during a 20 min. period. Either recovery after chromatography of α-amylase activity exceeding 100 per cent from crude extracts of the enzyme, or the occurrence of multiple pH optima for purified α-amylases are observations indicative of the presence of α-amylase inhibitors in the original tissue extracts.

The wheat and rye α-amylase inhibitors have been shown to specifically inhibit non-competitively only the mammalian salivary and pancreatic enzymes. For the red kidney bean the mode of action of the α-amylase inhibitor is also non-competitive. The inhibitor is claimed to form a 1 : 1 molar complex with the enzyme.

The mode of action of the protein inhibitors is unknown, but the interaction seems to be stoichiometric. K_i values of 10^{-10} M have been quoted for the binding of the kidney bean α-amylase inhibitor. For enzyme–inhibitor complexes small glucan chains are still hydrolysed and therefore the interaction between inhibitor and enzyme may not directly involve the active site of the enzyme. Furthermore, a greater inhibitory effect is often found when the enzyme alone has been pre-incubated with the inhibitor. In two instances, with wheat and oat inhibitors, thiols have inactivated the inhibitors which suggests that disulphide groups are required to maintain the essential tertiary struc-ture of either the inhibitors, or the enzyme–inhibitor complex. For three inhibitors obtained from wheat, sequence homologies have been found for peptides containing cysteine residues. Two protein inhibitors of α-amylase which retained 80 per cent of the inhibitory activity after heat-treatment at 100 °C for 10 min. have been obtained from an actinomycete (Goto *et al.* 1983). A large number of α-amylase inhibi-tors which are small oligosaccharides and contain one atom of nitrogen per mole have also been isolated from *Streptomyces sp N280* (Takeshi *et al.* 1983). Although some of the protein inhibitors are digested by pepsin, attempts have been made to use phaseolamin, the α-amylase inhibitor from *Phaseolus vulgaris* to inhibit the mammalian digestion of starch. However, for such 'starch-blockers' various unde-sirable side-effects, including intestinal flatulence and nausea, have been observed. Since 1982 the sale of 'starch-blockers' has been prohibited by the United States Food and Drug Administration.

The non-protein inhibitors of amylases are generally derivatives of small unusual oligosaccharides or monosaccharides (Table 2.8) and therefore probably act through association with the active site of the enzymes. The amylostatins, have been isolated from the culture filtrates of a *Streptomycetes diastaticus* (Fukuhara *et al.* 1982) and contain an N-substituted 4-amino-6-deoxy-D-glucose and an unsatu-rated cyclitol linked to small glucan chains (Fig. 2.6). Five different amylostatins have been obtained containing α-1,4-glucan chains which possess different inhibitory activities against various amylases.

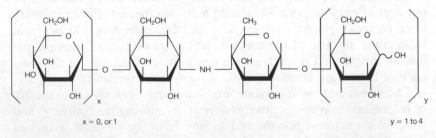

x = 0, or 1   y = 1 to 4

Fig. 2.6 The chemical structure of amylostatins (Fukuhara *et al.* 1982)

CELLULOSE

Cellulose is not a nutrient source for man, but it can be digested in the rumen of grass-eating animals. However as the main constituent of plant cell walls, cellulose is a substantial component of the diet. Moreover, in a microcrystalline form, and as chemical derivatives, cellulose is used by the food industry as a stabiliser and filler. Commercial microcrystalline cellulose is manufactured by partial hydrolysis of amorphous cellulose with dilute hydrochloric acid. The acid-insoluble material is essentially the natural crystalline component, with most crystallites having a particle size of 0.2 μm. Generally the product is used in conjunction with other water-soluble derivatives of celluloses and in the case of ice-cream in the presence of carrageenan and locust bean gum. The chemically modified celluloses and their uses by the food industry are listed in Table 2.9. With the exception of possible small degrees of hydrolysis by microorganisms in the large intestine, the cellulose derivatives are not hydrolysed by man. Consequently, all the cellulose derivatives are particularly valuable in dietetic foods as well as in special foods for diabetics, and for individuals allergic to wheat gluten. Cellulose, might be used for the manufacture of glucose syrups and more useful products if an efficient enzymatic process could be developed.

Table 2.9 Chemical derivatives of cellulose for the food industries

Cellulose derivative	Chemical substituent	Some common food uses
Carboxymethylcellulose	$-CH_2-CO_2H$	Soluble as the sodium salt Ice-cream stabiliser Ingredient in cream substitutes Reduce syneresis in starch gels Thickener and emulsifier Bulking agent in dietetic foods in conjunction with microcrystalline cellulose
Methylcellulose	$-CH_3$	Soluble on cold water-reversible gels formed at high temperatures Extruded impermeable films
Hydroxypropylcellulose	$-CH_2-CH(OH)-CH_3$	Soluble in cold water Good stabiliser of emulsions

Cellulose occurs naturally as an insoluble fibrous material which is not easily degraded by enzymes; it is a composite of linear residues of glucose which are linked by β-(1→4)-glycosidic bonds. The polymer chain of cellulose, because of the equatorial linkages, remains straight (Fig. 2.7) and therefore tends to form crystals. The molecules of cellulose, held together by hydrogen bonds and other non-covalent forces to form fibrils, may contain up to 10,000 residues of glucose. Along the fibril, there are intermittent highly ordered crystalline regions of approximately 50 nm interposed by more open amorphous regions. From electron micrographs it can be seen that cellulose from plants is composed of linear fibrils of 3.5 nm diameter which are calculated to contain approximately thirty-six chains of the β-D-glucan polymer. As the length of the fibrils is considerably greater than the length of the β-glucan chains, fibrils must also be made up of a series of β-glucan chains linked end-to-end (Fig. 2.7) with varying degrees of polymerisation. The β-glucan chains may also be folded which may extend and reinforce the crystalline regions transversely in directions perpendicular to the axis of the fibril.

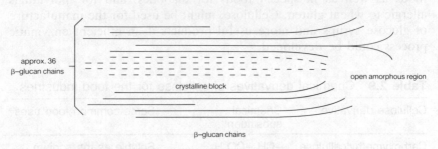

Fig. 2.7 Schematic representation of a cellulose fibre

The crystalline regions of cellulose react more slowly with acid and advantage is taken of this slow reaction for the manufacture of microcrystalline cellulose. However, in order to enhance hydrolysis of cellulose, physical and chemical pre-treatments are required. The physical treatments, which are energy-intensive, have included ball milling, wet milling and steam processing. Nevertheless, the chemical hydrolysis of cellulose is limited by both the low yield of glucose with many unwanted degradation products of monosaccharide and the high energy requirements.

For enzymatic hydrolysis catalysed by cellulases, susceptibility of the substrate to the enzymes can be increased by either first swelling in 0.5 M NaOH, or solubilisation in concentrated phosphoric acid followed by precipitation on dilution. Most extracellular preparations of cellulases can catalyse the hydrolysis of the chemical derivatives of cellulose like carboxymethylcellulose and phosphoric acid dispersed cellulose, but few cell-free preparations can hydrolyse native cellulose in a similar way to the whole microorganism. Generally, it is thought for the degradation of native cellulose that the amorphous regions are first hydrolysed followed by a slower hydrolysis of the crystalline parts of molecules. For a long time a unique enzymatic action (the C_1 enzyme or factor) has been suspected for 'opening up' the crystalline regions of native cellulose; it is possible that the C_1 factor splits the covalent bonds of cellulose chains at the crystallite surfaces to render cellulose fibrils more accessible to cellulases. For the complete degradation of native cellulose several enzymes are required to act sequentially or even synergistically.

Two types of enzymes, endo- and exoglucanases are believed to act cooperatively to produce the disaccharide cellobiose and glucose. The endoglucanase (1,4-β-glucanglucanohydrolase (EC 3.2.1.4) is believed to act randomly on the cellulose β-glucan chains. The exoglucanases (β-1,4-glucancellobiohydrolase and β-1,4-glucanglucohydrolase) produce cellobiose and glucose by catalysing the hydrolysis of the non-reducing terminal glucosidic bonds. Cellobiose can be further hydrolysed by β-glucosidase to produce glucose. However, maximum efficiency only occurs with either the crude enzyme extracts containing all three types of enzyme, or when the separated enzymes are recombined. β-Glucosidase is required to remove the cellobiose which is an inhibitor of the β-glucanases. Alternatively, cellobiose can be oxidised by either cellobiose dehydrogenase or cellobiose oxidase to relieve inhibition by cellobiose. The dehydrogenase enzyme requires an electron acceptor which may be one of several quinones. The oxidase enzyme uses molecular oxygen as electron acceptor.

Like many animal, plant and other microbial enzymes, the fungal cellulases exist in multiple forms in culture fluids and it is not yet clear whether these iso-enzymes are artefacts arising from extraneous proteolysis. Only limited progress has been made with the isolation of active cellulase preparations; and a better understanding of the kinetics, structure and function of cellulases is required before more efficient enzymes can be instituted through recombinant DNA technology.

GLYCOGENS

This polysaccharide is the carbohydrate reserve of animals and is mainly found in the liver and muscle tissue at concentrations of from 10 and 2 per cent, respectively. Glycogen, which is an α-1→4-glucan, is more highly branched than amylopectin and only contains approximately fifteen residues of glucose per chain length. The molecular weight is approximately 10^7. Glycogen is normally extracted from muscle tissue with concentrated potassium hydroxide solutions and recovered after precipitation with ethanol. The hydrolysis of glycogen is catalysed by phosphorylase to produce glucose-1-phosphate.

FRUCTANS

Polymers with molecular weights up to 8000 may contain from thirty to thirty-five residues of β-D-fructofuranoside which are linked by 1→2- or 6→2-glycosidic bonds. The fructans are essentially storage materials and may represent up to 80 per cent of the dry weight of some tubers or stems. Fructans are present in all cereals and form from 1 to 4 per cent of the dry weight. The polymer, is easily hydrolysed by acid and can be depolymerised enzymatically by β-fructan hydrolases. Fructan hydrolyases have been identified which cleave only the 1→2-β-glycosidic bonds between the fructose residues. Owing to the absence of these enzymes in the human small intestine it seems likely that fructans are not metabolised in man, although they are easily hydrolysed by dilute acid. For the food industry, fructans from plant tubers offer a more direct and alternative source of fructose syrups, without the need to use glucose isomerase.

The two types of polymeric fructans are higher fructose polymers of mainly two isomeric kestoses (Fig. 2.8). Grasses, including timothy grass (*Phleum protense*), contain the fructan phlein with a structure based on kestose. Inulin found in the tubers of dahlia or *Helianthus tuberosus* is a polymer based on the structure of isokestose. Inulin has been extracted from the roots of many plants including the Compositae and has been used as a diabetic food.

PECTINS

The plant cell walls of dicotyledons contain approximately 35 per cent of pectin. The middle lamella which lies between the primary cell walls is particularly rich in pectins. The crude content of pectin for a number of fruits and vegetables is given in Table 2.10. Pectins are a special group of substances responsible for the formation of gels in jam, preserves and fruit desserts. Pectin gel formation aids the long-term preservation by restricting the diffusion of water and other substances in an acidic product of low water activity. Commercially pectin is normally extracted from either apple waste by the manufacturers of cider or from citrus fruits.

Pectin is mainly a linear polymer composed of residues of esterified galacturonic acid which are linked by α-(1→4) axial–axial glycosidic

kestose-fructans

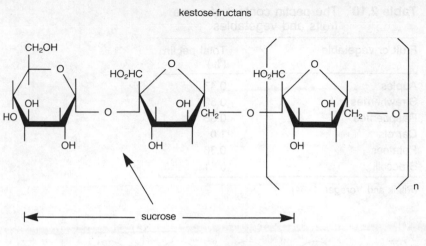

α–D–Glc*p*–(1 ⟷ 2)–β–D–Fru*f*–(6 → 2)–β–D–Fru*f*

isokestose-fructans

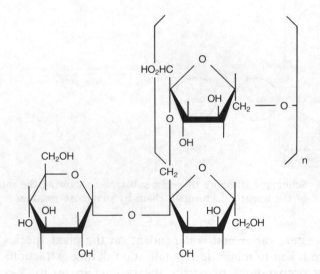

α–D–Glc*p*–(1 ⟷ 2)–β–D–Fru*f*–(1 → 2)–β–D–Fruf

Fig. 2.8 The chemical structure of fructans

bonds. For clarity the repeating chemical structure is given by the
Howarth configuration (Fig. 2.9). The precise molecular weight, like
that of other polysaccharides, is unknown and there may be as many
as 1000 monosaccharide residues per molecule. The amount of esterification of the carboxyl groups of the uronic acid residues, present as

Table 2.10   The pectin content of some
                 fruits and vegetables

Fruit or vegetable	Total pectin (%)
Apples	0.47
Strawberries	0.52
Raspberries	0.36
Carrots	1.0
Potatoes	0.36
Broccolli	0.51

(Pilnik and Voragen 1984).

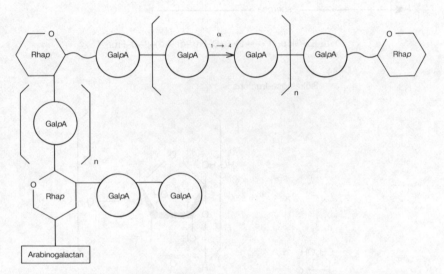

Fig. 2.9   Schematic structure of pectic substances, showing the interruption
              of the linear galacturonan chain by rhamnose residues

methyl ester, varies and is dependent on the plant species used and
the care taken to minimise saponification during extraction. As highly
purified preparations of pectin always contain up to 5 per cent of
neutral sugars, which include D-galactose, L-arabinose and L-rhamnose,
it is at present thought that the pectin polysaccharides consist
of mainly a rhamnogalacturonan backbone polymer with associated
side chains of arabinans and galactans. The rhamnose residues,
believed to be linked directly into the linear polymer of galacturonic
acid residues, form a kink in the chain through an α-(1→2)-bond at
the C-2 hydroxyl group of L-rhamnose. Other rhamnose residues may
form branch points for the arabinogalactans which in turn are covalently linked to xyloglucans. Thus the arabinogalactan interconnects
the linear galacturonans with xyloglucans (Dey and Brinson 1984).

Pectins can be de-esterified by dilute acid or alkali or by enzymes (pectin esterases) to produce pectic acid which is a polymer of α-D-galacturonic acid. Thus commercial preparations of pectin are mixtures of pectins with varying degrees of esterification and pectic acids. The gels formed with pectic acids are, like alginic acid gels, calcium dependent. It has been proposed that blocks of axially linked galacturonate residues form folded structures (Fig. 2.10) which are stabil-

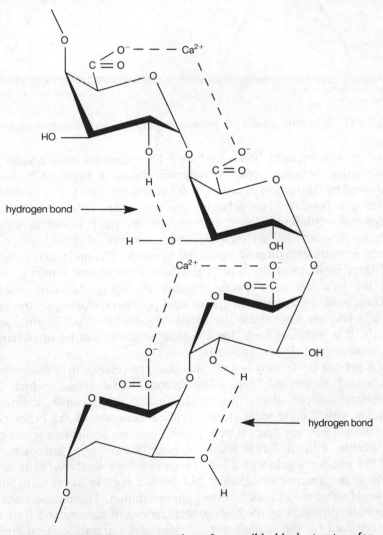

Fig. 2.10 Diagrammatic representation of a possible block structure for pectic acid. The galacturonic acid residues are linked by axial–axial bonds; such a structure may be stabilised by both hydrogen bonds and electrostatic bonds between the carboxylate anions and Ca²⁺

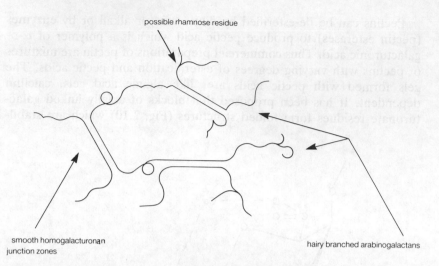

possible rhamnose residue

smooth homogalacturonan
junction zones

hairy branched arabinogalactans

Fig. 2.11 Schematic model for pectin gel junctions and branched regions

ised by non-covalent bonds and with Ca^{2+} through ionic bonds. The association between separate polymer chains is believed to be reinforced by interaction of either hydroxyl groups with Ca^{2+}, or through hydrogen bonding. For gelation, junction zones (Fig. 2.11) between segments of different linear polymer chains are believed to form at regular smooth (linear) regions, which are free of branch points, to form a continuous three-dimensional network. The molecular structure of three residues of the D-polygalacturonate is almost a mirror image of the structure of a similar number of L-polyguluronate residues (Thom *et al*. 1982) found in alginic acid polymers. Consequently, given a common mechanism for the mode of gelation of pectic and alginic acids, it is not surprising that the two polymers can be interchanged in a number of dessert products.

A gel can be defined as a product that can retain a firm recognisable structural shape imbibing a continuous liquid phase, which also contains a dispersed macromolecular matrix. Gels can be defined as liquids with a finite yield stress. Typical examples of the other polysaccharide gels are agar, starch, pectin, alginate and carrageenan gels.

Pectins with moderate levels of esterification (e.g. approximately 50 %) will form gels with Ca^{2+}. However, high methoxypectin forms gels in the absence of calcium, but both a high solids content and a low pH value are required in the gelling solution. These conditions are normally provided by the high concentrations of sucrose and fruit acid as required for the manufacture of jam and marmalade. Commercial preparation of rapid-set and slow-set pectins with high and lower esterification (70 % and 50 % respectively) are also available. Whether the araban and galactan side chains of pectins enhance gelation is unknown, but they may be important during the unwanted gelation of apricot nectar (Pilnik and Voragen 1984). At the low pH values and high methoxyl content, the electrostatic repulsion between polymer chains is likely to be minimal. Hence calcium-independent gelation of pectins is primarily due to interchain hydrogen bonds and it is known that urea, a hydrogen bond breaking reagent, weakens pectin gels. Nevertheless, at very high degrees of esterification (approximately 95 %) gelation does not occur, which also indicates that at low pH values a small number of un-ionised carboxyl groups might enhance intermolecular interactions for calcium-independent gelation of high methoxyl pectins. Pectin is stable under acid conditions, but it depolymerises under alkaline conditions by a β-elimination mechanism.

Enzymatic degradation

Although a pectinase is any enzyme capable of degrading pectin, the enzymes are classified by the now known mode of action of different types of enzymes on the substrates pectin and pectic acids.

Pectin esterase (EC 3.1.1.11)

This is a specific esterase only able to catalyse the hydrolysis of the esterified carboxyl groups of pectin. The enzyme is widely found in fruits and is produced by fungi and bacteria. The enzymatic activity can be determined by measurements of the titratable acid released, or alternatively where substantial hydrolysis occurs, by the precipitation of insoluble calcium pectate. Owing to the formation of blocks of carboxyl groups in pectinesterase-treated pectin, such pectins are highly sensitive to calcium ions. The pH optima for plant pectinesterases is approximately 6 to 8.0. The enzymes are activated by metal cations and quite high temperatures (70–90 °C) are required for inactivation. High concentrations of sugar inhibit pectinesterase and therefore prevent liquefaction of pectin gels in preserves.

Pectate hydrolases (EC 3.2.1.15)

Pectate hydrolases also act on high methoxyl pectin and therefore separate polymethylgalacturonases for specific hydrolysis of pectins probably do not exist. As for the hydrolysis of other polysaccharides or proteins, both endo- and exo-type enzymes for catalysing the hydrolysis of pectins and pectic acids have been distinguished. The endo-enzymes (Fig. 2.12) which inflict a large decrease in the molecular weight of the polymers can be assayed by changes in

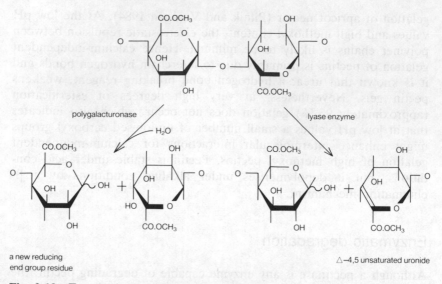

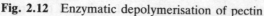

a new reducing
end group residue

△-4,5 unsaturated uronide

Fig. 2.12 Enzymatic depolymerisation of pectin

viscosity. The catalytic action of the exo-type enzymes (EC 3.2.1.67) results in the liberation of single residues of α-D-galacturonic acid or dimers which then can be detected chromatographically or with reducing group methods. For endo-enzymes it can be shown that only a few glycosidic bonds are hydrolysed for a large fall in viscosity, whereas for exo-enzymes large numbers of glycosidic bonds as determined by end-group methods are hydrolysed for small changes in viscosity. The hydrolase enzymes show optimum activity at pH 4.5 to 6.0 and are therefore active during the storage and processing of fruit.

Pectin lyases (EC 4.2.2.10)

The cleavage of the α-(1→4)-glycosidic bonds between residues of methylgalacturonate is catalysed by endopectin lyase. The exo-enzyme has not been described. The mode of action of the enzyme involves transelimination of a proton from the C-5 atom of a uronide residue and simultaneous cleavage of the adjacent glycosidic bond (Fig. 2.12). Owing to the production of the Δ,4,5-unsaturated uronide the extent of enzymatic degradation can be estimated at 235 nm. The enzyme has been found in higher plants and microorganisms. Although the optimum pH value is 8.0 in the presence of calcium, lower pH optima occur when lower methoxyl pectins are used as substrates. Hence the enzyme, despite the higher pH optima, may still catalyse the degradation of pectins during fruit processing.

Pectate lyases (EC 4.2.2.2 and 4.2.2.9)

Pectate lyases only cleave the glycosidic bonds adjacent to a free carboxyl group. The action of the exo-type of enzyme (EC 4.2.2.9) results in the liberation of dimers from the reducing end of the molecule. The enzymes are of microbial origin and require calcium. The pH optima is 8.0 to 9.5 and therefore they have an insignificant effect during fruit processing.

Although juices can be clarified and yields improved by the use of added pectinases, the natural occurrence of pectinases in fresh fruit can also give rise to inferior products during storage and processing. The very active pectin esterase of citrus fruits is responsible for the production of methanol and the loss of cloud suspension. The pectic acid formed is coagulated by naturally occurring calcium ions. This sediment causes a fall in viscosity, which then allows the further sedimentation of cloud particles. In concentrates a calcium pectate gel forms. The citrus pectin esterase is relatively thermostable and thus the required heat processing gives rise to a loss of flavour volatiles and possibly 'cooked' off-flavours. In fruit to be used for jam manufacture pectin esterase can cause the loss of pectin which is required for gelation in the presence of sugar. The hydrolysis of pectates by pectate hydrolases may cause a softening of fruit and vegetable products. During the isolation of pectins, either for commercial or laboratory purposes, enzymatic hydrolysis frequently takes place.

However, pectinases have been used to advantage for industrial purposes, but a greater knowledge of the occurrence and types of pectinases present in various cultivars is still required. Pectinases can be used for juice clarification with apple, grape and pear juices. The yield of juice and colour due to anthocyanins for blackcurrants and strong fruits can be improved by the use of pectin-degrading enzymes. The stabilisation of orange juice cloud suspension can be achieved by the hydrolysis of pectate which can no longer sediment with calcium ions. Degradation of pectin in citrus peel homogenates also facilitates the removal of essential oils. Commercial pectin lyase can be used to prevent the formation of pectate and methanol in apple and citrus juice products. For the manufacture of tomato concentrates the action of natural pectin esterase and polygalacturonase can be manipulated: by a cold 'break' process the natural tomato enzymes liquefy and lower the viscosity of the product, whereas the hot 'break' process is used to deactivate the enzymes to produce tomato juices of high viscosity. During the blanching of vegetables, or the canning of apple slices, peaches or tomatoes, advantage can be taken of limited pectin esterase activity to form pectate. Calcium pectate salts are formed within the tissues of such fruits and those of potatoes and carrots to produce firmer products. Calcium-dependent pectate gels can be used to replace the high sucrose-dependent pectin gels and thus bring about a reduction in dietary energy intake.

Pectin and pectate lyases have been used for structural studies on pectins. The analysis of pectins and the hydrolysed products, which result from acid-catalysed hydrolysis, is difficult due to the rapid degradation of liberated galacturonic acid by mineral acids. Consequently, pectinases have proved useful aids for the analysis of pectins. In particular the lyase enzymes are valuable as the Δ-4,5-unsaturated products formed are easily detected due to their absorbance at 235 nm. Analysis of pectin first by enzymatic degradation with poly-α-1,4-D-galacturonide lyase and subsequent separation by high performance liquid chromatography of unsaturated di- and trigalacturonic acid uronides has been described by Voragen *et al.* (1984).

EXUDATE AND SEED GUMS

In addition to pectins, starch and gelatin, the food industry uses a wider range of more chemically obscure polysaccharides sometimes described as gums, either as gelling agents or stabilisers. The term 'gums' arises originally from man's use of the rather sticky and viscous plant exudates and seed polysaccharides of high molecular weight. Gum ghatti, locust bean gum and others (Table 2.11) are typical natural plant products. The gums act as thickeners and stabilisers by increasing the viscosity of food suspensions and thus reducing sedimentation and coagulation.

Table 2.11 Types of polysaccharides used as gelling agents or stabilisers

Plant products		Microbial products
Starches		Xanthan
Pectins		Dextran
Arabic		Curdlan
Karaya	exudate	Pullulan
Ghatti	gums	
Tragacanth		Chemical derivatives
Guar		Carboxymethyl
Locust bean		celluloses
Psyllium seed	seed	Hydroxyethyl celluloses
Quince seed	gums	Hydroxypropyl
		celluloses
Seaweed products		Starch ethers and esters
Agar		Cross-linked starches
Alginic acids		Pectin amides
Carrageenans		Propylene glycol
		alginates

The molecular structure of the exudate and seed gums is more varied than that of either starch, cellulose or even pectins. Frequently, the natural exudate seed gums and the microbial polysaccharides contain many short branched structures superimposed on a linear core, or backbone, of repeating monosaccharide units.

The conformational structures of such molecules with side chains is important and it is apparent that the branched molecules do not pack and align easily in the solid state; thus their physical properties differ considerably from those of the linear cellulose and amylose molecules. The branched molecules are more soluble and due to steric restrictions and the intermolecular interactions may be weaker. Further, the occasional presence of uronic acid residues, containing carboxyl groups in the side chains, decreases the intermolecular interactions by electrostatic repulsion and also increases the solubility due to ionisation. The stability in aqueous solution of the gums is related directly to their molecular structure. The furanosyl glycosidic bonds are hydrolysed easily by dilute acids and extended heating in acidic solutions like fruit juices or sauces may also cause hydrolysis of other hexopyranosyl oligosaccharides. Thus the exudate and seed gums are generally not used where further heat-processing is required. Alternatively, the glycosidic bonds between uronic acids, as in pectins and alginates, are more stable and therefore are more suitable for use in heat-processed acidic foods, like jam preserves or pie fillings.

For the heteropolysaccharides, which contain several types of monosaccharides, structural information may now be obtained by analysis of hydrolysates of methylated and non-methylated polymers using gas chromatography–mass spectrometry (gc/ms). The free hydroxyl groups of the heteropolymer are first labelled as methoxy groups through methylation of the whole polysaccharide, while hydrolytically generated hydroxyl groups are later esterified as acetates (Fig. 2.13). Fast atom bombardment (FAB) and electron impact mass spectrometry can now be used for the determination of the molecular weight and sequence of oligosaccharide derivatives (O'Neill et al. 1986). However, for the heteropolysaccharides the number of possible derivatives is quite large and therefore other methods of structural analysis using periodate as an oxidising agent of diol groups are frequently also required. For hexuronate residues β-elimination reactions can be carried out with the organic base diazabicycloundecen (O'Neill et al. 1986). Enzymes which include the highly purified β-mannases, β-glucanases and α-galactosidases can also be used for partial degradation of the heteropolymers and separate modification of the molecular structure of food polysaccharides.

The generalised conformational structures for some of the heteropolysaccharides are shown in Fig. 2.14 (a)–(e).

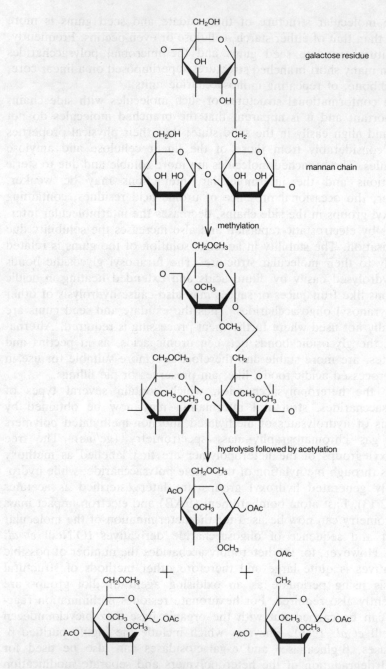

galactose residue

mannan chain

methylation

hydrolysis followed by acetylation

1,4–0–diacetyl,2,3,6–trimethoxy–2–D–mannopyranoside

Fig. 2.13 Scheme for analysis of the branch point in guar gum (a galactomannan). The derivatives are identified by gas chromatography–mass spectrometry. The acyl group marks the position of the previous glycosidic bonds

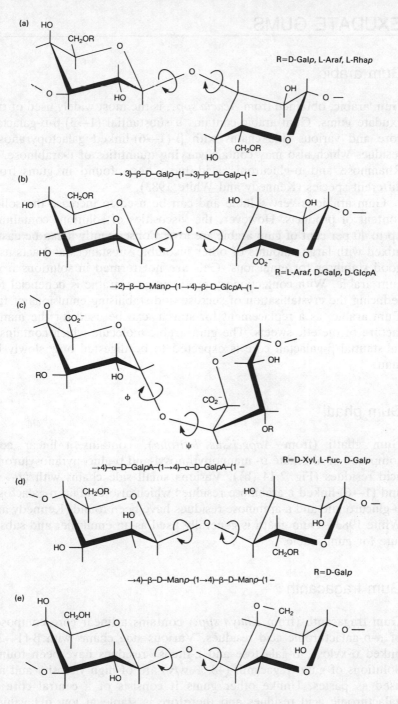

Fig. 2.14 Generalised main chain structures of gums and agarose (a) gum
arabic (b) gum ghatti (c) gum tragacanth (d) guar gum (e) agarose

EXUDATE GUMS

Gum arabic

Gum arabic, obtained from *Acacia spp.*, is the most widely used of the exudate gums. Gum arabic contains a substantial (1→3)-β-D-galactan core and various side chains with β-(1→6)-linked galactopyranosyl residues which also may contain varying quantities of L-arabinose. L-Rhamnose and D-glucuronic acid have been found in gums from different species (Kennedy and White 1983).

Gum arabic is very soluble and can be used to increase the solids content of products. However, the viscosities of solutions containing up to 40 per cent of gum arabic are low. Consequently it can be easily mixed with large amounts of other insoluble substances and acts as a good stabiliser for emulsions. Gels are not formed in solutions from gum arabic. With confectionery products gum arabic is beneficial for reducing the crystallisation of sucrose and stabilising emulsions of fat. Gum arabic, as a replacement for starch, can be used for the manufacture of dietetic sweets. The gum arabic molecule which contains a substantial β-galactan core is expected to be digested only slowly by man.

Gum ghatti

Gum ghatti (from *Anogeissus latifolia*), contains a linear core composed of alternate D- mannopyranosyl-and D-glucopyranosyluronic acid residues (Fig. 2.14 (b)). Various small side chains with (1→3)- and (1→6)-linked L-arabinose residues which also contain D-galactose, D-glucuronate and L-arabinose residues have been found (Kennedy and White 1983). Gum ghatti is generally used as an emulsifier and substitute for gum arabic.

Gum tragacanth

Gum tragacanth (from *Khaya spp.*) contains a linear core composed of α-D-galacturonic acid residues. Various side chains with β-(1→3)-linked D-xylose, D-galactose and L-fucose residues have been found. Solutions of gum tragacanth (48 % w/v) are of high viscosity and are used as pastes. Unlike other gums it consists of a central core of galacturonic acid residues and therefore is stable at low pH values. Consequently gum tragacanth can be used in salad dressings and fruit products. Recently it has been replaced by alginate esters, which have similar acid-resistant properties.

SEED GUMS

Guar gum (from the seed of *Cyamopsis tetragonoloba*) contains a linear linked β-(1→4)-D-mannan core (Fig. 2.14 (d)). Approximately one D-galactopyranosyl residue per two mannose residues is believed to occur as side chains on the linear mannan chain. Owing to the high frequency of side chains this type of galactomannan is described as hairy. Carob gum (locust bean gum) is also a galactomannan but possesses statistically only one galactose residue per four mannose units. The endosperm of carob seed contains up to 38 per cent galactomannan. The unbranched linear parts (smooth regions) of the mannan chain of carob gum are believed to interact with other polysaccharides like carrageenan and xanthan, to form gels. Both galactomannans in low concentrations (1 %) form highly viscous solutions and are therefore extensively used as thickening agents, but carob gum, which contains more unbranched region, aggregates and is relatively insoluble in cold water. Guar and carob gum solutions are stable over a wide range of pH values at ambient temperature and are not affected by fruit acids and salt. The gums are used as thickening agents and to bind water in sauces. For canned meat products, viscous solutions of the seed gums added to suspensions of meat reduce the migration of fat and the separation of an aqueous phase. Galactomannans are present in a wide range of leguminous seeds with properties similar to those of guar and carob galactomannans.

While the overall chemical structure of the exudate and the seed gum linear polymers are generally known, precise structural information for the side chains has not been presented here because of natural variations and incomplete knowledge. The side chain residues are readily accessible to enzymes and small differences in composition may merely be due to the catalytic action of various hydrolases and transferases. When the relationships between the rheological properties, such as viscosity and gelation, and the detailed chemical structure of highly purified gums at the monosaccharide residue level become known, then enzymes capable of modifying the chemical structure of gums will assume special importance. A number of galactomannan-degrading enzymes have been reported some of which can be isolated from the germinating seeds that contain galactomannans. McCleary and Neukom (1982) have shown that endo-β-mannanase (EC 3.2.1.78) catalyses random cleavage of the D-mannan chains in galactomannans and consequently reduces the viscosity. However, owing to steric factors, highly substituted galactomannans are only slowly hydrolysed. α-D-Galactosidase-modified guar galactomannans can be prepared which contain intermediate amounts of galactose. Unlike the native guar galactomannan, such enzymatically modified gums are able to form gels due to intermolecular interactions of the enzymatically generated smooth unsubstituted mannan regions in the modified galactomannan. However, if the action of the enzyme is not controlled, such that the concentration of galactose falls below 10 per cent, the smooth mannan chains interact further to form an insoluble precipitate: the proportion of branched units is now too small to maintain solubility and prevent extensive aggregation. In future other highly purified enzymes could be used for removing the neutral sugars, such as L-arabinose or L-fucose from gum exudates which might improve the gelation characteristics. Some of the properties of glucanases and xylanases have recently been collated (Matheson and McCleary 1985). Other mannans which are very soluble have been found in nuts and coffee beans. Many of these substances after suitable enzymatic modification may extend the range of substances that can be used in foods as thickeners, stabilisers and gelling agents.

SEAWEED AND ALGAL POLYSACCHARIDES

Glucans, mannans and xylans have been found in algae and seaweeds. For food purposes the most important group of seaweed polysaccharides include agar, the alginates and the sulphated carrageenans though there are, as yet, other uncharacterised algal polysaccharides.

Agarose

Agar (from the Rhodophyta), is a mixture of polysaccharides whose molecular structure is based on a galactan core (Kennedy et al. 1984) composed of alternate D-galactopyranosyl- and L-3,6-anhydrogalacto-pyranosyl residues. The glycosidic links are alternatively α-1$\rightarrow$4- and β-1$\rightarrow$3-bonds (Fig. 2.14 (e)). Owing to the occasional substitution of the 3,6-anhydrogalactose residues – in the linear backbone structure – by sulphated galactose residues, agar can be considered to be a heterogeneous mixture of different galactans. The polymer based on the alternate anhydro-structure (Fig. 2.14 (e)) is generally known as neutral agarose, which is the main gel-forming component. Agarose molecules are thought to aggregate to form double helical structures.

When the concentration of polymer is only 1.5 per cent, agar gels are extremely strong. A gel forms at approximately 30 °C and melts at approximately 85 °C and is therefore particularly valuable for canned products and pie fillings. Low concentrations of agar can be used to reduce diffusion and as a protective film against oxidative reactions. Stronger gels can be obtained by the inclusion of small amounts of carob gum, sucrose or dextrans, while weaker gels are obtained by the addition of starch or sodium alginate. Agar is not hydrolysed by mammalian digestive enzymes and therefore could be a useful adjunct to dietary fibre.

Alginates

Alginic acid can be obtained from the Rhodophyceae – brown algae which are primarily salt water plants. Production in the United States is mainly from *Macrocystis pyrifera*, the giant kelp. Each species produces a different type of alginate (Table 2.12), where the composition also depends on the time of harvesting and the anatomical part of the plant.

Table 2.12 The proportion of uronic acids in brown seaweeds

Type	High-M		High-G
	Ascophyllum nodosum	Macrocystis pyrifera	Laminaria hyberborea
Guluronic acid (%) (G)	35	40	70
Mannuronic acid (%) (M)	65	60	30

The molecule of alginic acid, unlike the galactomannans of the exudate and seed gums, is only linear and is composed of approximately 700 to 1000 residues of both D-mannuronic acid and L-guluronic acid in the $^4C_1$ and $^1C_4$ conformations, respectively. The L-guluronic acid residues arise from epimerisation at C-5 of D-mannuronic acid residues in biosynthesised mannuronan chains. Frequently the residues occur as twenty-residue homopolymer blocks of either D-mannuronic acid (M) or L-guluronic acid (G) units. Such M or G blocks are interspersed by polymer chains containing alternate D-mannuronic acid and L-guluronic acid residues:

$$- (M - M - M - M)_5 - M - G - M - G - (G - G - G - G)_5 -$$

The diaxial α-(1→4)-glycosidic bonds between the residues of L-guluronic acid confer a buckled conformation on the G-blocks (Fig. 2.15). The M-blocks are linked β-(1→4) and therefore possess a diequatorial linked ribbon-like structure.

Alginic acid is insoluble in water and therefore is used industrially as the sodium or potassium salt. The propylene glycol ester of alginic acid is prepared by reaction with propylene oxide. Up to 60 per cent of the carboxyl groups are normally esterified in the propylene glycol ester. However the esters, like those of pectin, are degraded in alkaline solutions by a β-elimination reaction. Alginates with predominant

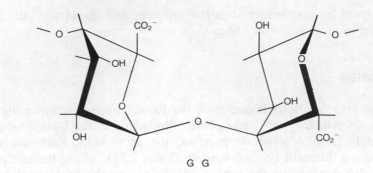

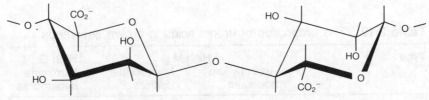

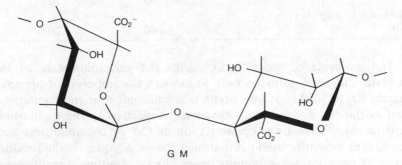

Fig. 2.15 Possible conformations of uronates in alginic acid (M = D-mannuronic acid, G = L-guluronic acid)

mannuronic acid form weak elastic gels, while those with substantial G-blocks give stronger and more thermostable gels. For gelation of un-esterified alginates, as with pectic acid, the presence of alkaline earth cations is required, which in foods is normally supplied as Ca^{2+}. An egg-box type structure of aligned polymer chains has been proposed, (Morris *et al.* 1978), to account for the binding of Ca^{2+} in G-blocks between two parallel polymer chains (Fig. 2.16). It seems probable that ionic bonds may be formed between the carboxyl groups and Ca^{2+} with hydrogen bonds between hydroxyl groups. Enzymes that depoly-merise alginate have been found to be of the lyase type (Matheson and McCleary 1985) in bacteria, where the hydrolysed products, anal-ogous to those formed by pectin lyase contain Δ-4,5-unsaturated uronate residues. Such enzymes will prove useful for structural studies

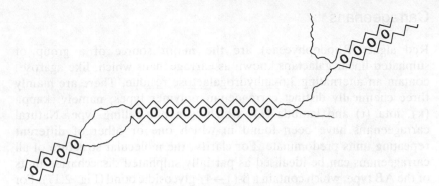

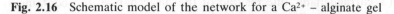

Fig. 2.16 Schematic model of the network for a Ca²⁺ – alginate gel

of alginates. However, more important from a practical point of view is the claim that for high molecular weight alginates enzymatic conversion of the D-mannuronic to L-guluronic acid residues can be achieved by the use of mannuronan C-5 epimerase (Skjåk-Braek 1984). Consequently, it is possible to carry out an enzymatic conversion of lower grade alginates to produce added value products with an enhanced ability to form gels.

Knowledge of the chemical structure of alginic acid has made it possible to control chemically by addition of Ca²⁺ the gelation of alginates in foods. The calcium for gelation can be selected from salts such as the phosphate, nitrate or tartrate; the pH value can be controlled; chelating agents can be used to allow a slow release of divalent metal ions. More homogenous and stable gels can be obtained by the slow cooling of hot solutions of alginate in the presence of Ca²⁺: the hot solutions do not form gels owing to the greater kinetic energy of the alginate molecules, which thus impairs intermolecular associations and the alignment of separate chains of the polymers. The gels formed during cooling are chemically set and do not melt on heating, although they are degraded at extreme pH values.

The propylene glycol esters are stable in acidic foods and therefore are used in fruit products, carbonated drinks and beer as foam stabilisers. Alginates are also used in desserts, milk products, ice-cream, marshmallows, meringues and also as a glaze on frozen fish. Often calcium complexing reagents, such as phosphates and citrates, are used in conjunction with alginates in order to control the formation of gels when other ingredients, such as milk, contain large amounts of Ca²⁺. Alternatively, extra calcium can be used in dry mix dessert powders to accelerate the rate of setting at room temperature. Artificial cherries are heat-stable alginate gels formed in a solution of a calcium salt. Artificial onion rings are manufactured from extruded calcium alginate gels containing small pieces of onion.

Carrageenans

Red algae (Rhodophyceae) are the major source of a group of sulphated linear galactans known as carrageenans which, like agarose, contain an alternating 3,6-anhydrogalactose residue. There are mainly three chemically distinct carrageenan polymer types, namely: kappa (κ), iota (ι) and lambda (λ), which is a non-gelling type. Natural carrageenans have been found in which one or other of different repeating units predominate. For clarity, the molecular structure of all carrageenans can be idealised as partially sulphated disaccharide units of the AB type, which contain a β-(1→4)-glycosidic bond (Fig. 2.17). For ι- and κ-carrageenans, one residue of the disaccharide unit contains a 3,6-anhydro group. The disaccharide units are linked together by α-(1→3)-glycosidic bonds and hence only the B-units can exist in the anhydro form. In λ-carrageenan, the 3,6-anhydro sugars are absent and are replaced by substantial amounts of α-D-galactose-2,6-sulphate. There is a sequential increase in the content of sulphate in the series (κ to ι to λ) carrageenans and the highly sulphated λ-carrageenan is unable to form gels. During the biosynthesis of carrageenans, the more highly sulphated B-residues (the 6-sulphate and the 2,6-disulphate) are precursors of the 3,6-anhydro-D-galactose residues, where the desulphation reaction at C-6 is catalysed by a 6-sulphoeliminase (Painter 1983). Therefore the distribution of λ- and ι-types of polymer chains is controlled by the activity of sulphatases and sulphoeliminases. κ-Carrageenan forms the strongest gels in the presence of potassium ions, while stronger gels for ι-carrageenan are obtained in the presence of Ca^{2+}. The ι-carrageenan is believed to exist as a double helix (Rees 1972) from which the sulphate groups protrude and the helical structure is thought to be reinforced by hydrogen bonds between the O-2 and O-6 hydroxyl groups of galactose residues. Isolation of carrageenans from seaweeds can involve air-drying in the sun followed by extraction with alkali. These are conditions in which enzymatic action and β-elimination reactions might result in desulphation and depolymerisation. κ-Carrageenase (EC 3.2.1.83), which is an endo-β-galactosidase, catalyses the hydrolysis of the β-1→4-linkages and has been found in marine bacteria (Matheson and McCleary 1985). The presence of the highly negatively charged sulphonic acid groups on all carrageenans indicates that intermolecular interaction with proteins will readily occur at low ionic strength. In this way 1.0 per cent of carrageenan can stabilise chocolate or produce gelling in cold milk products, such as milk puddings and possibly yoghurts and cheese-cake. The relatively high cost of carrageenan does not impede the use of such small amounts. Low concentrations of κ-carrageenan (0.05 %) are used in ice-cream as a secondary stabiliser to galactomannans or carboxymethylcellulose. κ-Carrageenan will react synergistically with carob gum to form a range of gels (Fig. 2.18) with variable textural properties where the galactomannan acts as a spacing agent. The

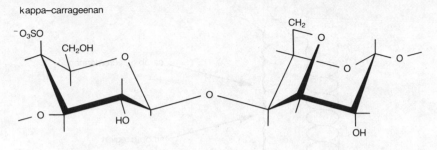

kappa–carrageenan

→3)–β–D–galactose–4–sulphate–(1→4)–3,6–anhydro–α–D–Galactose–(1 –

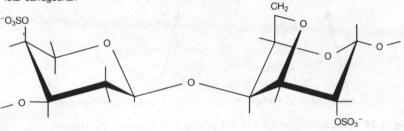

iota–carrageenan

→3)–β–D–galactose–4–sulphate–(1→4)–3,6–anhydro–α–D–galactose–2–sulphate–(1–

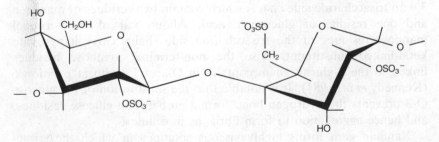

lambda–carrageenan

→3)–β–D–galactose–2–sulphate– (1→4)–α–D–galacto–2,6–sulphate–(1–

Fig. 2.17 Possible conformations of carrageenans

unsubstituted linear portion (smooth region) of the galactomannan is believed to interact with the carrageenan double helix.

MICROBIAL GUMS

Xanthan gum

This heteropolysaccharide is obtained from *Xanthomonas campestris*. The chemical structure of the molecule is mainly that of a linear β–

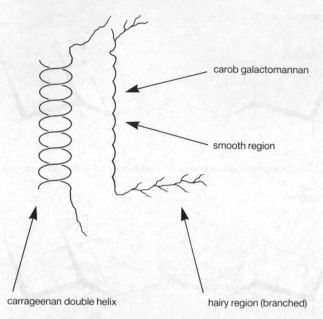

carob galactomannan

smooth region

carrageenan double helix   hairy region (branched)

Fig. 2.18 Schematic model for the interaction between carrageenans and locust bean galactomannan

glucan (Fig. 2.19). However, alternate residues are substituted at O-3 with trisaccharide side chains which contain two residues of mannose and one residue of glucuronic acid. About half of the terminal mannose residues of the trisaccharide side chains carry a pyruvate ketal-linked substituent. Also the non-terminal mannose residues linked to the β-glucan chain contain an O-acetyl group at position 6 (Kennedy *et al*. 1984). It is notable that the substitution of the glucose O-3 prevents the hydrogen bond formation between glucose residues, and hence aggregation to form fibrils as in cellulose.

Xanthan gum forms highly viscous solutions in which the trisaccharide side chains may align with themselves on the β-glucan core to form helical chains. Non-covalent interactions between supercoiled helixes are believed to be responsible for the high viscosity of xanthan

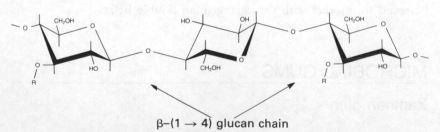

β–(1 → 4) glucan chain

Fig. 2.19 Generalised structure for xanthan from *Xanthomonas campestris*

gum solutions. Weak reversible gels are formed at low temperatures; the polysaccharide can be used as a stabiliser and as a thickening reagent to replace alginates or modified starches. Under shear stress the viscosity is rapidly reduced, but upon release of the shear, total recovery of the viscosity takes place. Xanthan gum is stable at temperatures up to 90 °C and is therefore used for batter coatings. Particulate suspensions like chocolate powder can also be stabilised by xanthan gum. Mixtures (0.3 %) of carob gum or debranched guar gums react synergistically with xanthan gum to form thermoreversible gels. The more linear nature of carob gum, and the galactose-depleted guar gum obtained after enzymatic modification with α-galactosidase, seems to permit an increased ease of association between regions of unsubstituted mannan chains and linear aggregates of xanthan gum. Mixtures of xanthan gum and carob gum are stable at temperatures up to 90 °C where there is very little fall in viscosity. Synergism between guar gum and xanthan gum results in an increased viscosity. Such mixtures are used in the manufacture of cottage cheese, ice-cream and sauces. On the basis of toxicological tests, xanthan gum has been approved for use in human foods by the United States Food and Drug Administration.

Pullulan

This α-D-glucan is obtained from *Aureobasidium pullulans* and is composed of three glucose units (maltotriose) linked by α-(1→6)-glycosidic bonds (Fig. 2.20). The hydrolysis of the molecule is only catalysed by the enzyme pullulanase, which hydrolyses the α, 1→6-glycosidic bonds. For food uses pullulan will form non-digestible films which may be used as a coating materials.

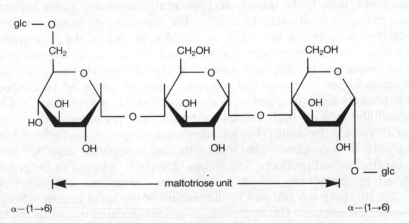

Fig. 2.20 The chemical structure of pullulan

Dextran

Dextrans are α-glucans where most of the glucose residues are linked by α-1→6-glycosidic bonds. Dextrans are synthesised by *Leuconostoc mesenteroides* through the action of the enzyme dextran sucrase (EC 2.4.1.5) acting as a transferase on sucrose. The fructose residues are released from sucrose by enzymatic action and the glucose residue transferred sequentially to an extending glucan polymer.

For the α-1,6-linked glucosides there is an additional covalent bond and an extra dihedral angle which gives the polymers increased flexibility. Therefore dextran is a neutral polymer which is readily soluble and forms clear viscous solutions. It can be used as a humectant – a moisture-holding material in bread and confectionery products – and as a syrup additive to increase the viscosity. It can also be used as a coating on fresh and frozen foods. Dextran may be slowly hydrolysed to release glucose during digestion, but it appears that the consecutive α-(1→6)-linkages are on the whole resistant to enzymes and micro-organisms in the intestinal tract.

$$(\alpha-1,6-\text{glucan})_n + \text{sucrose} \underset{\text{sucrase}}{\overset{\text{dextran}}{\rightleftharpoons}} (\alpha-1,6-\text{glucan})_n + \text{fructose}$$

chain

DIGESTION OF POLYSACCHARIDES

Starch is the main constituent of many foods of plant origin of which only a small proportion, approximately 8 per cent, is considered to be resistant to hydrolysis during mammalian digestion. Humans only synthesise enzymes that hydrolyse glucose polymers with α-glycosidic bonds such as starch and glycogen. In the mammal there are two α-amylases, namely the salivary and pancreatic amylases. As the salivary α-amylase is inactivated by acid in the stomach, its action on food starches is therefore limited to an initial softening of the hard starch granules to aid preliminary digestion and dispersion of the starch in the stomach. The second α-amylase secreted through the pancreatic duct catalyses extensive hydrolysis of ingested starch to yield short chain oligosaccharides and an α-amylase-resistant, α-limit dextrin. The small liberated oligosaccharides are hydrolysed to glucose at the intestinal surface by brush border membrane oligosaccharidases which include α-glucosidase. The small intestine completes digestion and absorbs the end products. The α-limit dextrin is believed to be hydrolysed by isomaltase, which as a sucrase–isomaltase complex (EC 3.2.1.10), is an integral part of the protein of the small intestinal brush border membrane. The hydrolysis of α-limit dextrins by the intestinal sucrase–isomaltase occurs by sequential removal of single residues of glucose from the non-reducing terminal of the glucan chains. The mode of action of the enzyme is similar to that of bacterial α-1,6-glucanhydrolases which remove glucose residues from the non-reducing ends of isomalto-oligosaccharides. However, although the mammalian enzyme is considered an isomaltase, the enzyme possesses a lower K_m value and thus a greater affinity for higher oligosaccharides, like the branched hexasaccharide 6-O-maltotriosylmaltotriose, and hence a somewhat lower affinity for maltose and maltotriose. Neither α-1,4-glucosidase nor isomaltase are able to catalyse the hydrolysis of starch itself.

Polysaccharides which contain β-glycosidic bonds are digested by ruminant mammals. In man, hydrolysis of such carbohydrates is impossible – with the exception of lactose. The dietary carbohydrates not hydrolysed by man are derived from the cell walls of plants that include cellulose, pectins, lignin and hemicelluloses (mainly pentosans) and are commonly classified as dietary fibre. Other materials which pass through the human intestines unchanged, like plant gums, chemically modified hydrocolloids, proteins resistant to proteolysis and similarly 'resistant starch', may have to be considered as adding to dietary fibre. However, some of these constituents may be digested by intestinal bacteria. Thus pectins, which in some fruit products may represent over 80 per cent of the dietary fibre, are not entirely devoid of calorific value, as they may be digested by bacteria in the colon. Colonic Bacteroides species can ferment several types of polysaccharides which include guar gum, xylans, pectins and arabinoxylans (Salyers *et al*. 1983). Thus dietary fibre may increase the mass of faecal bacteria, but this in turn may reduce the availability of essential minerals including zinc, magnesium, calcium and iron.

Thus, there is a continuing interest in all aspects of dietary fibre, which has developed from the proposal that many of the diseases of industrialised countries are due to a lack of fibre in the diet. It has been postulated that many of these diseases are due partly to the extra time and physical effort needed to transport low fibre–high density foods through the digestive system. However, the interactions between dietary fibre and other substances in the bowel is complex, although many beneficial claims have been made. Pectin and lignin constituents of dietary fibre have been said to bind unwanted cholesterol and steroids, while dietary fibre as a whole may reduce insulin requirements and prevent gallstones. For human subjects, mean faecal recoveries for cellulose (83 %), hemicelluloses (38 %) and lignin (92 %) have been recorded.

A qualitative composition for dietary fibre is given in Table 2.13. The three groups of compounds that are the most important and common in foods as components of dietary fibre are cellulose, hemicelluloses and pectin. Only small amounts of lignin and associated substances are likely to be present in most foods; there is very little

Table 2.13 The composition of dietary
fibre

Cellulose
Non-cellulosic β-glucans
Hemicellulose
Pectins (galacturonides)
Other uronides and gums
Lignin, plus small amounts of cutin, suberin
Maillard reaction products
Enzymic browning polymers

lignin in the human diet. Products from Maillard reactions are only present in cooked or processed foods. The products from enzymatic browning reactions are mainly found in dried fruits, tea, coffee and cocoa, where they make a minimal contribution to the diet. Mean values for the content of the total dietary fibre for some raw materials are given in Table 2.14. However, no agreed definition has been reached for which components should be included in a definition of dietary fibre. This makes a determination of dietary fibre difficult for the food analyst. The highest amount of dietary fibre is claimed for raspberries, but nearly half of this can be accounted for in a 'crude lignin' fraction which is surprising. During the cooking of vegetables there is an obvious further gain in dietary fibre content due to losses

Table 2.14 Dietary fibre values for some food
commodities[†]

Commodity	Total dietary fibres (g/100 g)
Apple pulp	10.0
Beans, haricot raw	31.9
Citrus pectin	93.5
Leek, cooked	36
Potato powder	17.6
Radish	40.8
Raspberries[‡]	55.0
Rye biscuit	19.8
	20.3
Rye flour	24.7
	23.4
Soya flour	11.1
Tomatoes	31.0
Wheat bran	39.8

([†] After Southgate and White 1981; [‡] Englyst 1981).

of water-soluble constituents.

Essentially, dietary fibre is derived from plant cell wall material: in the case of wheat bran the pericarp, the seed coat and the aleurone cells plus only a small amount of starchy endosperm, are collectively termed 'bran' and represent approximately 20 per cent of the mass of the wheat kernel. The hemicelluloses of wheat bran are pentosans where the main chain of the polysaccharides is composed of pyranose units of β-xylose with occasional side chains of α-L-arabinofuranosides. Cereal grains are much richer sources of dietary fibre than fruits or vegetables which contain large amounts of water. Thus an increase in dietary fibre is best achieved by increasing the consumption of cereal grains. In addition, cereal products are easily enriched by dietary fibre from other sources. The xyloglucans contain an α-(1→4)-β-linked D-glucan backbone:

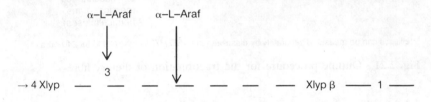

Fruits contain xyloglucans of the type shown above, glucuronoxylans and glucuronoarabinoxylans.

There are no perfect methods for quantifying the amount of dietary fibre in foods, due to the very heterogenous chemical nature of the material. An acid detergent method which uses 2 per cent cetyl trimethyl ammonium bromide in sulphuric acid leaves a residue which contains mainly cell-wall cellulose plus lignin to be measured gravimetrically. This is a rapid method and therefore useful, but water-soluble undigestible non-starch polysaccharides may be lost during the extraction with the detergent. The more complex methods which use various extraction techniques for the estimation of dietary fibre are derived from knowledge of the composition of plant cell wall material. The principle of such methods requires first, enzymatic solubilisation of starch, now generally using α-amylase and pullulanase, secondly, recovery of water-soluble non-starch polysaccharides by precipitation with ethanol, and then thirdly, further fractionation of the insoluble residue which contains cellulose, other non-starch polysaccharides and lignin (Fig. 2.21). Using the enzymatic digestion procedure, any starch which is resistant to the action of α-amylase ('resistant starch') is measured as dietary fibre. By chromatographic analysis the constituent sugars of the oligosaccharides in the non-starch polysaccharide fractions can be measured accurately (Englyst 1981) to provide valuable information on the components of dietary fibre products. Clearly errors in such methods can arise in a number of ways. The enzymes used must be free of any contaminating β-glucanases and not all

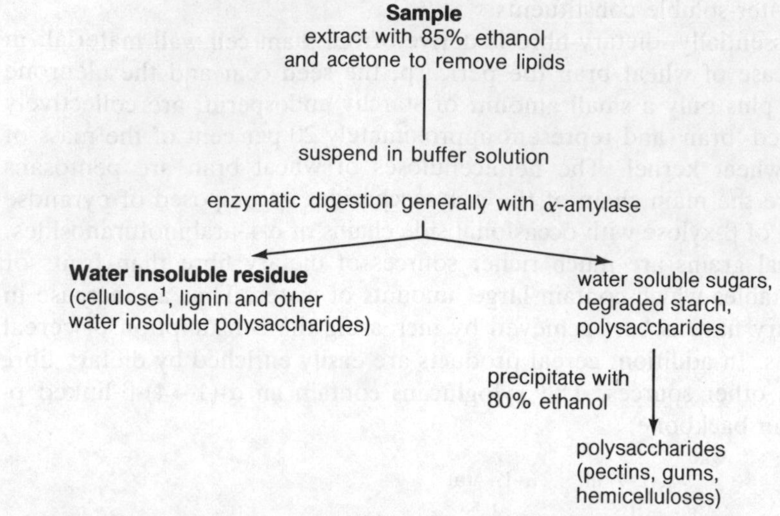

Sample
extract with 85% ethanol
and acetone to remove lipids

suspend in buffer solution

enzymatic digestion generally with α-amylase

Water insoluble residue
(cellulose[1], lignin and other
water insoluble polysaccharides)

water soluble sugars,
degraded starch,
polysaccharides

precipitate with
80% ethanol

polysaccharides
(pectins, gums,
hemicelluloses)

[1] cellulose can be measured separately by dissolving in H_2SO_4 (72% w/v) at 4°C for 24 hours

Fig. 2.21 Outline procedure for the fractionation of dietary fibre

soluble dietary fibre may be precipitated by 80 per cent ethanol. A more sophisticated method of extraction which uses aqueous sodium deoxycholate, dimethyl sulphoxide and a valuable phenol–acetic acid–water mixture has been advocated by Selvendran *et al.* (1981).

KEY FACTS

1.   Polysaccharides are used as thickeners and gelling agents in the food industry. Cellulose, mannans and xylans containing β-(1→4)-equatorial glycosidic bonds possess linear ribbon-like structures.

2.   The amylose component of starch containing an axial–equatorial bond forms coiled helical chains. Interchain hydrogen bonds in amylose enhance molecular association and gelation in starch pastes.

3.   In hard wheats used for bread manufacture there is strong adhesion between starch grains. Some additional amyloplast membrane proteins present in soft wheats may adversely affect these adhesive properties.

4.   The limited action of wheat α-amylase on wheat starch is beneficial for bread manufacture. Glucose and maltose syrups are manufactured by the selective use of starch-hydrolysing enzymes. The use of debranching enzymes which hydrolyse the α-(1→6)-glycosidic bonds increases the yield of products.

5.   Natural amylase inhibitors have been found in plant seeds and culture fluids of *Streptomyces spp.*

6.   The β-(1→4)-glucosidic bond of cellulose and the glycosidic bonds of pectin, galactomannon and pentosans are not hydrolysed by human enzymes. Only starch contains the amylase-susceptible glucosidic bonds.

7.   Pectins are required for gelation during the manufacture of preserves and are important for maintaining the viscosity of tomato paste. The action of pectin esterase results in loss of gelation and destabilises the desirable cloud in fruit juices. However, pectinases may be used to clarify juices and increase yields.

8.   Dietary fibre is a heterogeneous mixture of polysaccharides which are not hydrolysed by human enzymes. However, colonic micro-organisms may ferment several of these polysaccharides.

9.   The physical properties of seed and exudate gums can be modified by enzymatic hydrolysis to produce more linear polymers for use as thickeners and gelling agents.

10.   L-Guluronic acid-rich alginates can be produced by the action of mannuronan C-5 epimerase on mannuronate-rich alginates. The L-guluronic acid residue is responsible for folding of the alginate chain.

11.   Carrageenans are partially sulphated galactans. κ-Carrageenan forms the strongest gels and is synthesised by desulphation, catalysed by 6-sulphoeliminases, of λ-carrageenans. The carrageenans are used as stabilisers and gelling agents in foods.

REFERENCES

Couvain, S. P. (1987) Personal communication.

Dey, P. M. and Brinson, K. (1984) 'Plant cell-walls', *Adv. in Carbohydr. Chem. and Biochem.*, **42**, 265–382.

Englyst, H. (1981) 'Determination of carbohydrate and its composition in plant materials', in *The Analysis of Dietary Fiber in Food* (Eds James, W. P. T. and Theander, O.). Marcel Dekker, New York.

Fukuhara, K., Murai, H. and Murao, S. (1982) 'Isolation and structure–activity relationship of some amylostatins (F–1 b fraction) produced by *Streptomyces diastaticus* sub spp. *amylo-staticus* No. 9140', *Agric. Biol. Chem.*, **46**, 1941–5.

Goto, A., Matsui, Y., Ohyama, K., Arai, M. and Murao, S. (1983) 'Purification' and characterisation of an α-amylase inhibitor (Haim) produced by *Streptomyces griseosporeus* YM-25', *Agric. Biol. Chem.*, **47**, 83–8.

Gough, B. M., Greenwell, P. and Russel, P. L. (1985) 'On the interaction of sodium dodecylsulphate with starch granules', in *New Approaches to Research on Cereal Carbohydrates* (eds. Hill, R. D. and Munck, L.). Elsevier Science Publishers, Amsterdam.

Howling, D. (1980) 'The influence of the structure of starch on its rheological properties', *Food Chem.*, **6**, 51–61.

Jago, W. and Jago, W. C. (1911) *The Technology of Breadmaking*. Simpkin, Marchall, Hamilton, Kent and Co., London.

Kennedy, J. F., Griffiths, A. J. and Atkins, D. P. (1984) 'The application of hydrocolloids: recent developments, future trends', in *Gums and Stabilisers for the Food Industry* 2. *The Applications of Hydrocolloids* (eds. Philips, G. O., Wedlock, D. J. and Williams, P. A.). Pergamon Press, Oxford.

Kennedy, J. F. and White, C. A. (1983) *Bioactive Carbohydrates in Chemistry, Biochemistry and Biology*. Ellis Horwood, Chichester.

McCleary, B. V. and Neukom, H. (1982) 'Effect of enzymic modification on the solution and interaction properties of galactomannans', in *Progress in Food and Nutrition Science*, vol. 6 *Gums and Stabilisers for the Food Industry. Interactions of Hydrocolloids* (eds. Phillips, G. O., Wedlock, D. J. and Williams, P. A.). Pergamon Press, Oxford.

Manners, D. and Matheson, N. K. (1981) 'The fine structure of amylopectin', *Carbohydr. Res.*, **90**, 99–110.

Matheson N. K. and McCleary, B. V. (1985) in *The Polysaccharides*, vol. 3 (ed. Aspinall, G. O.). Academic Press, London.

Morris, E. R., Rees, D. A., Thom, D. and Boyd, J. (1978) 'Chiroptical and stoichiometric evidence of a specific primary dimerisation process in alginate gelation', *Carbohydr. Res.*, **66**, 145–54.

Norman, B. E. (1982) 'The use of debranching enzymes in dextrose syrup production', in *Maize: Recent Progress in Chemistry and Technology* (ed. Inglett, G. E.). Academic Press, London.

O'Neill, M. A., Morris, V. J. and Selvendran, R. R. (1986) 'Structural analysis of microbial polysaccharides which have potential commercial application', in *Gums and Stabilisers for the Food Industry* 3 (eds. Phillips, G. O, Wedlock, D. J. and Williams, P. A). Elsevier Applied Science Publishers, London.

Painter, T. J. (1983) 'Algal polysaccharides', in *The Polysaccharides*, vol. 2., (ed. Aspinall, G. O.). Academic Press, London.

Paul, A. A. and Southgate, D. A. T. (1978) *McCance and Widdowson's The Composition of Foods*, 4th edn. of MRC Special Report no. 297. HMSO, London and Elsevier, Amsterdam.

Pilnik, W. and Voragen, A. G. J. (1984) 'Polysaccharides and food', *Gordian*, **7** to **10**, 144–99.

Rees, D. A. (1972) 'Polysaccharide gels. A molecular view', *Chem. Ind. (London)* 630–6.

Robyt, J. F. (1984) 'Enzymes in the hydrolysis and synthesis of starch' in *Starch: Chemistry and Technology*, 2nd edn. (eds. Whistler, R. L., BeMiller, J. N. and Paschall, E. F.). Academic Press, London.

Salyers, A. A., O'Brien, M. and Schmetter, B. (1983) 'Catabolism of muco-polysaccharides, plant gums, and Maillard products by human colonic Bacteroides', in *Unconventional Sources of Dietary Fiber* (ed. Furda, I.). A.C.S. Symp. ser. 214, American Chemical Society, Washington D.C.

Selvendran, R. R., Ring, S. G. and Du Pont, S. (1981) 'Determination of the dietary fibre content of the EEC samples and a discussion of the various methods of analysis', in *The Analysis of Dietary Fiber in Food* (eds. James, W. P. T. and Theander, O.). Marcel Dekker, New York.

Shure, M., Wessler, S. and Fedoroff N. (1983) 'Molecular identification and isolation of the *Waxy* locus in maize', *Cell*, **35**, 225–33.

Skjåk-Braek, G. (1984) 'Enzymic modification of alginate', in *Gums and Stabilisers for the Food Industry* 2. *The Applications of Hydrocolloids*. (Eds.

Phillips, G. O., Wedlock, D. J. and Williams, P. A.). Pergamon Press, Oxford.

Snyder E. M. (1984) 'Industrial microscopy of starches', in *Starch: Chemistry and Technology*, 2nd edn. (eds. Whistler, R. L., BeMiller, J. N. and Paschall, E. F.). Academic Press, London.

Southgate, D. A. T. and White, M. A. (1981) 'Commentary on results obtained by the different laboratories using the Southgate method', in *The Analysis of Dietary Fiber in Food* (Eds. James, W. P. T. and Theander, O.). Marcel Dekker, New York.

Takeshi, T., Yojiro, K. and Seinosake, U. (1983) 'Amylase inhibitors produced by *Streptomyces sp.* No. 280', *Agric. Biol. Chem.*, **47**, 671–9.

Thom, D., Dea, I. C. M., Morris, E. R. and Powell, D. A. (1982) Interchain associations of alginate and pectins', in *Progress in Food and Nutrition Science*, vol. 6 *Gums and Stabilisers for the Food Industry. Interactions of Hydrocolloids* (Eds. Phillips, G. O., Wedlock, D. J. and Williams, P. A.). Pergamon Press, Oxford.

Voragen, A. G. J., Schols, H. A., Clement, A. J. J. and Pilnik, W. (1984) 'Enzymic analysis of pectins', in *Gums and Stabilisers for the Food Industry 2. The Applications of Hydrocolloids* (eds. Phillips, G. O., Wedlock, D. J. and Williams, P. A.). Pergamon Press, Oxford.

Whitaker, J. R. (1983) 'Protease and amylase inhibitors in biological materials', in *Xenobiotics in Foods and Feeds* (eds). Finley, J. W. and Schwass, D. E.). ACS Symposia 234. American Chemical Society, Washington DC.

ADDITIONAL READING

Avers, A. D. and Stevens, D. J. (1985) 'Starch damage', *Advances in Cereal Science and Technology*, vol. VII (ed. Pomeranz, Y.). American Association of Cereal Chemists, St Paul, Minesota.

Chang, M. M., Chou, T. Y. C. and Tsao, G. T. (1981) 'Structure, pretreatment and hydrolysis of cellulose in bioenergy', *Adv. in Biochem. Eng.*, **20**, 15–42.

James, W. P. T. and Theander, O. (1981) *Analysis of Dietary Fiber in Food*. Marcel Dekker, New York.

Kennedy, J. F. and White C. A. (1983) *Bioactive Carbohydrates; Chemistry, Biochemistry and Biology*. Ellis Horwood, Chichester.

Phillips, G. O., Wedlock, D. J. and Williams P. A. (1984) *Gums and Stabilisers for the Food Industry 2. The Application of Hydrocolloids*. Pergamon Press, Oxford.

Phillips, G. O., Wedlock, D. J. and Williams, P. A. (1986) *Gums and Stabilisers for the Food Industry*. 3. Elsevier Applied Science Publishers, London.

Whistler, R. L., BeMiller, J. N. and Paschall, E. F. (1984) *Starch: Chemistry and Technology*, 2nd edn. Academic Press, London.

Wilkie, K. C. B. (1979) The hemicelluloses of grasses and cereals *Adv. Carbohydr. Chem. and Biochem.*, **36**, 215–64.

Part II
Food proteins

INTRODUCTION

The requirements for proteins world wide are expansive because of the increasing human population. The food scientist and technologist can classify all the requirements simply under two common quality parameters; first, the fundamental need is for proteins of high nutritional value and secondly, a desirable textural quality, which is often provided by the protein constituent is important, as described in Chapter 5.

During the digestion of proteins by man and animals, the peptide bonds are rapidly hydrolysed in the stomach and the small intestine. Specific proteolytic enzymes, secreted by the stomach and pancreas, catalyse the hydrolysis of proteins. Rapid absorption of the liberated amino acids and small peptides into the blood of the portal vein takes place mainly from the small intestine. Thus from a nutritional point of view the real requirement is not for proteins, but for amino acids. In man and other animals these are then used for the biosynthesis of enzymes, structural proteins and non-protein nitrogen compounds like nucleic acids.

CHAPTER 3

The nutritional value of proteins

PROTEIN REQUIREMENTS OF MAN

The recent recommendations for total protein intake are greater than those recommended for the whole world population in 1973 (FAO/WHO 1973). The different recommended daily amounts published for various countries up to 1980 for all nutrients have previously been collated and reviewed (IUNS 1983). In 1981 the Food and Agriculture Organisation/World Health Organisation (FAO/WHO/UNU 1985), recommended levels of intake for protein which now approximate to the previous values recommended in both the United Kingdom and United States (Table 3.1).

The United Kingdom recommended values for dietary protein intake are for a range of ages, and are related to energy requirements. Whereas the recommended amounts for Canada and the United States are average values based on body weights.

Table 3.1(a) Examples of recommended daily amounts for proteins[†‡] United Kingdom

Age (years)	Energy intake (kcal)	Protein (g/day)
1	1200	30
7–8	1980	49
Males		
15–17	2880	72
35–64	2750	69
75+	2150	54

† The recommended amount of protein with a net protein utilisation value of 75 corresponds to 10 per cent of the recommended energy intake (i.e. 4 kcal = 1 g of protein in the United Kingdom).

(‡ DHSS 1981).

Table 3.1(b)   Examples of recommended daily amounts for proteins Canada

Age	Body weight (kg)	Protein (g/day)
9–11 months	9.5	18
7–9 years	25	31
Males		
16–18	62	54
25–49	74	57
75+	69	57

(After Department of National Health and Welfare 1983).

Table 3.1(c)   Examples of recommended daily amounts for proteins United States

Age	Body weight (kg)	Protein (g/day)
6–12 months	9.0	kg × 2.0 = 18
7–10 years	28	34
Males		
15–18	66	56
23–50	70	56
51+	70	56

(NRC/NAS 1980).

Table 3.1(d)   Abbreviated recommended daily amounts of protein by FAO/WHO/UNU[†]

Age (years)	Safe level (g protein/kg per day)
Infants and children	
0.25–0.5	1.86
0.75–1.0	1.48
2–3	1.13
9–10	0.99
Adolescents (male)	
10–11	0.99
14–15	0.96
17–18	0.86
Adults[‡§]	0.75

([†] FAO/WHO/UNU 1985).

[‡] For pregnancy it is recommended that the protein intake be increased by 6 g/day.

[§] For lactation an additional 16 g/day is recommended to the dietary protein amount.

The proposed adequate levels of protein are those considered necessary to maintain the health and physiological needs of most of the individuals in the population group. For the United Kingdom recommended daily amounts of protein have been calculated so as to represent 10 per cent of the total energy requirement where 4 kcal are provided per gram of protein. The factors 4 kcal per g protein (17 kJ), 9 kcal per g fat (38 kJ), 3.75 kcal per g available carbohydrate (16 kJ) predict the energy available from the dietary components in the United Kingdom (DHSS 1981).

However, the real dietary requirement is for α-amino acids and therefore the amino acid composition of dietary protein is extremely

	pK values	Molecular weight	
Valine	2.32, 9.67	117	$CH_3 - CH - CH - CO_2H$ (with CH_3 and NH_2 substituents)
Leucine	2.36, 9.60	131	$CH_3 - CH - CH_2 - CH - CO_2H$ (with CH_3 and NH_2 substituents)
Isoleucine	2.36, 9.68	131	$CH_3 - CH_2 - CH - CH - CO_2H$ (with CH_3 and NH_2 substituents)
Threonine	2.63, 10.43	119	$CH_3 - CH - CH - CO_2H$ (with OH and NH_2 substituents)
Phenylalanine	1.83, 9.13	165	(phenyl)$- CH_2 - CH - CO_2H$ (with NH_2 substituent)
Tyrosine	2.20, 9.11 10.07	181	$HO-$(phenyl)$- CH_2 - CH - CO_2H$ (with NH_2 substituent)
Tryptophan	2.38, 9.39	204	(indole)$- CH_2 - CH - CO_2H$ (with NH_2 substituent)
Lysine	2.18, 8.95 10.53 (ε–NH_2)	146	$H_2N - CH_2 - (CH_2)_3 - CH - CO_2H$ (with NH_2 substituent)
Cysteine	1.71, 8.33 (SH) 10.78	121	$HS - CH_2 - CH - CO_2H$ (with NH_2 substituent)
Methionine	2.28, 9.21	149	$CH_3 - S - CH_2 - CH_2 - CH - CO_2H$ (with NH_2 substituent)

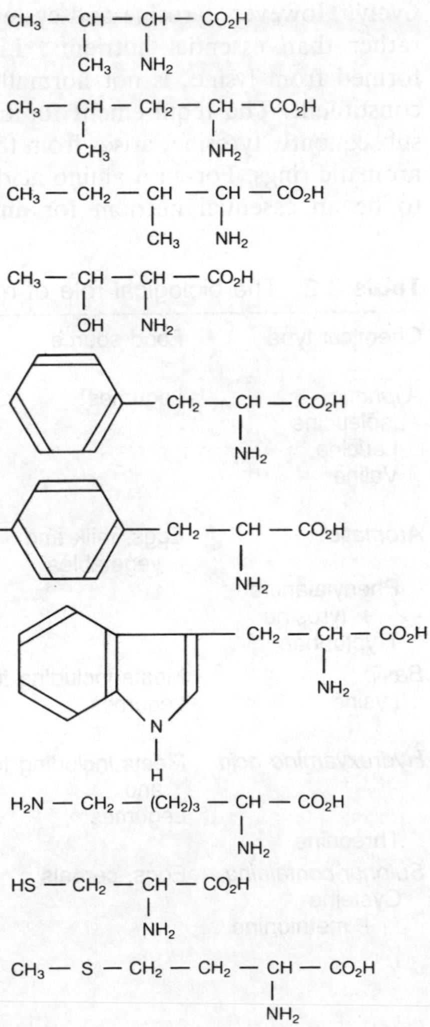

Fig. 3.1 The essential amino acids

important: eight α-amino acids are known to be strictly essential for adequate nutrition in adults (Fig. 3.1). While some of these essential amino acids, like tryptophan, are required directly for the biosynthesis of hormones and other metabolically active compounds (Table 3.2), the occurrence of a range of amino acids of differing charge, polarity and shape also determines the important tertiary structure of enzymes and structural proteins. However, of the eight strictly essential amino acids only five are likely to limit the protein quality of mixed human diets: these are lysine, the sulphur amino acids, threonine and tryptophan (FAO/WHO/UNU 1985).

Tyrosine and cysteine/cystine are also classified with the essential amino acids, as they cannot be synthesised in adequate amounts if there is a dietary deficiency of phenylalanine or methionine respectively. However, tyrosine and cysteine are really essential metabolites rather than essential nutrients. Likewise δ-hydroxylysine, which is formed from lysine, is not normally regarded as an essential dietary constituent. The requirement for tryptophan and phenylalanine, and subsequently tyrosine, arises from the inability of animals to synthesise aromatic rings. For an α-amino acid, or any other dietary constituent, to be an essential nutrient for animals, first, biosynthesis must be

Table 3.2 The biological role of essential amino acids

Chemical type	Food source	Special functions (precursors of)
Aliphatic Isoleucine Leucine Valine	Legumes	Hydrophobic regions or proteins
Aromatic Phenylalanine + tyrosine Tryptophan	Eggs, milk and vegetables	Tyrosine, epinephrine and thyroxin Seratonin, nicotinic acid
Basic Lysine	Meats including fish Legumes	Cross-links in collagen and elastin
Hydroxyamino acid Threonine	Meats including fish and Legumes	
Sulphur-containing Cysteine + methionine	Eggs, cereals	Tertiary structure of proteins and enzyme-active sites; keratin plus other structural proteins; methionine supplies methyl groups

impossible and secondly, the dietary component itself or a metabolic derivative must be necessary for normal growth and biochemical functions.

Arginine and histidine have not been included in Table 3.2, although these amino acids are considered to be essential for children. However, it has been thought that these two amino acids may be synthesised in sufficient amounts by adults, although recent investigations have indicated that histidine may be essential for adults and particularly for those with chronic disease. Nevertheless, it seems likely that during dietary deficiencies, sufficient histidine is mainly obtained from the degradation of common proteins, such as haemoglobin (Visek 1984). Arginine is a component of the urea cycle, where it is recycled and provides ornithine and citrulline for the removal of ammonia. Also arginine is an essential metabolite required for the synthesis of substantial amounts of creatine. Nevertheless it is generally thought that sufficient arginine is synthesised through the urea cycle to prevent deficiencies. Thus the distinction between essential and non-essential amino acids is still blurred. Also it should be noted that all the α-amino acids, except lysine and threonine, can be replaced in the diet of mammals by the synthetic α-keto acid analogues (Visek 1984). At all events, in general terms the two groups of essential and non-essential amino acids (Fig. 3.1, Fig. 3.2 and Table 3.2) will continue to be distinguished by the fact that one group are not normally synthesised by mammals, whereas the other group, the non-essential amino acids, are normally synthesised in sufficient amounts directly from commonly occurring metabolic intermediates. Plants and microorganisms, unlike animals, readily synthesise the essential amino acids through more complicated pathways (Stryer 1981).

Even though the essential amino acids form approximately 40 per cent of the tissue proteins, for adult man as little as 20 per cent of the total protein intake need be of the essential amino acids. For the human infant, approximately 35 per cent of the dietary protein must be provided as essential amino acids. The smaller than expected requirement arises because essential amino acids can be conserved within the body and are not rapidly excreted during protein turnover. Indeed only small amounts of nitrogen are lost in the urine, faeces, growing hair, nails and the sloughed cells. In adult man it has been suggested that the normal rate of protein turnover is approximately from 3.5 to 4.5 g per kg per day, whereas for young children the value may be from 6 to 7 g per kg per day (Waterlow 1980). For a 60 kg man such values amount to 240 g of protein being reutilised per day, which indicates that reused proteins are the major contributor to the daily requirement. However, as the human requirements are not easily measured, because of the changing needs through a relatively long life span, it is impossible to determine the absolute requirements for essential amino acids. It should also be noted that the essential amino acids,

Table 3.3 Estimated amino acid requirements for man

	Infants		Children 10–12 years	Adults
	FAO/WHO	NRC/NAS	FAO/WHO	FAO/WHO
	(mg/kg body weight/day)			
Ile	70	80	30	10
Leu	161	135	45	14
Lys	103	99	60	12
Met + Cys	58	49	27	13
Phe + Tyr	125	141	27	14
Thr	87	68	35	7
Trp	17	21	4	3.5
Val	93	92	33	10
His	28	33	—	—
Total:	742	721	261	83.5

(FAO/WHO 1973 and FAO/WHO/UNU 1985; NRC/NAS 1980).

phenylalanine, tyrosine, tryptophan, histidine and methionine, are toxic to some individuals if taken in excessive amounts. The estimated requirements for total protein are composites of the needs for specific amino acids, which have been intensively assessed by expert FAO/WHO and in the United States National Research Council authoritative committees (Table 3.3). The estimates have been arrived at by a comparison of results obtained from experiments involving the feeding of purified, α-amino acids to animals, and the composition of important proteins like those of cow's milk, human breast milk and egg. However, generally the methionine and cystine requirements are combined arithmetically, thus denying a separate value for methionine, from which cystine can be synthesised; likewise a separate value for phenylalanine is frequently not revealed.

The minimum dietary protein requirement for different food proteins is a variable quantity, which is determined by the relative proportions of the essential amino acids present in different proteins. Consequently, over-reliance on one source of protein could result in an insufficient dietary supply of some of the essential amino acids; for example, cereals are deficient in lysine while legumes are deficient in the sulphur amino acids. Likewise the nutritional benefit of bread and cheese combined is better than each consumed separately. Thus in order to meet the nutritional needs, man requires a mixed source of protein and therefore it is best to consider the nutritional contribution of the whole diet, rather than the contribution from separate items. From Tables 3.1 (d) and 3.4 for the infant and adult man, it is calcu-

Adults	$\dfrac{Adult}{Infant} \times 100$	
NRC/NAS	FAO/WHO	NRC/NAS
12	14.3	14.6
16	8.7	11.8
12	11.6	12.1
10	22.4	20.4
16	11.2	11.3
8	8.0	11.7
3	20.0	14.3
14	10.7	15.2
—	—	—
91		

lated that approximately 39 per cent and 11 per cent, respectively, of the dietary intake of the ideal protein should be composed of essential amino acids.

Overall the recommended daily amount of protein proposed by FAO/WHO/UNU (1985) declines exponentially with age from a high value of 1.86 g per day per kg for infants, to approximately 0.75 g per day per kg body weight for the adult man. The recommended daily amounts for protein (per kilogram of body weight) fall by approximately 40 per cent during the first 2 years of human development. These changes correspond to the phases of rapid growth in infants to the no 'net growth' position in the adult, where 70 per cent or more of the α-amino acids utilised for protein synthesis are provided by a breakdown of other body proteins. From Table 3.3, it is evident that the requirement for the sulphur amino acids is deemed to fall less rapidly than for other essential amino acids with increasing age. This could indicate that the requirement by adults is relatively greater for the very important sulphur amino acids which are required substantially for the synthesis of skin in adults: alternatively the requirements by the infant for the sulphur amino acids may have been underestimated.

As shown in Table 3.4, the total recommended daily amount by FAO/WHO/UNU (1985) for essential amino acids (E) falls with increasing age at a greater rate than the recommended daily amount for total dietary protein (T). Thus the recommendations imply that the need for a protein to supply all the essential amino acids in the

Table 3.4 The relationship for men between recommended amounts of essential amino acids and total protein[†]

Age (years)	Essential amino acids (E, g/day/kg body weight)[‡]	Protein (T, g/day/kg body weight)	Ratio E/T
0.25–0.5	0.742	1.86	0.39
10–12	0.261	0.99	0.26
Adult man	0.083	0.75	0.11

([†] FAO/WHO/UNU 1985 data per kg of body weight/day).

[‡] From Table 3.3.

amounts required declines substantially with increasing age.

Although it is now widely accepted that the dietary E/T ratio falls with increasing age, the information is incomplete as the precise magnitude and rate of fall for the essential amino acids is not established. Furthermore, there are many variations such as body composition (including the skeletal ratio), race and physiological state, which can affect the estimated requirements for α-amino acids. The proportion of different organs of the body varies not only with age, but with height; for example, the surface area to volume ratio and hence the proportion of skin tissue is considerably different for the Eskimo and African populations. Furthermore, the nitrogen requirements of the different organs such as the heart and liver are certainly very different, as determined by just their biological function. Also it has been suggested that adaptation can occur where people living on low protein intakes may adapt their dietary requirement by increasing their efficiency to recycle protein. For example, albumin synthesis/breakdown and oxidation of amino acids may decrease; additionally, the recapture of amino acids may increase.

Lacking precise information on both the average amino acid and protein requirements, the FAO/WHO committee have used the upper ranges of dietary amino acid and protein requirements: the recommended daily allowances are placed two standard deviations above the calculated mean requirements. For this subject the student must be aware that the present recommended daily amounts (RDA values) and amino acid scores (p. 133) are based on estimates for population groups and not the absolute needs of individuals. Although in the 1985 FAO/WHO/UNU report there is a shift towards greater emphasis and consideration of the needs of individuals. The methods used to assess the requirements have depended on both the creation of deficiency states for individual nutrients, and determinations of the minimum amounts of nutrient required to cure the deficiency state in animals. Such methods are subject to considerable errors during scaling up to estimate man's needs and assume equal needs for men and experimental animals. Moreover, during nutritional experiments any excess of dietary energy consumed with protein may also have increased the efficiency of the total digestive and assimilation processes for the amino acids, whereas in reality most of the world's population may be deprived of an adequate source of energy. Such deficiencies of energy can give rise to utilisation of body protein and eventually marasmus, whereas a protein deficiency alone causes kwashiorkor. For a moderately active adult man (65 kg) in the United States the energy requirement estimated by FAO/WHO/UNU (1985) to be of approximately 3468 kcal per day can be met, if necessary, from starch or glucose syrups or alternatively from larger quantities of cereals (approximately 0.9 kg). However, through the consumption of such quantities of cereals or legumes to satisfy the energy need, the total dietary protein requirements are also easily achieved, unless the protein has been chemically damaged by incorrect drying or processing.

Non-essential amino acids (Fig. 3.2) (ten for humans) are each synthesised from metabolic intermediates by one- or two-step enzyme-catalysed reactions. The liver is the site for such biochemical conversions, where the amino groups of many of the non-essential α-amino acids are obtained from the α-amino group of glutamic acid by transamination reactions which are catalysed by various transaminases. For the synthesis of glutamate, the citric acid cycle (App. IV) intermediate, α-ketoglutarate, is aminated through the catalytic action of glutamate dehydrogenase: NADPH is the cofactor.

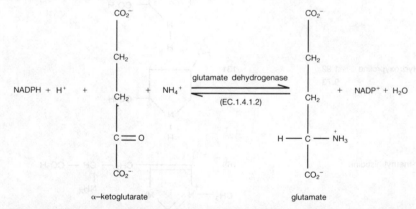

However, for the deamination of glutamate, NAD is the oxidant. Glutamate can also be synthesised from glutamine which acts as amino group donor to α-ketoglutarate:

$$\alpha\text{-ketoglutarate} + \text{glutamine} + \text{NADPH} + \text{H}^+ \underset{\substack{\text{synthase} \\ \text{(EC 1.4.1.13)}}}{\overset{\substack{\text{glutamate}}}{\rightleftharpoons}} 2 \text{ glutamate} + \text{NADP}^+$$

For the synthesis of the other non-essential amino acids, simple transamination reactions are required where glutamate provides the

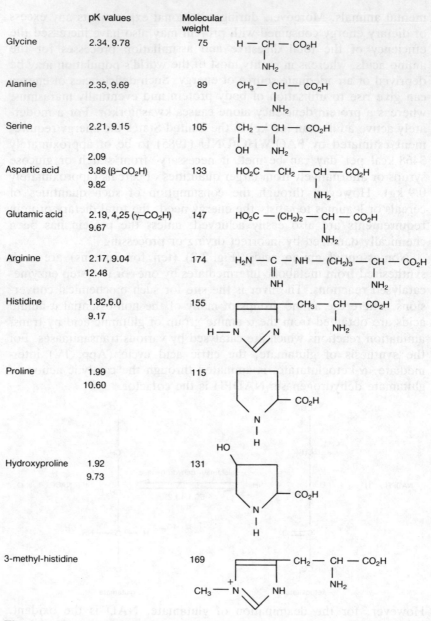

	pK values	Molecular weight	
Glycine	2.34, 9.78	75	H — CH — CO₂H, NH₂
Alanine	2.35, 9.69	89	CH₃ — CH — CO₂H, NH₂
Serine	2.21, 9.15	105	CH₂ — CH — CO₂H, OH NH₂
Aspartic acid	2.09, 3.86 (β–CO₂H), 9.82	133	HO₂C — CH₂ — CH — CO₂H, NH₂
Glutamic acid	2.19, 4,25 (γ–CO₂H), 9.67	147	HO₂C — (CH₂)₂ — CH — CO₂H, NH₂
Arginine	2.17, 9.04, 12.48	174	H₂N — C — NH — (CH₂)₃ — CH — CO₂H, NH NH₂
Histidine	1.82, 6.0, 9.17	155	CH₂ — CH — CO₂H, NH₂
Proline	1.99, 10.60	115	
Hydroxyproline	1.92, 9.73	131	
3-methyl-histidine		169	CH₂ — CH — CO₂H, NH₂

Fig. 3.2 Non-essential amino acids

amino group, for example as shown on page 128 for the synthesis of aspartate.

Likewise pyruvate is the precursor for alanine. Similarly 3-phosphoglycerate is transaminated to form serine, which also acts as a precursor of glycine. Proline (Fig. 3.3) is synthesised from glutamate

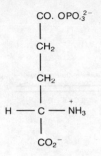

glutamyl   phosphate

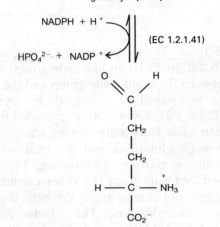

NADPH + H$^+$

(EC 1.2.1.41)

HPO$_4^{2-}$ + NADP$^+$

glutamate-γ-semialdehyde

H$_2$O

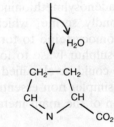

pyrroline-5-carboxylate

H$^+$ +NADPH

NADP$^+$ pyrroline-5-carboxylate reductase

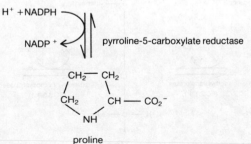

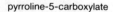

proline

Fig. 3.3 Biosynthesis of proline

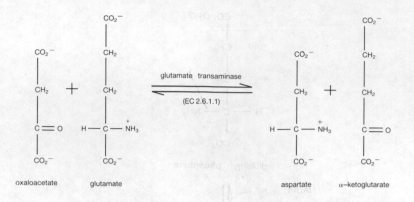

by three consecutive reactions. These require first, phosphorylation and reduction of the carboxyl group to an aldehyde group, secondly, subsequent cyclisation between the γ-aldehyde group and the α-amino group followed thirdly, by reduction catalysed by pyrroline-5-carboxylate reductase (EC 1.5.1.2). Clearly NH_4^+ provided by the de-amination of dietary amino acids is assimilated into synthesised non-essential amino acids through glutamine and glutamate which are therefore two key molecules in nitrogen metabolism. Tyrosine and cysteine can be synthesised, but only from two other essential amino acids, namely phenylalanine and methionine. Tyrosine is normally formed by hydroxylation of phenylalanine. The cofactor is dihydro-biopterin which is reduced by NADPH, and therefore the overall reaction results in the formation of NADP and tyrosine (Fig. 3.4). For the synthesis of cysteine, S-adenosylmethionine is first demethylated to form homocysteine. Secondly serine, which is the precursor of cysteine, is combined with homocysteine to form cystathionine which is then cleaved by a carbon–sulphur lyase to form cysteine.

Thus tyrosine and cysteine could be classified as indirectly essential, to distinguish them from the simpler non-essential amino acids formed by more direct transamination of the main metabolic intermediates of the citric acid cycle.

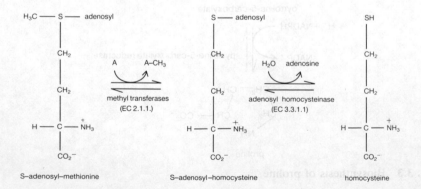

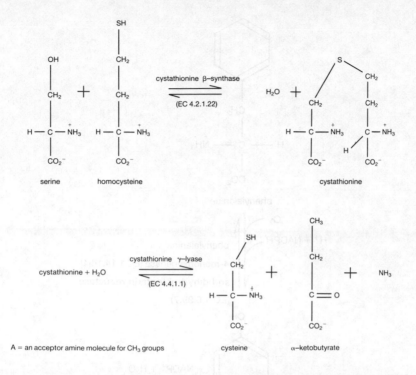

serine   homocysteine

cystathionine

A = an acceptor amine molecule for CH₃ groups   cysteine   α–ketobutyrate

EVALUATION OF FOOD PROTEIN QUALITY

Biological values

All biological measurements of protein quality are determined by the concentration of the limiting α-amino acid and do not provide any information on the other essential amino acids. The biological value (BV) of a protein is the fraction of its nitrogen retained in the body for growth and maintenance of cell synthesis. The biological value of proteins can be determined by nitrogen balance experiments:

$$BV = \frac{IN - UN - FN}{IN - FN}$$

where IN = nitrogen intake
         UN = urinary nitrogen output
and   FN = faecal nitrogen output.

In practice the test animal is first fed a very low nitrogen-containing diet to attain a minimum nitrogen output. Dietary addition of the test protein increases nitrogen output in the urine, only when the protein is of poor quality and is not efficiently utilised. The apparent biological value is expressed as a ratio where BV = 1.0 for 100 per cent retained nitrogen, when urinary nitrogen is unchanged (i.e. UN = 0).

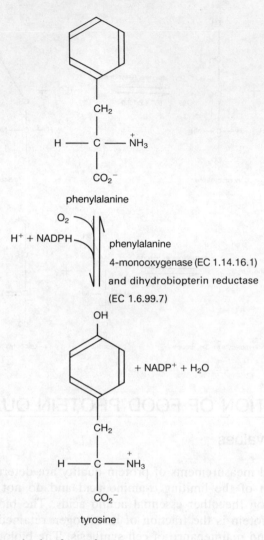

phenylalanine

phenylalanine
4-monooxygenase (EC 1.14.16.1)
and dihydrobiopterin reductase
(EC 1.6.99.7)

tyrosine

Fig. 3.4 Biosynthesis of tyrosine

Table 3.5 The biological value of proteins

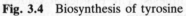

Food	BV
Egg (soft boiled) or human milk	1.0
Skim milk	0.85
RHM myco-protein	0.84
Meat, fish protein	0.75
Wheat protein	0.50
Peanut	0.40
Gelatin†	0.0

† Pure gelatin does not contain any sulphur amino acids.

Such experimentally determined biological values, although of limited use for human foods – because the experimental measurements are normally made with rats – permit numerical comparisons for different proteins.

Other biological methods used for evaluating the nutritional value of proteins include the use of the proteolytic microorganisms *Streptococcus faccilis* subsp. *zymogenes* and *Tetrahymena pyriformis*, and the nitrogen balance technique. The latter method is used to determine both the supply of essential amino acids and the total nitrogen required to achieve equilibrium where the intake equals the output for nitrogen.

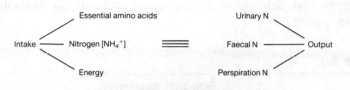

In order to determine the essential whole body amino acid requirements, there must be both an adequate intake of nitrogen in the form of ammonia or non-essential amino acids, and an adequate intake of energy to permit the normal synthesis of non-essential amino acids from metabolic intermediates. Thus the variable minimum protein requirement is affected by the amounts of essential and non-essential amino acids. Therefore this method of assay may be criticised when the total nitrogen intake is low. Also specific amino acids may be preferentially retained by adaptation of metabolic processes within cells and individual tissues. Moreover, the nitrogen balance technique, like the biological value assay, cannot measure the needs of individual cells, and so changes in metabolism in separate tissues as well as the uneven distribution of supplied protein within the test animal are not accounted for. However, despite these shortcomings the nitrogen balance technique has remained popular.

Protein efficiency ratios (PER) is an index of gain in weight over mass of protein intake (MpI), which is generally measured over a 10 to 28 day period.

$$PER = \frac{W_2 - W_1}{MpI}$$

This index has been very widely used but is not precise; it can be influenced substantially by the energy intake, and furthermore no allowance is made for the normal maintenance requirements of the test animals for protein. The relationship between PER values and the ability of a protein to supply all the essential amino acids in the amounts needed is non-linear: a PER value of 1.5 does not represent a 50 per cent efficiency of a PER value of 3.0. Moreover, the PER value varies with the amount of food eaten, and the weight gain by the test animal is not restricted to protein. Nevertheless, the method is rapid, not too expensive to carry out and hence popular.

Net protein utilisation (NPU) is the ratio of nitrogen retained to total protein nitrogen intake and is thus influenced by the biological value of a protein and its digestibility. The nitrogen retained can be determined by analysis of the carcase. However, the determination can yield a positive value when one or more essential amino acids are completely absent from the test food. Further the method is time-consuming and expensive if carcases are used to determine nitrogen retention. The NPU values for some common foods and mycoprotein are given in Table 3.6, where the order of values for commodities is similar to that determined by the other methods for evaluation of protein quality.

Table 3.6

Food	Biological assessment (NPU)
Egg	100
Fish	83
Beef	80
Cow's milk	75
Mycoprotein	60
Wheat flour	52
Beans	47

(With permission from Edelman *et al*. 1983).

Generally for all the biological methods of assay for protein quality, it should be noted that the various values obtained mainly reflect the content of the limiting essential amino acid. For most human and animal foods this is generally lysine, the sulphur amino acids or thre-onine. An alternative and more direct method of assay for estimating the biological value of proteins is by amino acid analysis. Such analysis now uses routine, inexpensive and rapid methods. Amino acid analysis affords a much more direct means of assessing the adequacy of a protein. The data obtained can be compared directly to the amino acid composition of a reference protein, such as egg or human milk.

AMINO ACID REQUIREMENTS

The expert committees of the Food and Agricultural Organisation/World Health Organisation or National Research Council/National Academy of Sciences have attempted to estimate the infant's requirements for essential amino acids (Table 3.3) from data reported for feeding experiments. However, despite the decreasing requirement for essential amino acids with increasing age – a relationship which is poorly understood – the recommendation by FAO/WHO for adults has been based until recently on the recommendation for pre-school children. However, recently although the estimates for amino acid requirements are unchanged (Table 3.3), the patterns of amino acid requirements per gram of protein are based now on the differing amino acid requirements of humans from infancy to adulthood (Table 3.7). Also the recommendation for total protein intake has been increased, and therefore the essential amino acids required per gram of protein are lower than those suggested for the FAO/WHO 1973 reference protein. The pattern which includes histidine indicates a requirement for infants of 460 mg of essential amino acids per gram of reference protein and a decreasing requirement with increasing age for high quality protein. Therefore by using the 1985 FAO/WHO/UNU patterns the adequacy of proteins for consumption by infants, pre-school children (2–5 years) and adults can now be estimated separately from their amino acid composition. For this purpose chemical scores related to the FAO/WHO pattern are determined for individual amino acids by simple ratio:

$$\text{Chemical score} = \frac{\text{mg of essential amino acid per g of test protein}}{\text{mg of essential amino acid per g of reference protein}} \times 100$$

For test proteins the most limiting amino acid is the component which determines the overall score of the protein. However, there are a number of disadvantages associated with the use of the chemical score method. First, the efficacy is dependent on the choice of reference protein (Table 3.7), which is based on estimates of the composition of human milk. Secondly, the reference pattern still combines the sulphur-containing amino acids as well as the aromatic amino acids: thus any deficiencies of the strictly essential individual amino acids, methionine or phenylalanine, may be obscured. Thirdly, amino acids measured by chemical analysis may be biologically unavailable: in animals proteins have to be digested and assimilated before they are effective sources of nutrients. Nevertheless, scoring patterns based on amino acid requirements allow comparative predictions of the effectiveness of various proteins to meet human needs.

Data for the comparative digestibility of proteins is available (FAO/WHO/UNU 1985). Therefore adjustments can be made for safe levels of intake for various individual dietary proteins, although the values may be substantially changed by the presence of other constituents like dietary fibre. Consequently the amino acid score value can be adjusted for poor digestibility and values of some proteins are given in Table 3.8. Numerical values for amino acid scores of plant and animal proteins are not given here, as there are significant variations for the amino acid composition of various cultivars grown under

Table 3.7 FAO/WHO/UNU suggested patterns of human amino acid requirements[†]

Amino acid (mg/g crude protein)	Suggested pattern of requirement			
	Infant Mean (range)[‡]	Pre-school child (2–5 years)	School-child (10–12 years)	Adult
Histidine	26 (18–36)	19	19	16
Isoleucine	46 (41–53)	28	28	13
Leucine	93 (83–107)	66	44	19
Lysine	66 (53–76)	58	44	16
Methionine + cystine	42 (29–60)	25	22	17
Phenylalanine + tyrosine	72 (68–118)	63	22	19
Threonine	43 (40–5)	34	28	9
Tryptophan	17 (16–17)	11	9	5
Valine	55 (44–77)	35	25	13
Total				
including histidine	460 (408–588)	339	241	127
minus histidine	434 (390–552)	320	222	111

([†] FAO/WHO/UNU 1985).

[‡] Amino acid composition of human milk.

For adults, safe level taken as 0.75 g/kg; children (10–12 years) 0.99 g/kg; children (2–5 years) 1.10 g/kg. (This age range is chosen because it coincides with the age range of the subjects from whom the amino acid data were derived. The pattern of amino acid requirement of children between 1 and 2 years may be taken as intermediate between that of infants and pre-school children.)

Table 3.8 Digestibility of proteins in man

Plant proteins	
Whole wheat	86
Maize	85
Millet	79
Rice, polished	88
Soyflour	86
Beans	78
Animal proteins	
Egg, milk, meat	94–7

(FAO/WHO/UNU 1985).

different conditions. Hence amino acid scores should be calculated for individual samples of protein for assessment of their nutritional value.

Sample calculation for a cereal diet

A wheat diet contains 9 g of nitrogen and 1.1 g of lysine per 100 g of cereal. For wheat the nitrogen conversion factor is 5.83 (Table 3.9). The reference protein for the infant contains 66 mg of amino acid per gram of protein (Table 3.7) (FAO/WHO/UNU 1985). The digestibility factor for wheat is 86 per cent (Table 3.8).

Calculate the protein value of the diet.

The total protein content of the diet = 5.83 × 9
$$= 52.47 \text{ g per 100 g of cereal}$$

$$\text{The amino acid score} = \frac{\text{mg of lysine per g of cereal protein}}{\text{mg of lysine per g of reference protein}}$$
$$= \frac{1100/52.47}{66}$$
$$= 0.318$$

Calculated protein value of the wheat diet

= protein content × amino acid score digestibility
= 52.47 × 0.318 × 0.86
= 14.35 g

100 g of the wheat cereal is only equivalent to 14.35 g of the reference protein (human milk protein).

The total protein content and amino acid composition of food raw materials and whole foods has been determined by a variety of methods. Crude protein can be estimated from the percentage nitrogen

Table 3.9 The factors for converting
total nitrogen in foods to protein

Food commodity	Nx factor
Wheat	5.83
Rice	5.95
Barley, oats, rye	5.83
Soybean	5.71
Milk	6.38
Meat, eggs	6.25

(From FAO/WHO 1973).

using factors to convert to per cent protein. The FAO/WHO Committee on Energy and Protein Requirements (1973) has suggested the use of specific factors for food commodities (Table 3.9). However, such estimations fail to account for extraneous non-protein nitrogen which is present in some carbohydrates, nucleic acids and non-protein amino acids. Concentrates of food proteins may also be contaminated with ammonium salts, and thus the nitrogen values obtained may result in overestimates for the concentration of protein. The calculated data reported in The First Supplement to *McCance and Widdowson's The Composition of Foods* (Paul *et al.* 1980) is based on both the nitrogen content of food items and the amounts of amino acids related to 1 g of nitrogen. Other errors for moisture values can also give rise to incorrect estimates of the amino acid content of foods.

For soluble extracts and concentrates an approximate value for crude protein can be obtained simply and quickly by spectrophotometric measurements at 276 nm, although slight contamination (3–4 %) with nucleic acids or other ultraviolet light absorbing materials, will cause a serious overestimate for protein. Alternatively, electrophoresis of the concentrate on polyacrylamide gels and subsequent dye staining specifically for proteins will indicate quickly the proteinaceous nature and authenticity of concentrates. If dye-binding techniques are used for the estimation of total protein, calibrations for the type of protein being analysed should be used (e.g. for barley proteins, standard barley prolamins or total barley protein should be used for calibration purposes).

More accurate values for protein content may be obtained from summation of the amounts of all the amino acids present in a protein. However, concentrated acid required for hydrolysis of proteins destroys the hydroxyamino acids, serine and threonine, and the peptide bonds of valine, leucine and isoleucine, are only hydrolysed slowly. Therefore accurate results can only be obtained from analyses of a series of hydrolysates obtained for different hydrolysis periods with extrapolation of the results obtained back to zero hydrolysis time.

Separate analyses for alkaline hydrolysates are required for trypto-phan, which is destroyed by acid. Accurate values for cysteine and cystine can be obtained by oxidisation with performic acid followed by measurements of the original sulphur-containing amino acids as cysteic acid. Nevertheless, unfortunately many results have not been reported in a consistent manner and therefore comparisons of amino acid content for different raw materials is often difficult. In nutritional studies the hydrated amino acid content is often expressed per 16 g of nitrogen, or per 100 g of total amino acids. Occasionally it has to be assumed that the weights of amino acids reported refer to hydrated amino acids. However, as the amino acids mainly occur naturally as anhydrous residues in proteins, the most accurate method for expression of results should be either as molar residue per 1000 moles or moles per cent. Such data can be derived from just the amino acid analyses charts and need not depend on separate determinations of nitrogen or accurate weighing of hygroscopic material. From such data the number of residues of amino acids per mole for pure proteins of known molecular weight can also be calculated.

PROTEIN SOURCES

Plant proteins

In developed countries the main sources of dietary protein have been milk, animal meats including fish, eggs, cereal and legume seeds. Based on a knowledge of the amino acid composition of proteins, dietary sources have been described as good, adequate or poor. Good sources of protein are legume seeds, dairy products, meat, eggs and fish. Adequate sources of protein are rice, corn and wheat. Whereas poor sources of protein are cassava, potato and sweet potato, along with many fruits. The nutrient composition of more than 2700 fresh and cooked foods of varying type has been published by Leveille *et al.* (1983).

For humans, cereals which are members of the grass family have provided universally the bulk of the protein needs. Legumes provide approximately 2 per cent of man's total needs, while surprisingly the potato, owing to consumption of relatively large quantities, may supply approximately 3 per cent of the protein requirement. For different parts of the world the type of cereal grown depends on the climate; in the tropics and subtropics rice and maize are grown extensively; for tropical regions with limited rainfall sorghum and millet are the main crops; wheat is grown in temperate zones; oats are grown in cold climates with a high rainfall. The soybean and peanut are also grown for their oil content, but like other legumes contain larger amounts of protein than cereals. However, other legumes such as the field pea, owing to the variable yields of protein, are not at present good choices for alternative sources of protein. On the other hand the protein content of the fababean is usually less variable (28–32 %), and thus after dehulling and pin milling, intact starch granules can be removed by air classification to yield a fababean fraction containing 65 per cent protein. The average amounts of protein reported for some selected import-

Table 3.10 Average protein content of cereal grains[†]

Cereal grain	Protein (% of dry weight)
Wheat	12.2
Rye	11.6
Triticale[‡]	12.8–17.9
Barley	10.9
Oats	11.3
Maize	10.2
Millet	10.3
Sorghum	11.0
Rice	8.1

([†] After Lásztity 1984).

[‡] Hybrid cereal species of wheat and rye.

Table 3.11 Averaage protein content of some animal foods

Animal food	Protein (%)
Whole cow's milk, 3 % fat	3.3
Skimmed cow's milk, 1 % fat	3.3
Dried non-fat milk powder	36.2
Whole goat's milk	3.6
Chicken's egg, whole raw	12.1
Chicken's egg albumen, raw	9.4
Chicken's egg yolk, raw	16.1
Chicken's egg, whole dried	45.2
Beef, roast, no visible fat	30.6
Lamb, leg roast	28.8
Pork, leg roast	29.7
Chicken, roast, light meat	27.2
Hen turkey, roast, light meat	28.7
Cod fillet, cooked	28.5
Salmon, broiled	25.7

(Leveille *et al*. 1983).

ant raw food materials are given in Tables 3.10 to 3.13. The average protein content of cereals ranges from 8 to 13 per cent which is less than that for animal proteins and considerably less than the protein content of legume seeds. The proteins derived from oil-producing seeds listed in Table 3.13 are obtained after the extraction of oil with organic solvents

Table 3.12 Average protein content of some plant raw materials (other than cereals)

Plant raw material	Protein (%)
Cassava	0.7
Fababean	28
Kidney bean, red raw	22.1
Lupin seed	34
Peas, dried raw	21.6
Peanuts, no shells	24.3
Potato, dried	9.1
Potato, raw	2.1
Rapeseed	25
Sesame seed	20
Soybean	36
Sunflower	28.7
Yeast, dried	47

(Paul and Southgate 1978).

Table 3.13 Average protein content of some commercial refined products

Refined product	Protein (%)
Soya, defatted soya flour[†]	54
Soya, protein concentrate[†]	70
Soya protein isolate[‡]	92
Winter rapeseed defatted meal[‡] (Brassica napus)	40
Oriental rapeseed defatted meal[‡] (Brassica juncea)	47.4
Winter rapeseed protein isolate	83.0
Oriental rapeseed protein isolate	93.2
Rapeseed flour, dehulled	46.9
Wheat gluten	80
Mycoprotein[§]	48
Peanut meal, defatted	57.0

([†] Pearson 1983; [‡] Sosulski 1983a; [§] Edelman et al. 1983).

such as n-hexane. Soybeans are dehulled and cracked before oil extraction. Whereas for the manufacture of rapeseed defatted meal, where the seed is very small, the hulls are not removed due to the potential loss of oil. Mycoprotein is the name for a new commercial protein-rich product obtained from the fungus *Fusarium graminearum*. The mycoprotein product which contains less than 2 per cent of ribonucleic acids can be manufactured into texturised frozen food products.

For nutritional assessment it is only necessary in the first instance to know the amounts of both total protein and the essential amino acids. While the total protein acts as a source of nitrogen for synthesis of non-essential amino acids, the low content of the sulphur amino acids normally limits the nutritional value of proteins. Therefore it is often necessary first, to consider the content of sulphur amino acids and secondly, the amounts of lysine and tryptophan. However, for cereal grains, lysine is the limiting amino acid, except for maize where both lysine and tryptophan are limiting. In Table 3.14, for comparative purposes amounts of amino acids are expressed on a common basis per 100 g of total amino acids.

For cereals, the endosperm proteins or the total seed proteins contain only small amounts of lysine, tryptophan and threonine. The lysine content of wheat, maize and sorghum is particularly low. The content of tryptophan in maize is also small and consequently the biological values for many cereal proteins are low with the possible exception of rice where biological values of from 67 to 89 have been found (Lásztity 1984). For oats, the proportion of lysine is higher than

Table 3.14   The important amino acids of some cereals (mean values g/100 g of total protein)

Amino acid	Wheat grain[†]	Maize grain[†]	Maize[†] high Lys opaque-2 mutant	Oats[†]
Arg	4.6	3.8	5.1	6.4
Cys	2.2	1.1	2.1	1.7
His	2.2	2.8	3.4	2.4
Ile	3.6	3.7	4.3	4.2
Leu	6.8	13.6	12.1	7.5
Lys	2.5	2.6	3.5	4.2
Met	2.1	1.8	2.7	2.3
Phe	4.7	5.1	6.0	5.4
Thr	2.9	3.6	4.4	3.3
Trp	1.3	0.7	0.8	1.7[†]
Tyr	3.2	4.4	5.2	2.6
Val	4.2	5.3	5.9	5.8

([†] See Lásztity 1984; [‡] after Seyed Rasheduddin and McDonald 1974; [§] after Bressani *et al.* 1971).

that present in other cereals (Table 3.14). The more favourable chemical composition of oats coupled to the need for a lower proportional mass of hulls is receiving increased attention.

The data for the amino acid composition of isolated storage and cytoplasmic proteins of cereals has been reviewed by Lásztity (1984). In the endosperm, the storage proteins form a matrix of protein surrounded by starch granules and the concentration of protein ranges from 6.2 per cent in the innermost layers of the endosperm to 13.7 per cent close to the aleurone layer. The aleurone layer itself contains approximately 20 per cent protein. The protein content of the whole grain is higher than that of the endosperm, and the total amount of essential amino acids present in the whole grain varies with changes in the mass ratio of the main morphological parts of the grain. For wheat, the proportion of protein is generally negatively correlated with the total yield of grain. Furthermore, the proportion of lysine present decreases with increased yield of the total protein. Thus 'high-lysine', opaque-2 maize which contains a smaller proportion of endosperm has a lower content of the storage protein.

All cereals contain a very large number of different proteins as shown by gel electrophoresis and isoelectric focusing (Fig. 5.30). The distribution of and intensity of the stained proteins on electrophoretograms can be used for varietal identifications. Nevertheless, generally the proteins are still named and classified as by Osborne in 1907. Wheat proteins were divided into four classes: albumins, globulins, alcohol-soluble gliadins and insoluble glutenins and glutelins. Cyto-

Sorghum[†]	Millet[†]	Barley[†]	Triticale[‡]	Milled rice[§]
3.2	4.7	5.0	4.8	7.5
1.7	2.2	2.2	2.7	1.5
1.7	2.3	2.3	2.2	2.3
3.8	4.5	3.8	3.4	4.8
13.1	10.3	7.4	6.4	8.1
2.2	3.0	3.6	3.0	3.6
1.2	1.8	1.8	1.5	2.5
4.9	4.9	5.4	4.5	5.5
3.6	3.2	3.4	2.9	3.7
1.2[†]	1.4	1.4	0.9	1.1
3.4	3.7	3.6	2.9	5.1
4.5	5.3	5.4	4.2	6.3

Table 3.15 Distribution of cereal proteins

Cereal	Cytoplasmic proteins	Storage/endosperm proteins	
		Alcohol-soluble: low molecular weight	Insoluble glutelins: high molecular weight
Wheat	(17 %)	Gliadins (28 %)	Glutenin (30 %)
Rye	(45 %)	Secalin, prolamins (19 %)	Glutelin (21 %)
Barley	(13–25 %)	Hordeins (35–45 %)	Glutelins (35–40 %)
Maize	(17 %)	Zeins (39 %)	Glutelins (40 %)
Oats	(30 %)	Avenins (20 %)	Glutelins (15 %)
Rice	(10–20 %)	Prolamins (2–10 %)	Oryzenin (37–91 %)
Sorghum	(3–16 %)	Kafirin (32–59 %)	Glutenin (19–37 %)
Millet	(25 %)	Prolamins[1]	Glutenins[1]

The figures in parentheses represent the approximate proportional amounts of the total seed protein

[1] Prolamins and glutenins total >60 % of all proteins.

plasmic proteins correspond approximately to the albumin–globulin group, while storage proteins represent the gliadin–glutelin group. Arising from a greater knowledge of the molecular structure of the wheat proteins, the gliadins and glutenins are now thought to form a larger class of prolamins (see Ch. 5). However, for all cereals common names are still frequently used to describe the storage proteins (Table 3.15).

Table 3.16 Some important amino acids of legume flours

Amino acid	Lentil[†]	Field pea[†]	Navy bean[†]	Soya[†]	Lima bean[†]
g/100 g of total amino acids					
Arg	7.7	8.1	6.4	7.5	5.5
Cys	1.0	1.5	0.8	1.1	1.0
His	2.4	2.4	3.2	2.2	3.0
Ile	4.7	4.3	4.6	4.8	5.1
Leu	7.8	7.4	8.4	7.6	8.7
Lys	7.8	7.7	7.2	6.5	6.7
Met	0.8	0.9	1.2	1.4	1.2
Phe	5.1	4.6	5.5	5.0	6.1
Thr	3.7	3.9	4.0	3.8	4.2
Trp	1.0	1.0	1.0	1.3	1.3
Tyr	3.6	2.9	3.0	3.5	3.0
Val	5.2	4.8	5.2	5.0	5.5

([†] Recalculated after Sosulski 1983b); [‡] after Duranti and Cerletti 1979; [§] Lusas 1979).

The cereal cytoplasmic proteins with a higher lysine content and a lower content of glutamic acid (or glutamine) are richer than the storage proteins in essential amino acids. However, rich sources of metabolisable nitrogen are provided by large amounts of glutamic and aspartic acids, which generally occur as amides. For barley grain the low lysine content can be explained by the small content of lysine in the main endosperm storage proteins. While for the lysine-enriched maize opaque-2-mutants, biosynthesis of the storage protein (zein) is suppressed when compared to the low-lysine varieties of maize. Thus in the maize opaque-2 variety a lower content of glutamic acid (or glutamine) is found with a corresponding increase in lysine. Consequently it is now accepted that a change in the total amino acid composition of cereal grains can only be achieved if the proportion of the different types of proteins is altered. For example, a thicker aleurone layer (20 % protein), germ content (30 % protein), or conversely a lower prolamin content would favour a higher content of lysine in cereals.

For most legume proteins the content of the essential amino acids lysine and leucine, together with arginine, is substantial (Table 3.16), whereas the amounts of methionine, cysteine and tryptophan are small. However, for peanut protein meal, the values for lysine and threonine are also low. For lupin seed, the fababean and peanut, arginine represents more than 10 per cent of the total protein. Like cereal grains, all legumes contain substantial amounts of glutamine and asparagine, but due to the greater amounts of lysine in legumes, supplementation of cereal products with legume flours increases the nutritional value: for example, the nutritional value of bread can be

Fababean[‡]	Lupinus albus[‡]	Peanut meal[§]
10.6	11.1	11.3
1.2	2.1	1.3
2.5	2.1	2.3
4.2	4.3	4.1
7.8	7.3	6.7
6.7	4.4	3.0
0.8	0.5	0.9
4.2	3.9	5.2
3.5	3.9	2.5
1.1	0.4	1.0
3.1	4.6	4.1
4.9	3.5	4.5

improved by supplementation of wheat flour with legume flour. Legume flours from fababean and field pea can be prepared, after pin milling, by air classification due to the greater size and uniformity of the starch granules. However, all legumes generally contain significant quantities of antinutritional factors, like trypsin inhibitors and haemagglutinins which can reduce digestion and utilisation of proteins generally.

For *Brassica spp.*, rapeseed owing to its increasing use as a source of vegetable oil offers a viable source of protein, even though the seeds are very small with the hulls forming approximately 25 per cent of the oil-free proteinaceous residue. The amounts of the nutritionally important amino acids present in rapeseed flours are given in Table 3.17. The amount of methionine is comparable to that for oats and wheat. The amount of lysine present also compares favourably with the lysine content of legumes. Thus the overall nutritional value of total rapeseed protein is superior to that of many other seed proteins. Therefore rapeseed protein might be used to enrich new cereal-based foods now being manufactured increasingly by extrusion processes. Unfortunately, rapeseed may also contain up to 2 per cent of thio-glucosides, which when hydrolysed by myrosinase may result in the formation of thiocyanate and other goitregenic factors, thus making some rapeseed flours unfit for human consumption. However, cultivars which are low in glucosinolates and erucic acid are becoming increasingly available and a continual breeding programme to lower the contents of thioglucosides should produce more valuable protein products.

A number of other plant proteins have been frequently suggested as alternative sources of protein for human consumption. These have included cottonseed, peanut, leaf and microbial proteins. For cottonseed protein, the nutritional value is only moderate, due to deficiencies in lysine, isoleucine and methionine (Table 3.18). Sesame proteins may become an important source of high quality protein food, because of

Table 3.17 Some important amino acids in winter rapeseed (*Brassica napus*) flours

Amino acid		Amino acid	
(g/100 g of total amino acids)			
Arg	6.27	Met	1.7
Cys	2.1	Phe	4.2
His	3.0	Thr	4.3
Ile	3.9	Trp	1.1
Leu	7.5	Tyr	2.7
Lys	6.2	Val	4.9

(Sosulski 1983a).

Table 3.18 Important amino acids of leaf and some oil seed proteins

Amino acid	Leaf[t]	Cottonseed[‡]	Sesame[§]	Sunflower[§]
			(g/100 g total amino acids)	
Arg	6.5	13.1	12.8	8.5
Cys	1.2	2.3	1.9	1.6
His	2.4	3.2	2.6	2.4
Ile	5.7	3.2	3.8	4.6
Leu	9.5	6.2	7.1	6.8
Lys	6.1	5.0	2.8	3.8
Met	2.4	0.7	3.0	2.0
Phe	6.1	5.7	4.6	4.8
Tyr	4.9	2.1	3.3	2.0
Thr	5.2	3.8	3.8	3.9
Val	6.5	4.8	4.9	5.4
Trp	—	2.1	1.6	1.5

([t] Kuzmicky and Kohler 1977; [‡] Zarins and Cherry, 1980; [§] Bodwell and Hopkins 1985).

the unique amino acid composition with higher amounts of the sulphur amino acids. However, of all the various suggested new sources of plant protein, leaf protein probably has the greatest potential in the long term. Although the levels of protein in individual leaves is low (4–5 % of dry mass), large quantities of protein could be made available from prolific plants grown in tropical regions. Furthermore, the process for the preparation of concentrates by crushing of green leaves is relatively simple and the energy requirements are small. The leaf protein can be recovered from pressed leaf juices by precipitation to yield a concentrate containing 60 per cent protein. In the temperate regions, investigations have been carried out on crops like *Medicago sativa* (alfalfa) which can be grown quickly within the seasons on a large scale. For the tropical regions a large number of plant leaves from tropical legumes and grasses have been investigated. The amino acid composition of most leaf protein concentrates is similar and close to those reported for rapeseed protein (Table 3.17), although there is a slight underprovision of methionine and cysteine. However, as leaves contain a very diverse mixture of other substances, such as phenols and quinones, and are metabolically active, loss of essential amino acids can occur rapidly before processing.

Mycoprotein is a fibrous protein-rich food derived from a strain *Fusarium graminearum* (Schwabe) by continuous fermentation of a carbohydrate energy source supplemented with trace minerals. After full nutritional and toxicological testing clearance has been given in the United Kingdom by the Ministry of Agriculture, Fisheries and Food

Table 3.19   Amino acid analysis of RHM mycoprotein

Amino acid		Amino acid	
(g/100 g total amino acids)			
Lys	8.1	His	3.9
Met	2.2	Arg	7.7
Cys	0.8	Tyr	3.9
Thr	5.5	Asp	9.9
Trp	1.7	Ser	5.1
Val	5.9	Glu	11.5
Leu	8.3	Pro	4.7
Ile	5.1	Gly	4.6
Phe	4.8	Ala	6.3

(Mycoprotein Technical Data Sheet, June 1983, with the kind courtesy of RHM Research Ltd, High Wycombe, England.)

for marketing of products containing mycoprotein. The complete amino acid composition of the RHM mycoprotein is given in Table 3.19. The content of the essential amino acids, is superior to most vegetable proteins and more comparable to meat protein, especially with respect to threonine. Hence mycoprotein, which has been approved for human consumption, could find widespread use as a protein supplement and as a complete protein food in its own right.

Table 3.20   Important amino acids of some animal foods

Amino acid	Whole cow's milk[†]	Lean pork[†]	Fish[†] (cod)
g per 100 g of total amino acids			
Arg	3.6	6.1	6.2
Cys	0.9	1.3	1.1
His	2.7	4.4	2.8
Ile	4.9	4.6	5.2
Leu	9.0	7.2	8.3
Lys	7.4	9.8	9.6
Met	2.6	2.8	2.8
Phe	4.9	3.9	4.1
Thr	4.4	4.4	4.7
Trp	1.3	1.1	1.1
Tyr	4.1	3.8	3.4
Val	6.6	4.9	5.6

† By summation of the values for amino acids in the First Supplement to *McCance and Widdowson's The Composition of Foods* (Paul *et al.* 1980).

Animal proteins

The main edible portions of animal tissues consist substantially of muscle made up of proteins of high nutritional value. Substantial amounts of lysine and sufficient amounts of methionine and tryptophan are consumed from meats and fish although, as shown in Table 3.20, methionine and tryptophan in fact occur quite infrequently in animal proteins. However, in turn this means that the requirement by animals, including man, for these amino acids is not very high.

Egg and milk proteins have often been considered for nutritional purposes as reference proteins. However, human milk (Table 3.21) is now frequently used as a reference protein for the estimation of the nutritive value of foods and is the basis for the FAO/WHO/UNU reference amino acid pattern. Human milk contains the least amount of protein of all milks (Table 3.22). The whey proteins account for 70 per cent of the human milk protein, whereas in bovine milk approximately 80 per cent of the protein is derived from the caseins. Nevertheless, the bovine whey proteins do represent a very valuable source of protein of high nutritive value due to the high content of essential amino acids. In particular, the amounts of Lys, Ile, Thr and Trp are high in bovine whey protein, whereas the amounts of the aromatic amino acids are low. In the United States it is claimed that 70 per cent of produced whey proteins are used for human consumption. It is possible to prepare infant feeds enriched with bovine whey proteins thus

Whole egg[†]	Egg white[†]	Egg yolk[†]
6.1	5.4	7.3
1.8	1.8	1.6
2.4	2.2	2.6
5.6	5.5	5.8
8.3	8.1	8.6
6.3	5.8	7.3
3.2	3.5	2.6
5.1	5.8	4.1
5.1	4.8	5.6
1.8	1.8	1.8
4.0	4.0	4.1
7.6	7.9	7.0

Table 3.21   The amino acid composition of human breast milk[†]

Amino acid		Amino acid	
(g/100 g of total amino acid)			
Lys	6.9	Gly	2.0
Arg	3.5	Ala	3.4
His	2.3	Cys	2.3
Asp	9.2	Met	1.6
Glu	20.3	Val	6.0
Pro	10.4	Leu	9.6
Ser	4.6	Ile	5.2
Thr	4.6	Phe	3.5
		Tyr	4.5

[†] Excluding Trp, calculated from Hambraeus (1982). A value of 1.7 g is given for Trp by FAO/WHO/UNU (1985).

Table 3.22   The occurrence of protein in milks from various species

Animal species	Total protein (g/100 g of milk)
Cow	3.4
Goat	2.9
Man	0.9
Sheep	5.5
Seal	8.9

(Hambraeus 1982).

Table 3.23   Whey protein composition of human and cow's milk

Protein	Human milk (mg/cm³)	(g/100 g of whey protein)	Cow's milk (mg/cm³)	(g/100 g of whey protein)
α-Lactalbumin	1.6	29	0.9	23.4
β-Lactoglobulin	—	—	3.0	61.5
Lactoferrin	1.7	30.8	0.012	0.25
Lysozyme	0.4	7.2	0.0001	2.05×10^{-3}
Serum albumin	0.4	7.2	0.3	6.2
Immunoglobulins	1.42	25.7	0.66	13.5

(From Hambraeus 1982).

imitating the ratio (7 : 3) of whey proteins to caseins found in human milk. However, human whey protein contains 100 times more lactoferrin, an iron-binding protein and lysozyme, a bactericidal protein (Table 3.23) than bovine whey protein. Therefore, although the content of casein can be reduced to 30 per cent in such bovine whey protein-enriched milks, the bound iron content of the fabricated milk may be insufficient. There are substantial amounts of unused whey proteins available as a by-product from the manufacture of cheese and, therefore, the proper use of this protein source may depend largely on the development of economic ways of fractionating the proteins to produce nutritionally valuable and safe protein supplements.

KEY FACTS

1.   The total protein required by humans falls with age from a high value of almost 2 g per kg body weight per day for infants to 0.75 g for adults.
2.   For adults more than 70 per cent of the essential amino acids are provided by recycling. Histidine and arginine may be synthesised' in sufficient amounts by adults. For the biosynthesis of many non-essential amino acids, glutamate provides the amino group.
3.   The FAO/WHO/UNU 1985 reference protein patterns are based on the differing amino acid requirements for humans from infancy to adult. The nutritional needs of the infant are estimated from the amino acid composition of human milk.
4.   Animal proteins provide the highest quality protein. However, for adults most sources of protein, with the exception of cottonseed protein, can provide adequate amounts of essential amino acids.
5.   Only the essential amino acids, i.e. lysine, the sulphur amino acids, threonine and tryptophan, are likely to limit the nutritional quality of plant proteins.

REFERENCES

Bodwell, C. E. and Hopkins, D. T. (1985) 'Nutritional characteristics of oilseed proteins', in *New Food Proteins*, vol. 5 *Seed Storage Proteins* (eds. Altschul, A. M and Wilcke, H. L.). Academic Press, London.

Bressani, R., Elias, L. G. and Juliano, B. O. (1971) 'Evaluation of the protein quality of milled rices differing in protein content', *J. Agric. Food Chem.*, **19**, 1028–34.

DHSS (1981) Department of Health and Social Security. *Recommended Daily Amounts of Food Energy and Nutrients for Groups of People in the United*

Kingdom. Report by the Committee on Medical Aspects of Food Policy, no. 120. HMSO, London.

Department of National Health and Welfare (1983) *Recommended Nutritional Intakes for Canadians*. Bureau of Nutritional Sciences Food Directorate, Health Protection Branch, Ottawa.

Duranti, M. and Cerletti, P. (1979) 'Amino acid composition of seed proteins of *Lupinus albus*', *J. Agric. Food Chem.*, **27**, 977–8.

Edelman, J., Fewell, A. and Solomons, G. C. (1983) 'Myco-protein – a new food', *Nutr. Abstr. and Revs*, **53A**, 471–80.

FAO/WHO (1973) Food and Agricultural Organisation/World Health Organisation. *Energy and Protein Requirements*, WHO Tech. Rep. ser. no. 522, WHO Geneva, FAO Nutr. Meet. Rep. ser. No. 52, FAO, Rome.

FAO/WHO/UNU (1985) *Energy and Protein Requirements*, Report of a Joint FAO/WHO/UNU Expert Consultation. World Health Organisation Technical Report series 724. WHO, Geneva.

Hambraeus, L. (1982) 'Nutritional aspects of milk proteins' in *Developments in Dairy Chemistry* 1. *Proteins* (ed. Fox, P. F.). Applied Science Publishers, London.

IUNS (1983) 'Recommended dietary intakes around the world', *Nutr. Abstr. & Revs.*, series A, **53A**, 939–1015.

Kuzmicky, D. D. and Kohler, G. O. (1977) 'Nutritional value of alfalfa leaf protein concentrate (Pro–Xan) for broilers', *Poult. Sci.*, **56**, 1510–16.

Lásztity, R. (1984) *The Chemistry of Cereal Proteins*. CRC Press, Boca Raton, Florida.

Leveille, G. R., Zabik, M. A., Morgan, K. J. (1983) *Nutrients in Foods*. The Nutrition Guild, Cambridge, Massachusetts.

Lusas, E. W. (1979) 'Food uses of peanut protein', *J. Am. Oil Chem. Soc.*, **56**, 425–30.

NRC/NAS (1980) National Research Council Committee on Dietary Allowances. *Recommended Dietary Allowances*, 9th edn. National Academy of Sciences Press, Washington DC.

Paul, A. A. and Southgate, D. A. T. (1978) *McCance and Widdowson's The Composition of Foods*, 4th edn. of MRC Special Report no. 297. HMSO, London and Elsevier, Amsterdam.

Paul, A. A., Southgate, D. A. T. and Russell, J. (1980), First Supplement to *McCance and Widdowson's The Composition of Foods*. HMSO, London and Elsevier, New York.

Pearson, A. M (1983) 'Soy proteins', in *Developments in Food Proteins*, vol. 2 (ed. Hudson, B. J. F.). Applied Science Publishers, London.

Seyed Rasheduddin, A. and McDonald, C. E. (1974) 'Amino acid composition, protein fractions and baking quality of triticale', in *Triticale: First Man-Made Cereal* (ed. Isen, C. C.). American Association of Cereal Chemists, St. Paul, Minnesota

Sosulski, F. W. (1983a) 'Rapeseed proteins for food use', in *Developments in Food Proteins*, vol. 2 (ed. Hudson, B. J. F.). Applied Science Publishers, London.

Sosulski, F. W. (1983b) 'Legume protein concentration by air classification', in *Developments in Food Proteins*, vol. 2 (ed. Hudson, B. J. F). Applied Science Publishers, London.

Stryer, L. (1981) *Biochemistry*, 2nd. edn. W. H. Freeman and Co., San Francisco, California.

Visek, W. J. (1984) 'An update of concepts of essential amino acids', *Ann. Rev. Nutr.*, 4, 137–55.

Waterlow, J. (1980) 'Protein turnover in malnutrition, obesity and injury', in *Nutrition and Food Science, Present Knowledge and Utilisation*, vol. 3 (eds. Santos, W. S., Lopes, N., Barbosa, J. J. and Chaves, D.). Plenum Press, New York.

Zarins, Z. M. and Cherry, J. P. (1980) 'Storage proteins of glandless cottonseed flour', *J. Food Sci.*, 46, 1855–59.

ADDITIONAL READING

Bushak, W. and Larter, E. N. (1980) 'Triticale: production, chemistry and technology', in *Advances in Cereal Science and Technology*, vol. III (ed. Pomeranz, Y.). American Association of Cereal Chemists, St Paul, Minnesota.

FAO/WHO/UNU (1985) *Energy and Protein Requirements*, Report of a Joint FAO/WHO/UNU Expert Consultation. World Health Organisation Technical Report Series 724. WHO, Geneva.

Hudson, B. J. F. (1983) *Developments in Food Proteins* 2. Applied Science Publishers, London and New York.

Kasarda, D. D., Bernardin, J. E. and Nimmo, C. C. (1976) 'Wheat proteins', in *Advances in Cereal Science and Technology*, vol. I (ed. Pomeranz, Y.), American Association of Cereal Chemists, St Paul, Minnesota.

Lásztity, R. (1984) *The Chemistry of Cereal Proteins*. CRC Press, Boca Raton, Florida.

Wilcke, H. L., Hopkins, D. T. and Waggle, D. H. (1979) (eds,) *Soy Protein and Human Nutrition*. Academic Press New York.

Wolf, W. J. (1976) 'Chemistry and technology of soybeans', in *Advances in Cereal Science and Technology*, vol. I (ed. Pomeranz Y.). American Association of Cereal Chemists, St Paul, Minnesota.

CHAPTER 4

Enzyme-catalysed hydrolysis of proteins

The true nutritional value of dietary proteins irrespective of source is only realised after digestion in animals. In mammals, hydrolysis of proteins, catalysed by the enzymes pepsin, trypsin, chymotrypsin and other proteinases, to liberate amino acids and small peptides takes place consecutively in the stomach and small intestine. Although limited hydrolysis of proteins catalysed by other proteinases can also occur during the storage and processing of both traditional foods (e.g. yoghurt and cheese, tenderisation of meat) and newer food products (fortified soups and beverages). Studies of the mode of action of proteinases have shown that the enzymes can be classified simply by the chemical nature of the enzyme's active site residue (Table 4.1).

Previously enzymes such as trypsin, chymotrypsin, carboxypeptidases and elastases which possess maximum enzymatic activity at neutral pH values have been described as neutral proteinases. Likewise the enzymes pepsin, chymosin (rennin) and cathepsin D are still sometimes referred to as acidic proteinases, because they possess maximum enzymatic activity at pH values below 5. However, as it is now known that two carboxyl groups form part of the active sites of the acidic

Table 4.1 Classification of proteinases

Proteinase		Active site constituents
Carboxyl endoproteinases	EC 3.4.23	Carboxyl groups of two aspartic acid residues
Serine endoproteinases	EC 3.4.21	Hydroxyl group of serine and imidazole group of histidine
Cysteine endoproteinases	EC 3.4.22	Sulphydryl group of cysteine
Metalloendoproteinases	EC 3.4.24	Divalent metals, generally Zn^{2+} or Mn^{2+}
Metalloexocarboxypeptidases	EC 3.4.17	Generally Zn^{2+}, Glu and Tyr
Metalloexoaminopeptidases	EC 3.4.11	Generally Zn^{2+} or Mn^{2+}
Metallodipeptidases	EC 3.4.13	Generally Zn^{2+} or Mn^{2+}

proteinases the more specific term 'carboxyl proteinase' is now widely used; the group includes lysosomal proteinases, pepsin, chymosin and mould proteinases.

The enzymatic activity of proteinases can be determined easily by any of a number of methods which use scrum albumin or casein as test substrates. For enzymes, like pepsin, papain and pronase which catalyse the hydrolysis of proteins substantially, precipitation by trichloroacetic acid to remove any residual unhydrolysed protein followed by subsequent measurement in the clear supernatant of solubilised aromatic amino acids at 280 nm affords a particularly rapid and useful general assay method. Although care must be taken to reduce contamination with other UV-absorbing substances, and in particular nucleic acids. Alternatively, a reaction with ninhydrin or titration with sodium hydroxide can be used to follow the increase in concentration of liberated amino and carboxyl groups during proteolysis. However, for kinetic measurements and the detection of specific proteinases, it is necessary to use substrates which contain only one susceptible bond. For this purpose a number of nitroanilide derivatives of different L-amino acids are available, so that the amide bond between the carboxyl group and the nitroanaline residue is hydrolyzed specifically by different proteinases.

For many food proteins, including those of egg, meat and plant seeds, heating and the consequent denaturation increases the digestibility. Denaturation of the total protein exposes buried amino acids and peptide bonds and thus enables substantial hydrolysis by enzymes. For cereals and legumes, cooking also causes the denaturation of many naturally occurring proteinase inhibitors which results in an improved biological value. For other proteins, such as milk proteins, heat denaturation is not necessary prior to consumption; the caseins of milk exist naturally in a readily digestible form and are susceptible to the catalytic action of all known proteinases. The ease by which milk proteins are attacked by proteinases is exemplified for the calf, where the very specific hydrolytic action of chymosin (rennin), on one susceptible peptide bond destabilises the native micellar caseins, after which further hydrolysis occurs which is then catalysed by other less specific proteinases. In some milk products, such as cheese and yoghurts, partial proteolysis readily occurs during their manufacture.

During the digestion of foods in man the first stage of hydrolysis is carried out in the stomach through the catalytic action of the carboxyl proteinase pepsin, followed later by proteolysis catalysed by the pancreatic neutral proteinases – trypsin, chymotrypsin and carboxypeptidases. Pepsin, in the presence of stomach acid, catalyses the rapid hydrolysis of large protein molecules to smaller polypeptide fragments. Likewise, chymosin, the carboxyl proteinase present in the calf's stomach, catalyses the partial hydrolysis of milk proteins and causes coagulation of the caseins, and renders them more susceptible to further degradation by the other proteinases. The more specific pancreatic-secreted proteinases pass through the duodenum and then catalyse the further hydrolysis of the pepsin-produced polypeptide fragments, so that rapid absorption from the lumen of the small intestine of di- and tripeptides and free α-amino acids can occur.

MAMMALIAN PROTEINASES

Pepsin, chymosin, trypsin, chymotrypsin, carboxypeptidases and elastase (Table 4.2) are synthesised and secreted by mammals as inactive enzyme precursors (zymogens). The biosynthesis of zymogens, in the stomach and pancreas, no doubt serves to protect the secretory organs themselves against destruction by the very same enzymes they are required to synthesise. Also present in the pancreas are a number of natural mammalian proteinase inhibitors, which further protect the organ from self-destruction by inadvertent formation of active proteinase. However, for catalysis the zymogens are specifically and rapidly activated by very limited hydrolysis to yield active enzyme (Table 4.2).

Table 4.2 Zymogens of digestive enzymes

Zymogen	Active enzyme	Site of synthesis
Pepsinogen (MW 42,000)	Pepsin (MW 35,500)	Stomach
Trypsinogen (MW 23,800)	Trypsin (MW 23,100)	Pancreas
Chymotrypsinogen (MW 25,000)	Chymotrypsin (MW 25,000)	Pancreas
Procarboxypetidase (MW 70,000)	Carboxypeptidase (MW 34,500)	Pancreas
Prochymosin (MW 36,500)	Chymosin (MW 30,700)	Calf stomach

CARBOXYL PROTEINASES

Pepsin (EC 3.4.23.1)

Understanding of the structure and function at the molecular level of the carboxyl proteinases, such as pepsin and chymosin, has been relatively slow but now important structural and mechanistic information is emerging. The enzymes are specifically inhibited by the peptide analogue, pepstatin. The inactive zymogen, pepsinogen, secreted in the stomach is a single polypeptide chain and composed of 371 α-amino acid residues. Various isopepsinogens are also believed to be synthesised. The zymogens contain three intrachain disulphide bonds and one phosphate O-substituted serine residue. Irreversible activation of pepsinogen and conversion to pepsin occurs spontaneously at low pH values as found in the stomach. For activation of porcine pepsinogen forty-four α-amino acids are removed from the N-terminal region of the zymogen to liberate Ile-45 as the new amino terminal residue of the pepsin. It is thought that the release of forty-four residues from pepsinogens takes place stepwise through first acid hydrolysis of the peptide bond between Leu-16 and Ile-17, to give rise to an intermediate active pepsin containing Ile-17 as the amino terminus (Fig. 4.1) Formation of the final porcine pepsin with Ile-45 at the amino terminus from the intermediate is believed to be a bimolecular reaction catalysed by the activated pepsinogen. However, conversion of all pepsinogen molecules to porcine pepsin can occur in less than 10 sec. For different animal species there is an extensive degree of homology of amino acid sequences for the activation peptides (residues 1 to 45) of the pepsinogens, and in both porcine pepsinogen and bovine pepsinogen residue 16 is Leu and residue 45 is either Ile or Val, respectively. Thus for both porcine and bovine pepsins the N-terminal residue is a hydrophobic amino acid.

Generally, pepsin has been described as a wide spectrum enzyme capable of catalysing the hydrolysis of a number of different kinds of peptide bonds. However, the peptide bonds of proteins consisting of the α-amino groups of aromatic amino acids and other hydrophobic amino acids are normally hydrolysed first, followed by the hydrolysis

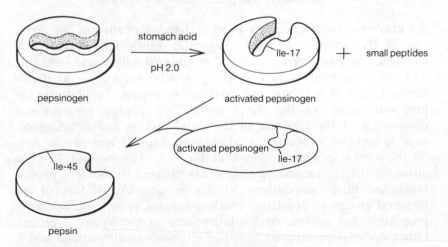

Fig. 4.1 Formation of pepsin from pepsinogen

of peptide bonds, composed of leucine, histidine, valine and alanine residues. A group of synthetic peptides of the type:

$$Z - His - \overset{\downarrow}{X} - Y - OMe$$

have been used to study the mode of action of pepsin. The residues X and Y of the sensitive bond (↓) are normally aromatic amino acids. Spectrophotometric methods can used to follow the hydrolysis of the susceptible bond when X = *p*-nitro-L-phenylalanine. Hexapeptides have also been recommended as test substrates for the assay of carboxyl proteinases:

$$Leu-Ser-Phe-NLe-Ala-Leu-Me,$$
$$\underset{NO_2}{|}$$

NLe = L-norleucine

The pH value for optimum enzymatic activity for natural substrates is between 2 and 3. Kinetic studies have indicated that the pK values of the active site residues of pepsin are approximately 2 and 5 which correspond to Asp-32 and Asp-215 in porcine pepsin.

During catalysis it is proposed that one of the carboxyl groups is protonated and the other is in the form of a carboxylate anion. A phosphate group attached to a serine residue in the pepsin molecule does not affect the enzymatic activity as the phosphate group can be removed without loss of activity. Pepsin also catalyses transpeptidation reactions, which result in the transfer of amino acid residues between peptides. Such transpeptidation reactions have been claimed to indicate that

$$Leu-Tyr-Leu + Enzyme \rightleftharpoons Leu-Enzyme + Tyr-Leu$$
$$Leu-Enzyme + Leu-Tyr-Leu \rightleftharpoons Leu-Leu-Tyr-Leu + Enzyme$$
$$Leu-Leu-Tyr-Leu \overset{pepsin}{\rightleftharpoons} Leu-Leu + Tyr-Leu$$

the enzyme-substrate complex is an acylated derivative of the active site of the enzyme. Pepstatin (Fig. 4.2) which is a hexapeptide analogue containing two residues of an unusual amino acid, 4-amino-3-hydroxy-6-methylheptanoic acid (generally known as a statine residue), acts as a competitive inhibitor of pepsin. To illustrate the proposed action of the statyl residue on pepsin, diagrammatic comparison of the structure of the statyl residue and a susceptible peptide bond of a protein placed between Asp-215 and pepsin–Asp-32 of porcine pepsin is shown in Fig. 4.3. The α- and β-carbon atoms of the central statine residue are claimed to mimic a peptide bond and bind competitively to the pepsins. Acetylation of the hydroxyl groups of pepstatin, which drastically reduces its inhibitive properties, has established the importance of the hydroxyl groups. Other carboxyl proteinases including chymosin, cathepsins D and E and mould proteinases from *Penicillium janthinellum* are inhibited by

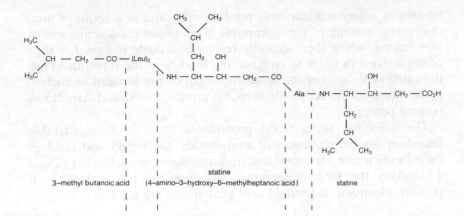

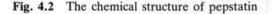

Fig. 4.2 The chemical structure of pepstatin

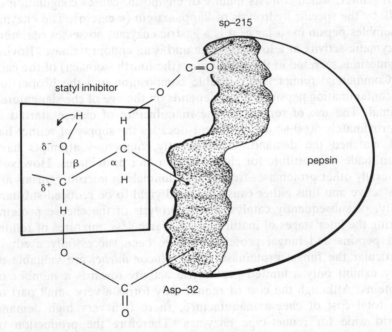

Fig. 4.3 Schematic diagram of interaction of the α- and β-carbon atoms of a statyl residue with pepsin

pepstatin, which is now used as a 'detective' inhibitor for the presence of the carboxyl proteinases.

From studies of the kinetic properties of porcine pepsin using a series of substrates containing Z–(Gly)$_n$–Phe–Phe when $n = 0$ to 4, it is concluded that porcine pepsin may accommodate and bind up to seven amino acid residues, adjacent to its active site. Such secondary binding of adjacent amino acid residues may arise as a result of first, the specific binding of the susceptible bond to the main active site of the enzyme, which then secondly results in a conformational change of the enzyme in order to enhance the binding of the substrate. Thus the susceptible bond of the substrate would be predisposed to nucleophilic attack by the active site carboxyl groups Asp-32 and Asp-215 of porcine pepsin.

Generally for all carboxyl proteinases there is a considerable homology for the sequences of amino acids: the amino acid residues close to the active site aspartates are homologous to each other (Table 4.6). Also the three-dimensional structures of the molecules of pepsins, chymosin and mould acid proteinases are similar.

Chymosin (EC 3.4.23.4)

Calf rennet, which consists mainly of chymosin, causes coagulation of milk by the specific hydrolysis of kappa-casein (κ-casein). The enzyme resembles pepsin in so far as it is a gastric enzyme, possesses optimum enzymatic activity at a low pH value and is an endoproteinase. Bovine chymosin is secreted in the abomasum (the fourth stomach) of the calf.

Commercial rennet is of variable composition and the proportion of contaminating pepsin present depends on the age of the slaughtered animal. The use of rennet for the manufacture of cheese started in approximately 5000 BC and in recent decades the supply of rennet has not matched the demand. Consequently, numerous attempts have been made to substitute for chymosin by other proteinases. However, generally other proteinases from plants, animals or microorganisms are too active and thus either cause the curd yield to be reduced substantially, or subsequently catalyse the hydrolysis of the cheese proteins during the later stages of maturation. Nevertheless, mixtures of rennet and pepsins and fungal proteinases have been successfully used: in particular the fungal proteinases from *Mucor miehei* are valuable as they exhibit only a limited proteolytic activity towards a number of proteins. Although the cost of rennet only forms a very small part of the total cost of cheese manufacture, there is a very high demand world wide for rennet-type enzymes. Therefore the production of chymosin by genetically modified microorganisms seems economically sound and superior to the costly isolation and testing needed for substitute enzymes from *Mucor spp*.

The coagulation of milk proteins catalysed by chymosin occurs in two stages. First, κ-casein which stabilises the casein micelles is hydrolysed very specifically by rennin: a Phe_{105}–Met_{106} peptide bond is cleaved and the original C-terminal macropeptide (residues 106–169) of κ-casein, which is negatively charged and contains an oligosaccharide, is liberated from the casein micelles. Secondly, when approximately 85 per cent of the κ-casein has been hydrolysed partially in this way the changed micelles coagulate.

The enzyme chymosin is a typical carboxyl proteinase: the enzyme contains two catalytic aspartic acid residues and is inhibited by pepstatin. However, unlike pepsin, chymosin is stable up to pH 6.5 (the approximate pH value of fresh milk), whereas pepsins are generally denatured and undergo self-digestion at pH 5.0. Calf chymosin is optimally active at pH 5.5 but inactive at pH values of 2.0 and 7.0. The bovine chymosin molecule consists of 323 amino acid residues and like pepsin it is secreted as an inactive zymogen, prochymosin (approximate MW 36,500). Active chymosin is formed by limited proteolysis and the release of forty-two residues from the amino terminal end of the zymogen. Asp-76 and Asp-261 of the enzyme are the catalytic residues that react with epoxides and diazo compounds, respectively. As with other carboxyl proteinases the two catalytic residues are located pointing towards a cleft within the enzyme. Additionally, a high degree of structural homology (Table 4.6) has been found between the carboxyl proteinases. Comparison with penicillopepsin (EC 3.4.23.6), from *Penicillium janthinellum* gives eighty-nine common sequences. Generally the molecules are bilobal with an extended hydrophobic interior. Of the carboxyl proteinases, chymosin is claimed to be the most specific enzyme (Table 4.3), but the comparability studies have been determined using the B-chain of insulin and not milk proteins as substrate. By the use of various short chain peptides as substrates for chymosin, it has been shown that the k_{cat}/K_m ratio of 2.5×10^3 (s^{-1} mm^{-1}) is greatest for a tridecapeptide (residues 98 to 111) derived from κ-casein:

–His–Pro–His–Pro–His–Leu–Ser–Phe–Met–Ala–Ile–Pro–Pro–Lys–

98   103   105 106   108   111

Table 4.3 Comparative specificity of some acid proteinases. Peptide bonds hydrolysed in the B-chain of insulin

Chymosin	Pepsin	*Mucor miehei*
	Asp–Glu	
	Glu–His	
Leu–Val	Leu–Val	
	Glu–Ala	Glu–Ala
	Ala–Leu	ALa–Leu
Leu–Tyr	Leu–Tyr	Leu–Tyr
Tyr–Leu	Tyr–Leu	
		Gly–Gly
	Gly–Phe	
Phe–Phe	Phe–Phe	Phe–Phe
Phe–Tyr	Phe–Tyr	Phe–Tyr

(Dalgleish 1982).

Table 4.4 The kinetic properties of chymosin

Substrate	K_m	k_{cat}	k_{cat}/K_m
	(mM)	(s⁻¹)	(s⁻¹ mM⁻¹)
Leu–Ser–Phe–Met–Ala–Ile	0.85	18.3	22
Leu–Ser–Phe–Met–Ala–Ile–Pro	0.7	38	55
Leu–Ser–Phe–Met–Ala–Ile–Pro–Pro	0.4	43	105
Ser–Phe–Met–Ala–Ile	8.5	0.33	0.04
Ser–Phe–Met–Ala–Ile–Pro	9.2	1.0	0.1
Ser–Phe–Met–Ala–Ile–Pro–Pro	3.2	0.75	0.2

(Dalgleish 1982).

Small tri- and tetrapeptides which contain a Phe–Met bond are not hydrolysed. Data for the catalytic efficiency of chymosin towards certain other peptides is shown in Table 4.4. The best substrates seem to contain hydrophobic amino acids at residues 103 and 108.

The repeating (His–Pro) sequence from residues 98 to 102 also seems to be important. Thus the binding of a large part of the substrate to the enzyme is considered to be necessary for the hydrolysis of the Phe–Met bond, which must also be accessible to the enzyme.

In milk it has been suggested that κ-casein molecules lie on the surface of the casein micelles and impart negative charges to prevent coagulation. The negative charge is due to the presence of a κ-casein oligosaccharide containing sialic acid, which is liberated as part of the C-terminal macropeptide (residues 106 to 169). Removal of the hydrophilic glycopeptide which contains N-acetylgalactosamine, galactose and sialic acid residues by cleavage of the Phe_{105}–Met_{106} bond creates a more hydrophobic micellar surface and reduction of the zeta-potential by from 5 to 7 mV such that coagulation of the casein micelles occurs (Dalgleish 1982).

For cheese manufacture, the milk clotting process which involves the aggregation of the casein micelles is coupled to a physical contraction of the curd, expulsion of water (syneresis) and further but very limited proteolysis of the caseins (Table 4.5). Most of commercial rennet constituents added to coagulate the milk caseins are soluble in the whey supernatant, although a small proportion of chymosin imbibed and adsorbed to the curd continues to slowly hydrolyse the α_{s1}- and β-caseins. However, as the catalytic efficiency of chymosin towards these caseins is 100 times less than its specific action towards the Phe–Met bond of κ-casein, only minimal proteolysis of the cheese curd occurs. Nevertheless, previous contamination of milk by microbial proteinases may also cause considerable proteolysis of the curd which in turn can cause the formation of bitter hydrophobic peptides from β-casein during maturation of cheese. The microbial proteinases and other enzymes can arise from psychotrophic bacteria which

Table 4.5 The action of chymosin on caseins; peptide bonds hydrolysed

α_{s1}-casein	β-casein
Phe$_{23}$–Phe*$_{24}$	Leu$_{139}$–Glu$_{140}$
Phe$_{24}$–Val$_{25}$*	
Phe$_{28}$–Pro$_{29}$	Leu$_{163}$–Ser$_{164}$
Leu$_{169}$–Gly$_{170}$	Ala$_{189}$–Phe$_{190}$*
Phe$_{150}$–Arg$_{151}$	Leu$_{192}$–Tyr$_{193}$*

* Primary site of enzymatic hydrolysis by chymosin
  (Dalgleish 1982).

multiply in fresh milk at temperatures greater than 4 °C. Additionally, in some instances the microbial proteinases are thermostable and survive ultra-high temperature processing (UHT) at 130 °C. The natural milk proteinases (proteinases I and II) produce γ-caseins by catalysing the limited hydrolysis of β-casein which may reduce curd yield and also result in texture defects in cheese.

Chymosin is also used for the manufacture of rennet casein from skim milk, where the κ-casein is partially hydrolysed and the casein micelles consequently destabilised. In the past, continuous processes have been used for the supply of rennet caseins to the plastics industry, but now there is an increasing use of rennet caseins by the food industry for the manufacture of new cheese-like products with various textures and flavour. While there has been a long-standing requirement for chymosin, more recently attempts have been made to use other proteinases and lipases to hasten the slow ripening processes which take place during the maturation of cheese. Nevertheless, such a development is only viable if a substantial decrease in the costs of production can be easily achieved alongside improvements in quality.

Cathepsin D (EC 3.4.23.5)

Cathepsins are generally thought of as intracellular proteinases contained within lysosomes. Like pepsin or chymosin, cathepsin D is a carboxyl proteinase. Although the action of cathepsin D to date has been of little interest to the food sciences, cathepsin D (approximate MW 42,000) is a major mammalian lysosomal proteinase and occurs in cartilage, kidney, liver, lung and muscle tissues of various animals (Barrett 1977). The enzyme is sensitive to the carboxyl proteinase inhibitors, such as pepstatin and diazo compounds. Cathepsin D is active over the pH range 3 to 5, but like pepsin is unstable in solution in the absence of substrate. However, in view of the low pH optima of 3.5, cathepsin D is unlikely to catalyse hydrolysis of muscle proteins

Table 4.6 Homologous sequences at the active sites of
carboxyl proteinases

Pepsin[†]	Ile–Val–Asp*–Thr–Gly–Thr–Ser–Leu
Penicillopepsin[†]	Ile–Ala–Asp*–Thr–Gly–Thr–Thr–Leu
Chymosin[‡]	Ile–Leu–Asp*–Thr–Gly–Thr–Ser–Lys
Cathepsin D[†]	Ile–Val–Asp*–(Thr,Gly,Thr,Ser)

* Active site residue required for catalysis.
([†] Barrett 1977. [‡] Flotman *et al.* 1979).

in post-mortem meat. Collagen, gelatin, serum albumin, myosin and casein are only slowly hydrolysed by cathepsin D. The enzymatic action of cathepsin D on the oxidised chain of insulin is similar to that of pepsin or chymosin: the most susceptible types of peptide bonds are Leu–Tyr, Tyr–Leu, Phe–Phe and Phe–Tyr as shown in Table 4.3. The amino acid sequences adjacent to one of the catalytic aspartate residues for cathepsin D, and other carboxyl proteinases are given in Table 4.6.

SERINE PROTEINASES

Many of the well known digestive enzymes together with some of cathepsins and microbial enzymes, possess an activated serine residue which acts as the catalytic site during proteolysis. The range of serine proteinases is listed in Table 4.7.

Trypsin (EC 3.4.21.4)

During digestion in mammals, the partially hydrolysed products present in the stomach stimulate the secretion of the hormone cholecystokinin, which increases pancreatic secretion of the proteinase zymogens trypsinogen, chymotrypsinogen, pro-elastase and procarboxypeptidases. Trypsinogen is a single polypeptide chain looped together by six disulphide bonds. The secreted trypsinogen is activated to form

Table 4.7 Serine proteinases

Trypsin, chymotrypsin
Thrombin, elastase
Subtilisin, plasmin
Cathepsins A, C and G
Rat skeletal muscle proteinases
Alkaline proteinase from *Aspergillus spp.*

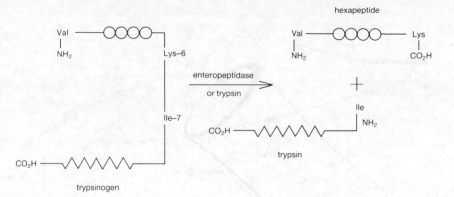

Fig. 4.4 Activation of trypsinogen

the enzyme trypsin through the catalytic action of the enzyme entero-
peptidase which is secreted by intestinal cells. The initial hydrolysis of
trypsinogen (Fig. 4.4) involves cleavage of the peptide bond Lys-
6→Ile-7 in trypsinogen, to release a hexapeptide. Ile-7 is the new
amino terminal group of active trypsin. Additional quantities of trypsin
are then formed by the action of trypsin itself on further quantities of
trypsinogen. In the presence of calcium ions, activation to form trypsin
is nearly 100 per cent, which is believed to be due to the stabilisation
of the active enzyme by Ca^{2+}. Also trypsin has a wider use as a digestive enzyme because it activates the formation of the other mammalian
pancreatic proteinases from their zymogens.

During digestion trypsin acts as a very specific endoproteinase, as
it catalyses only limited hydrolysis of food proteins. In proteinaceous
substrates only the peptide bonds on the C-terminal side of Lys or Arg
residues are hydrolysed by the enzyme. Recognition by trypsin of the
larger positively charged side chains of either Lys or Arg residues is
thought to reside in the structure of the enzyme molecule, where the
side chains fit into appropriate clefts or pockets (Fig. 4.5). For
formation of the enzyme–substrate complex the positively charged
amino groups of the Lys or Arg residues and the anion of Asp-189 of
trypsin interact by electrostatic attraction. The hydrogen atoms of the
glycyl groups of trypsin which line the pocket of the enzyme offer no
steric hindrance to either the lysyl or arginyl side chains of the
substrate. For the catalysed hydrolysis of the peptide bond on the C-
terminal side of the Lys or Arg residue protonation is facilitated by
the concerted action of the hydroxyl group of Ser-195, an imidazole
group of a His residue and the carboxyl group of an aspartic acid
residue: His-57 is believed to be responsible for the ionisation of the
hydroxyl group of Ser-195, which thus facilitates nucleophilic attack
at the carbonyl groups of the peptide bonds of the Lys or Arg residues.

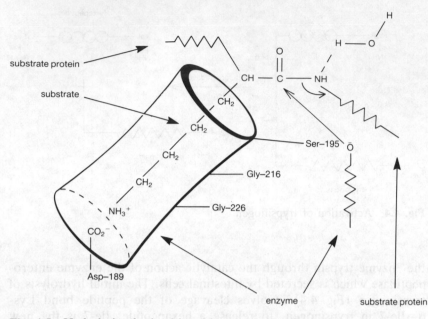

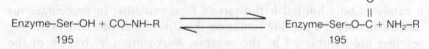

Fig. 4.5 Hydrolysis of a lysyl bond by trypsin Ser-195

An enzyme–substrate complex containing an acyl derivative of Ser-195 is believed to exist as an intermediate during the enzymatic-catalysed hydrolysis. The peptide (NH_2–R) contains the N-terminal amino acid, which previously formed the peptide bond on the N-terminal side to the susceptible Lys or Arg residues of the substrate:

$$\text{Enzyme–Ser–OH} + \text{CO–NH–R} \rightleftharpoons \text{Enzyme–Ser–O–}\overset{\displaystyle O}{\overset{\displaystyle \|}{C}} + NH_2\text{–R}$$
$$\quad\quad\quad 195 \quad\quad\quad\quad\quad\quad\quad\quad\quad\quad\quad\quad\quad\quad\quad\quad\quad 195$$

The esterified OH-group of Ser-195 of the enzyme–substrate complex is hydrolysed to release active trypsin and a peptide containing Lys or Arg in the C-terminal position.

Di-isopropylphosphofluoridate (DFP) is an inhibitor of trypsin and the other serine proteinases, chymotrypsin, elastase and microbial subtilisin, where again a serine residue is part of the active site of the enzyme. DFP forms a covalent derivative with the active site serine residues. Trypsin is also specifically inhibited by ovomucoid present in egg albumen and the soybean trypsin inhibitor. These proteinaceous inhibitors form stable enzyme–inhibitor complexes which are not readily hydrolysed to product and free enzymes.

Owing to the highly selective catalytic action of trypsin for hydrolysis of proteins at the C-terminal side of only Lys and Arg peptide bonds, the enzyme has proved extremely useful for structural studies of proteins where limited proteolysis is required to produce a small

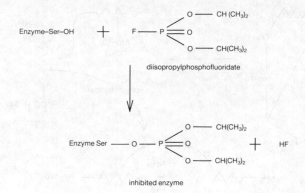

diisopropylphosphofluoridate

inhibited enzyme

number of large polypeptide fragments. The polypeptides are easily separated by either electrophoresis to produce tryptic peptide maps, or by chromatography for preparative purposes. Suitable synthetic test substrates for assay of trypsin include benzoyl-L-arginine methyl ester, tosyl-L-arginine methyl ester where the enzyme specifically acts as an esterase and various nitroanilide derivatives (Table 4.8).

Table 4.8 Nitroanilide substrates for assay of proteinases

Enzyme	Synthetic substrate
Trypsin	L-Lysine-4-nitroanilide
	N-α-Benzoyl-D,L-lysine-4-nitroanilide
	N-α-Benzoyl-D,L-arginine-4-nitroanilide
Chymotrypsin	L-Phenylalanine-4-nitroanilide
	L-Tyrosine-4-nitroanilide
Pepsin,chymosin and other proteinases	L-Leucine-4-nitroanilide
	L-Alanine-4-nitroanilide

Chymotrypsin and elastase (EC 3.4.21.1 and 3.4.21.36–37)

Chymotrypsinogen is activated to form π-chymotrypsin through the catalytic action of trypsin. The susceptible peptide bond of chymotrypsin is between Arg-15 and Ile-16: thus the activation of chymotrypsinogen depends on the highly specific catalysed hydrolysis by trypsin of a peptide bond on the C-terminal side of the Arg-15 residue. The further autodigestive action of π-chymotrypsin (Fig. 4.6) results in the formation of the more stable α-chymotrypsin. The residues Leu-13, Tyr-146 and Asn-148 are sites for autohydrolysis by π-chymotrypsin to yield the two dipeptides. The polypeptide parts of α-chymotrypsin are held together by five disulphide bonds.

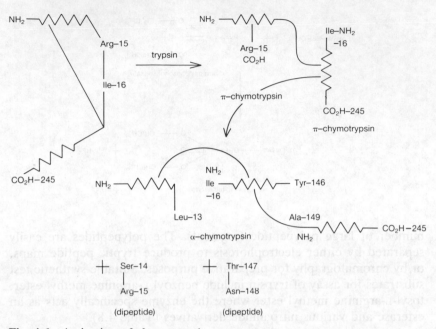

Fig. 4.6 Activation of chymotrypsinogen

For all serine proteinases, the mechanism of catalysis is similar. However, the various serine proteinases exhibit different specificities towards the peptide bonds of mainly the basic, the aromatic and the hydrophobic amino acids. Unlike trypsin, chymotrypsin catalyses the hydrolysis of the peptide bonds on the C-terminal side of mainly aromatic amino acids, whereas elastase catalyses the hydrolysis of peptide bonds mainly on the C-terminal side of hydrophobic amino acids. The different specificities of these enzymes are due to small variations in the molecular structure of the clefts or pockets of the different serine proteinases into which the side chains of the suscep-tible amino acids fit. In α-chymotrypsin and elastase the pocket residue, Ser-189, has been substituted for the Asp-189 of trypsin (Fig. 4.5), whereas in elastase the pocket residues, Gly-216 and Gly-226 of trypsin are substituted by the more bulky Val-216 and Thr-226 residues. Therefore for steric reasons the access of the bulky side chains of Lys, Arg and aromatic amino acids is prevented.

For trypsin, chymotrypsin and elastase the sequence of amino acid residues adjacent to the active site Ser-195 are identical:

Gly–Asp–Ser*–Gly–Gly–Pro

195

For studies of the kinetic properties of the serine proteinases a series of synthetic substrates which contain only one susceptible amide bond have proved useful. In particular, substrates which contain the susceptible residues of either Lys and Arg residues or Phe and Tyr are used for the assay of trypsin or chymotrypsin, respectively (Table 4.8). N-Substituted nitroanilides are commercially available for the assay of endo-type proteinases where the enzymatic activity is determined at 405 nm by following the release of 4-nitroaniline.

Through the use of both such test substances and the availability of specific avian and plant seed inhibitors, it is now possible quickly to detect the presence of serine proteinases in foods. Such enzymes (proteinases I and II) have been found in fresh bovine milk and are now known to be identical to the bovine blood serum enzymes thrombin and plasmin. In fresh milk these enzymes appear to be adsorbed to the casein micelles but they are generally denatured by pasteurisation.

Metalloproteinases

The carboxypeptidases, aminopeptidases and collagenases belong to a group of enzymes which contain divalent metal ions in their active sites (Table 4.9). The enzymes are inhibited by the chelating agent 1,10-phenanthroline, a potato inhibitor and glycyltyrosine.

Table 4.9 Metal-containing proteinases

Carboxypeptidases	Zn^{2+}
Collagenases Zn^{2+}	
Gly–Gly–dipeptidase	Zn^{2+}
Leu–aminopeptidase	Mn^{2+}
Prolidase	Mn^{2+}
Iminodipeptidase	Mn^{2+}
Thermolysin, Gelatinase	Zn^{2+}

Carboxypeptidases (EC 3.4.17)

Enzymatically active carboxypeptidases (MW 34,500) are formed by substantive catalytic action of trypsin on procarboxypeptidases (MW approximately 70,000). An active α-form of carboxypeptidase A consists of 307 amino acid residues arranged in helical and β-sheet structures. The carboxypeptidases contain one atom of zinc per mole,

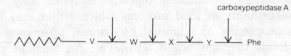

and catalyse the hydrolysis of peptide bonds in sequence at the C-terminal ends of proteins and polypeptides. Thus carboxypeptidases are classified as exopeptidases as they catalyse the hydrolysis of the terminal peptide bonds and release single amino acids from the substrate. There are two types of pancreatic carboxypeptidases, A and B (EC 3.4.17.1–2), which can also catalyse the hydrolysis of the esters like cinnamoyl L-α-phenyllactate. The carboxypeptidase A enzyme exhibits the greatest enzymatic activity towards the terminal peptide bonds derived from C-terminal aromatic and branched side chain amino acids. The binding of the substrate and enzyme have been deduced from studies of the enzyme–inhibitor complexes between carboxypeptidase and glycyltyrosine and spin-labelled substances (Makinen *et al.* 1985).

The substrate is held in position within a cleft of the enzyme through an ionic bond between the C-terminal carboxyl group of the substrate and Arg-145 of carboxypeptidase A (Fig. 4.7). The adjacent carbonyl group of the peptide bond is believed to be polarised by the Zn atom which is tetrahedrally coordinated to His-69, His-196, Glu-72 residues of the enzyme and a molecule of water. A mixed anhydride is believed to be formed by interaction with the carboxylate oxygen atom of Glu-270, which results in cleavage of the C–N bond to release the terminal amino acid bound to Arg-145. The metal hydroxide formed by loss of H^+ from the Zn-bound water molecule by nucleophilic attack hydrolyses the mixed anhydride to liberate the polypeptide with its new C-terminal amino acid residue. Pancreatic carboxypeptidase B, where the mode of action at the molecular level is likely to be similar, exhibits a greater enzymatic activity towards peptides which contain lysyl and arginyl residues. Whereas the plant carboxypeptidase enzymes are able to catalyse the release of proline residues from the C-terminal positions of peptides.

Because of the liberation during mammalian digestion of single amino acids, and preferentially the aromatic amino acids, by carboxypeptidase A, the enzyme catalyses the further hydrolysis of chymotrypsin-produced polypeptides to release some important essential amino acids for assimilation. Similarly, carboxypeptidase B has a special role for the liberation of arginine and the important essential basic amino acid, lysine, present in the C-terminal positions of trypsin-produced peptides. Thus the sequential actions of the serine proteinases and the carboxypeptidases results in the preferential liberation of some of the essential amino acids from ingested proteins and peptides.

In the laboratory, mammalian digestive enzymes may be used to assess the digestibility of food proteins which either may have been affected by processing or inhibited by natural proteinase inhibitors present in foods of plant origin. However, for such purposes it is important to use the enzymes sequentially in the order in which they

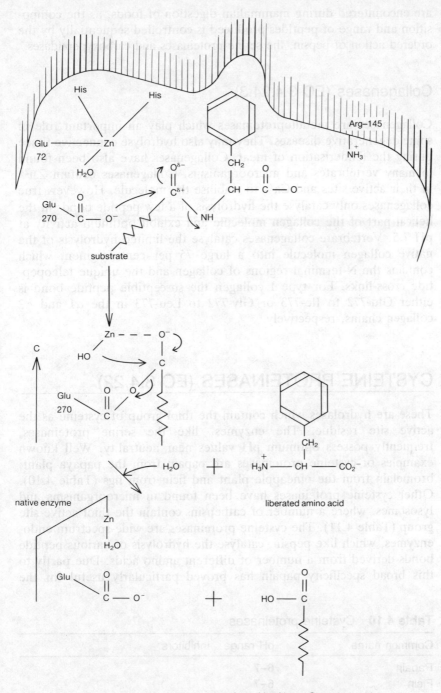

Fig. 4.7 Schematic diagram of metal ion assisted hydrolysis by carboxypeptidase (The mechanism is after Makinen *et al.* 1985)

are encountered during mammalian digestion of foods, as the composition and range of peptides produced is controlled sequentially by the ordered action of pepsin, the serine proteinases and carboxypeptidases.

Collagenases (EC 3.4.24.3)

Collagenases are metalloproteinases which play an important role in some degenerative diseases. They may also hydrolyse connective tissue during the tenderisation of meat. Collagenases have also been found in many vertebrates and microorganisms. Collagenases contain Zn^{2+} in their active sites and Ca^{2+} to stabilise the molecule. However, true collagenases only catalyse the hydrolysis of a few peptide bonds in the helical part of the collagen molecule and exhibit optimum activity at pH 7.5. Vertebrate collagenases catalyse the limited hydrolysis of the native collagen molecule into a large 75 per cent fragment which contains the N-terminal regions of collagen and the unique teleopeptide cross-links. For type I collagen the susceptible peptide bond is either Glu-772 to Ile-773 or Gly-772 to Leu-773 in the $\alpha1$ and $\alpha2$ collagen chains, respectively.

CYSTEINE PROTEINASES (EC 3.4.22)

These are hydrolases which contain the thiol group of cysteine as the active site residue. The enzymes, like the serine proteinases, frequently possess optimum pH values near neutrality. Well known examples of cysteine proteinases are papain from the papaya plant, bromelain from the pineapple plant and ficin from figs (Table 4.10). Other cysteine proteinases have been found in microorganisms and lysosomes, where a number of cathepsins contain the thiol active site group (Table 4.11). The cysteine proteinases are wide-spectrum endoenzymes, which like pepsin, catalyse the hydrolysis of various peptide bonds derived from a number of different amino acids. Due partly to this broad specificity papain has proved particularly useful for the

Table 4.10 Cysteine proteinases

Common name	pH range	Inhibitors
Papain	6–7	
Ficin	6–7	
Bromelain	6–7	
Cathepsin B, H, L, N and S	3–6	Sulphydryl reagents, and leupeptins

tenderisation of meat, where the meat can be impregnated with papain prior to cooking or infused prior to slaughter of cattle. Papain is particularly useful for the tenderisation of meat as it remains active up to 60 °C.

As a group of enzymes cysteine proteinases are inhibited by simple chemical reagents which react with the –SH group: these include Hg^{2+}, 4-chloromeruribenzoate, N-ethylmaleimide and iodoacetic acid. A covalent derivative of cysteine, S-carboxymethylcysteine, is formed by reaction of the active –SH group with iodoacetic acid in aqueous solution at pH values greater than 7.0 where the alkylation of the thiol group is irreversible.

$$Protein–SH + ICH_2CO_2H \rightarrow Protein–S–CH_2CO_2H + HI$$

For papain the active site sulphydryl group is at Cys-25, which lies close to a longitudinal cleft in the enzyme molecule. The mode of action of the enzyme is thought to be similar to that of the serine proteinases, but for cysteine proteinases the nucleophilic attack on the carbonyl carbon atom of the peptide is by a polarised –SH group. The second stage of the reaction involves hydrolysis of a thio-acyl intermediate. The sequences of amino acids adjacent to the active cysteine residues of papain, bromelain and ficin are almost identical:

Cys–Gly–Cys*$_{25}$–Trp, papain, ficin
Cys–Gly–Ala–Cys*–Trp, bromelain

Although many of the cathepsins are cysteine proteinases, frequently the enzymes isolated to date have been given arbitrary names (Table 4.11). Cathepsin B is widely distributed in mammalian tissues and is the most thoroughly investigated lysosomal cysteine proteinase. The enzyme shows optimum activity at pH 5.5 to 6.0 although it also catalyses the hydrolysis of collagen at pH 3.5. The

Table 4.11 Lysosomal cysteine proteinases

Common name	Molecular weight	pH range	Suitable test substrates
Cathepsin B	24,000–28,000	3.0–6.0	Synthetic arginine dipeptide derivatives, collagen, azocasein
Cathepsin H	26,000–28,000	3.0–6.0	Amino-terminal regions of peptides
Cathepsin L	21,000–24,000	3.0–6.0	Azocasein, cytosol proteins
Cathepsin N	18,000–20,000 also 36,000	3.5–6.0	Soluble collagen
Cathepsin S	14,000 and 19,000–25,000	3.6–6.0	Haemoglobin

(From Kirschke *et al.* 1980).

enzyme catalyses the hydrolysis of a number of different peptide bonds in the insulin B chain and is therefore of the wide-spectrum type. Cathepsins N and L also degrade insoluble collagen. A number of synthetic substrates have been used for differentiating the cathepsins, but there is a lack of sufficient substrates and inhibitors for each type of cysteine proteinase to permit the elucidation of the fundamental process which each cathepsin plays in catabolism of proteins in animals and particularly in muscle tissue.

ASSIMILATION OF AMINO ACIDS AND PEPTIDES

The final hydrolysis of small peptides is partly intracellular and may be completed in the cytosol of the intestinal cells. Hydrolysis of small oligopeptides may take place in the membrane of the cells of the intestinal microvilli to produce tri- and dipeptides. Some of the enzymes responsible for hydrolysis of small peptides, such as glycylglycine, and glycineleucine dipeptidases, prolinase and prolidase only catalyse the hydrolysis of certain peptides. Less specifically, leucine aminopeptidase (EC 3.4.11.1) catalyses the hydrolysis of the N-terminal peptide bond of all amino acids with the exception of lysine and arginine. However, because of the previous action of trypsin during mammalian digestion the latter two amino acids are unlikely to be found in N-terminal positions of small peptides.

The physiological process for amino acid transfer through the intestinal wall is extremely efficient and requires separate carrier systems for four groups of amino acids and small peptides (Table 4.12). Only small amounts of protein are excreted by mammals and even the amino acids of pepsin and the pancreatic enzymes, rich in sulphur amino acids, are also assimilated and thus recycled together with the degraded products of intestinal cells. The efficient absorption of amino acids requires a source of energy, generally provided by ATP where the transport processes are coupled to the transport of sodium ions.

Table 4.12 Transport groups for assimilation of amino acids

(1)		(2)	(3)	(4)
Met	Ala	Lys	Pro	Glu
Ile	Ser	Arg	OHPro	Asp
Leu	His	Orn		
Val	Tyr	Lys		
Thr	Phe			
Gly	Trp			

However, separate carrier systems for separate groups of amino acids help to ensure transport of a well balanced mixture of amino acids from the intestinal lumen to the portal vein. For example, a predominance of Glu and Asp arising from the digestion of plant proteins does not influence the rate of uptake of essential amino acids like methionine and lysine, due to the existence of independent transport mechanisms (Table 4.12). Di- and tripeptides are also transported across the intestinal wall and again a coupled transport of Na^+ is probably required. However, the relative quantitative importance of the absorption of peptides as opposed to amino acids is unknown.

PROTEINASE INHIBITORS

Of particular concern to both human and animal nutritionists is the presence of substantial amounts of proteinase inhibitors and phytohaemagglutinins in well known plant foods. Both these groups of substances can impair the mammalian digestion of proteins.

The proteinase inhibitors – which in many cases are themselves proteins – can be detected systematically by the addition of extracts of seeds, plants or microorganisms to solutions containing known amounts of test enzymes and substrates. For example, trypsin inhibitors can be detected by their inhibition of tryptic hydrolysis of synthetic substrates, like N-benzoyl-L-arginine ethyl ester. Also screening tests can be carried out on solidified substrate media by sequential application of strips of suspected inhibitory substances and enzymes. By such means zones of inhibitory substances can be detected by non-clearing of opaque media. The inhibitors can often be isolated by affinity chromatography using solid support-bound enzymes that are specific for which the inhibitory activity is being sought. For example, trypsin inhibitors can be isolated and purified by affinity chromatography using sepharose-bound trypsin. Improvements in the biological value of heat-treated protein foods is also indicative of the presence of antinutritional factors, which primarily inhibit the test animals' digestive enzymes. In the dormant seeds of legumes and cereals, proteinase inhibitors which inhibit the enzymes trypsin and chymotrypsin as well as other proteinases are found in quite large quantities as families of isohibitors. Proteinase inhibitors can account for from 0.2 to 2 per cent weight of soluble legume proteins. Trypsin inhibitors have been found in all species of the Leguminosae of which a large number also possess inhibitors of chymotrypsin. For cereals, proteinase inhibitors have been found in wheat, rye, barley, maize, rice and sorghum. Wheat, rye and triticale seeds contain at least four inhibitors in the embryo, and two similar but immunologically different inhibitors in the endosperm. Proteinase inhibitors have also been found in the leaves of plants, like the potato and tomato. Most proteinase inhibitors from plants inhibit trypsin, although others can simultaneously inhibit other serine proteinases, such as chymotrypsin or elastase. The precise biological role of proteinase inhibitors in plants is unknown, although clearly they can impede digestion of the main seed proteins by mammals or insects. Proteinase inhibitors are also found in many animal tissues which include blood plasma and the pancreas: thus the pancreas is afforded protection by its own proteinase inhibitors against inadvertent activation of the zymogens, trypsinogen, chymotrypsinogen and procarboxypeptidase. The α1-trypsin inhibitor of human plasma also inhibits chymotrypsin and elastase. The role of such inhibitors in animals seems clearly to be the protection of the tissues against digestion by the species natural occurring enzymes. The presence of a trypsin inhibitor, ovomucoid, in egg albumen has been known for a long time. Together with other more recently discovered egg albumen cysteine proteinase inhibitors the presence of ovomucoid affords one means by which the egg embryo can be protected against attack by proliferating microorganisms. Significant amounts of the proteinase inhibitor of bovine blood serum have also been found in milk.

Owing to the presence, particularly in plants, of significant amounts of proteinase inhibitors, considerable quantities of these substances are consumed by man and other animals. In some instances infant foods containing soybean have been found to possess residual trypsin inhibitor activity. Raw soybean meal or purified trypsin inhibitors can cause enlargement of the pancreas together with overstimulation of the secretion of pancreatic enzymes, inhibition of growth and a loss of metabolisable energy. The proteinase inhibitors, by means of a feedback mechanism, seem to stimulate the pancreas to synthesise greater amounts of trypsin and chymotrypsin. However, heating of legume flours and soybean meal can improve the nutritional value to produce a higher quality protein supplement. Nevertheless, in some legumes trypsin inhibitor activity can be detected after 1 hour at 100 °C. Alternatively, the proteinase inhibitors can be removed by aqueous extraction. Thiol reagents have been shown (Friedman et al. 1982) to enhance the inactivation of trypsin inhibitors of soybean at lower temperatures: such increased susceptibility to heat denaturation may be caused by cleavage of the disulphide bonds present in the trypsin inhibitors. Also the trypsin inhibitor from kintoki beans (Phaseolus vulgaris) which is very stable to heat at pH 5 to pH 7 can be completely destabilised to heat by stoichiometric quantities of other proteins like serum albumin, gelatin or cytochrome-c.

Proteinase inhibitors are best classified by the type of enzyme which is inhibited. Not surprisingly it has been found that individual inhibitors only inhibit a single type of proteinase. For example, inhibitors for serine proteinases cannot inhibit cysteine, acid proteinases or metalloproteinases. However, trypsin inhibitors may block the action of other serine proteinases, such as chymotrypsin or elastase. Only the α2-macroglobulins of blood plasma show a general inhibitory property to all proteinases, where such action is thought to be due to the enzyme being trapped within the large macroglobulin (MW 720,000) after very limited hydrolysis of a small number of susceptible macro-globulin peptide bonds. The most widely studied group of proteinase inhibitors are for the serine proteinases.

Serine proteinase inhibitors

The serine proteinase inhibitors are of two distinct types, which are classified as either Kunitz inhibitors, or the Bowman–Birk inhibitors. The Bowman–Birk inhibitors are uniquely held together through seven disulphide bonds to form a compact symmetrical molecule, whereas the Kunitz inhibitors possess a more flexible molecular structure with only two disulphide bonds per molecule. In some cases the serine proteinase inhibitors are able to inhibit either trypsin alone, both trypsin and chymotrysin or even three different serine proteinases. Therefore such inhibitors are described as single-headed, double-headed or triple-headed and contain separate inhibitory sites (domains), specific for each serine proteinase. The inhibition of proteinases is competitive, and independent for the different enzymes. The inhibitors from a large number of legumes can inhibit bovine trypsin stoichiometrically at 1 : 1 molar ratio, but in some cases (such as for navy beans) 2 moles of trypsin are inhibited per mole of inhibitor. Multiheadedness in inhibitors generally arises from duplication of the active inhibitor sites within a protein molecule, as shown in Fig. 4.8. where active site A is responsible for the inhibition of trypsin, while active site B inhibits chymotrypsin. Triple domains have been found

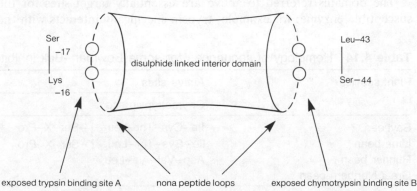

Fig. 4.8 Schematic diagram of the active site domains of Bowman–Birk soybean inhibitor

Table 4.13 Amino acid sequences of the five reactive sites of
Japanese quail ovoinhibitor[†]

Reactive site	Amino acid sequence	Enzyme potentially inhibited
1	... Val–Ala–Cys–Pro–Arg ↓ –Asn– Met–Lys–Pro–Val–Cys ...	Trypsin
2	... Val–Ala–Cys–Pro–Arg ↓ –Asn– Leu–Lys–Pro–Val–Cys ...	Trypsin
3	... Ala–Ala–Cys–Pro–Tyr–Ile–Leu– His–Glu–Ile–Cys ...	Chymotrypsin–elastase
4	... Met–Ala–Cys–Thr–Met–Ile–Tyr– Asp–Pro–Val–Cys ...	Chymotrypsin–elastase
5	... Pro–Val–Cys–Thr–Met–Glu–Tyr– Ile–Pro–His–Cys ...	Chymotrypsin–elastase

([†] Adapted from Laskowski and Kato 1980).
↓ indicates the susceptible bond.

in ovomucoids obtained from duck egg albumen where 2 moles of
trypsin and 1 mole of chymotrypsin per mole of inhibitor are inhibited
simultaneously. The ovoinhibitor from Japanese quail egg albumen
possesses six separate domains for the inhibition of trypsin, chymotrypsin and elastase (Table 4.13).

Each of the domains for the avian ovoinhibitor which are composed
of nonapeptide loops is enclosed within cystine residues. There is a
considerable degree of amino acid sequence homology between the
inhibitory active sites. Sequence homology is also found in other
groups of inhibitors, which can be further classified by the nature of
the active inhibitory site of the proteinase inhibitor (Table 4.14). A
very small number of dipeptide groups have been shown to be
important for inhibition for a large number of plant inhibitors (Table
4.15).

The domains referred to above are essentially target sites for the
susceptible enzyme: for example, trypsin specifically interacts with the

Table 4.14 Homology of sequences for some Bowman–Birk inhibitors[†]

Plant species	Active sites
	Chymotrypsin site
Soybean	Ile–Cys–Thr–Leu$_{55}$ ↓ –Ser–X–Pro
Lima bean	Ile–Cys–Thr–Leu$_{55}$ ↓ –Ser–X–Pro
Runner bean	Asp–Val–Ala–Leu
Great Northern bean	

([†] From Sgarbieri and Whitaker 1982).
↓ indicates the susceptible bond.

Table 4.15 Active site dipeptide units of plant proteinase inhibitors

Plant species	Enzyme inhibited	Active site group
Wheat	Trypsin	Arg–Ala
Soybean	Trypsin	Arg–Ala
Maize	Trypsin	Arg–Leu
Soybean	Trypsin	Lys–Ser
Lima bean	Trypsin	Lys–Ser
Potato	Trypsin	Lys–Ser
Soybean	Chymotrypsin	Leu–Ser
Potato	Chymotrypsin	Leu–Val
Potato	Chymotrypsin	Lys–Ser
Potato	Chymotrypsin	Leu–Asp
Potato	Chymotrypsin	Met–Asp
Soybean	Elastase	Ala–Ser
Garden bean	Elastase	Ala–Ser

(With permission from Richardson 1981).

Lys or Arg residues exposed on the surfaces of the inhibitor molecules (Fig. 4.9). Likewise soybean Bowman–Birk inhibitor possesses an exposed Ser–Leu (Fig. 4.8) peptide bond for reaction with chymotrypsin. The overall reaction between enzyme and inhibitor can be represented by

$$E + I \rightleftharpoons EI$$

which does not rapidly proceed to hydrolysis of the inhibitor. Indeed an equilibrium mixture is obtained where the mass ratio of hydrolysed inhibitor to native inhibitor is close to unity. Thus, proteinase inhibitors exist in two forms (I, EI) in the presence of target enzyme. Such a facile interaction of inhibitor and target enzyme, which depends on the dynamic formation and reversible dissociation of the enzyme–inhibitor complex, explains first, why native inhibitors can still

Trypsin site

Cys–Thr–Lys_{16} ↓ –Ser–X–Pro
Cys–Thr–Lys_{26} ↓ –Ser–X–Pro
Ile–Tyr–Lys ↓ –Ser–X–Pro
Cys–Thr–Arg_{55} ↓ –Ser–X–Pro

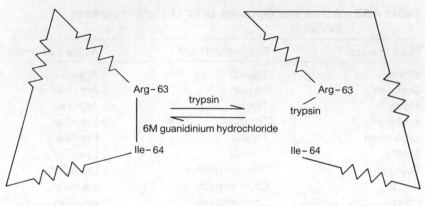

Fig. 4.9 Partial proteolysis of a soybean Kunitz-type inhibitor

be recovered after treatment of the enzyme–inhibitor complex with denaturing agents, and secondly, how a susceptible site residue, such as Arg-63, can be replaced chemically by other target residues and still regenerate active inhibitors. For example replacement of Arg-63 by tryptophan, followed by reversion with the denaturing agent, converts the Kunitz trypsin inhibitor to a chymotrypsin inhibitor. However, the molecular events taking place during such reactions are not fully understood and it is not known why the inhibitors are not just excellent substrates.

Many other inhibitor families for serine proteinases are known (Laskowski and Kato 1980). An inhibitor from corn (Mahoney *et al.* 1984) has been shown to contain a unique reactive site sequence consisting of four proline residues:

$$Pro–Arg–Pro–Arg*_{36}–Leu–Pro–Trp–Pro$$

In such a sequence the imino acid residues must restrict the flexibility of the susceptible domain region of the corn inhibitor and therefore predispose the known target Arg–Leu bond to a favourable position for association with trypsin. Additionally the paired proline residues, on either side of the target Arg–Leu bond impart two 180 ° turns on either side of the hydrolysed bond which restrict the dissociation of the enzyme–corn inhibitor complex.

Aldehyde peptides which inhibit papain, trypsin, chymotrypsin, elastase and cathepsins have been found in culture filtrates of *Streptomyces spp.*: these have been designated antipain, chymostatin and elastinal (Umezawa and Aoyagi 1977) but their use does not permit an unambiguous distinction between the different cathepsins.

Cysteine proteinase inhibitors

Protein inhibitors of the cysteine proteinase group of enzymes have received less attention than the protein inhibitors of the serine proteinases. The specific protein inhibitors of cysteine proteinases have been found in pineapple, egg white and mammalian skin. These inhibitors are active against papain, ficin, bromelain and cathepsin B. Two forms of the chicken egg albumen cysteine proteinase inhibitor have been isolated which are immunologically identical (Anastasi *et al.* 1983). These inhibitors in view of their action on cysteine proteinases have been renamed cystatins, which are active against a number of proteinases including the cathepsins (Table 4.16). Cysteine proteinease inhibitors, in addition to human α2-macroglobulin have also been reported to be present in human plasma.

Table 4.16 Inhibition of proteinases by egg albumen cystatin

Common name	K_i value (m)
Papain	8×10^{-11}
Cathepsin B	8×10^{-10}
Cathepsin H	2×10^{-8}
Cathepsin L	3×10^{-12}

(Anastasi *et al.* 1983).

Recently a class of unusual small peptides, which contain an important aldehyde group (Umezawa and Aoyagi 1977), have proved very useful inhibitors for cysteine proteinases. Their action is typified by leupeptins which are secreted by some *Streptomyces spp.* Leupeptin is a group name for a series of peptides which contain the aldehyde argininal in the C-terminal position.

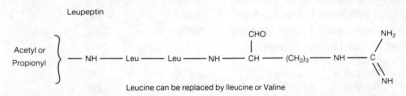

Leupeptin

Leucine can be replaced by Ileucine or Valine

Although leupeptins are frequently used to test for the presence of cysteine proteinases, they also inhibit some serine proteinases including trypsin. The aldehyde group of the inhibitor is essential for inhibitory activity which arises from the formation of a hemithioacetal derivative in the enzyme–inhibitor complex. The leupeptins seem to have low toxicity and exist in solution mainly in hydrated and cyclic forms.

PHYTOHAEMAGGLUTININS

Ingested phytohaemagglutinins, sometimes known as lectins, cause the clumping of mainly red blood cells and sometimes leucocytes. In some instances outbreaks of food poisoning have been attributed to the agglutination action of lectins (Bender 1983) and therefore these substances are of special interest. The plant lectins, often called phytolectins, are generally glycoproteins which contain approximately 5 per cent of covalently-bound carbohydrate. Lectins are proteins of non-immunoglobulin nature capable of specific recognition and reversible binding to carbohydrate moieties of complex carbohydrates without altering the covalent structure of any of the recognised glycosyl ligands. In the Leguminosae over 600 species contain lectins which may represent from 2 to 10 per cent of the total legume seed protein. Various cultivars are believed to contain several isolectins (Table 4.17). The lima bean lectins agglutinate specifically blood group A cells, whereas lectins of *Phaseolus vulgaris* varieties react unspecifically with human erythrocytes of all blood groups. Assays for lectins are carried out on trypsin-treated erythrocytes. The lectins of some seeds are also mitogenic, which is determined by their ability to stimulate *in vitro* DNA synthesis of mouse spleen lymphocytes. Lectins

Table 4.17   Lectin content of a number of legumes[†]

Name	HU[‡] per gram (dry weight)	Removed after soaking in water 18 h (%)
Red lentils (*Lens esculenta*)	7700	22
Green lentils (*Lens esculenta*)	1800	19
Garden peas (*Pisum sativum*)	5100	65
Yellow split peas (*Lens culinaris*)	1600	11
Green split peas (*Lens culinaris*)	1000	11
Black eye beans (*Vigna sinensis*)	1000	100
Red kidney beans (*Phaseolus vulgaris*):		
Sample 1	53,000	66
Sample 2	44,000	29
Sample 3	37,000	22
White kidney beans (*Phaseolus vulgaris*):		
Sample 1	43,500	36
Sample 2	17,000	18
Rose coco beans (*Phaseolus vulgaris*)	39,000	18

([†] With permission from Bender 1983).

[‡] HU = haemagglutinin unit.

present in some potato cultivars have been reported not to be activated after cooking for 45 min. Bender (1983) has shown that the agglutination activity can be reduced substantially for kidney beans by soaking in water or by heat-treatment at 100 °C. However, heating at lower temperatures of 70 °C and 80 °C enhanced the agglutination activity and in one instance by a factor of seven. Consequently it is clear that the ingestion of improperly cooked, as well as fresh, grains and pulses may result in food poisoning. Nachbar and Oppenheimer (1980) found lectin-like activity in seeds from pomegranates, grapes, blackberries, tomato and cucumber and claimed that 30 per cent of fresh foods are able to aggregate erythrocytes. Lectins have also been detected in preparations of wheat gluten solubilised in dimethyl sulphoxide.

Biochemical studies have shown that red kidney bean lectin can be inhibited by oligosaccharides isolated from erythrocytes after proteolysis or by a chemically synthesised trisaccharide (Sgarbieri and Whitaker 1982). Therefore haemagglutination is believed to be due to an interaction with small oligosaccharides present in cell wall glycoproteins and lectins are now often classified by their ability to bind different carbohydrates (Table 4.18). Pea seed lectins belong to a group which includes concanavalin (from *Canavalia ensiformis*), lentil and broad bean lectins which all bind to mannose and glucose residues.

Table 4.18 Properties of food lectins

Name	Carbohydrate binding residue[†]	Mitogen
Broad bean (*Vicia foba*)	D-Mann, D-Glc	+
Castor bean (*Ricinus communis*)	D-Gal	+
Kidney bean (*Phaseolus vulgaris*)	NANA	+
Lentil (*Lens culinaris*)	D-Mann, D-Glc	+
Lima bean (*Phaseolus limensis*)	D-Gal NAc	+
Pea (*Pisum sativum*)	D-Mann, D-Glc	+
Potato (*Solanum tuberosum*)	GlcNAc	—
Soybean (*Glycine max*)	D-GalNAc	—
Wheat (*Triticum vulgaris*)	GlcNAc	—

[†] GalNAc = 2,N-acetygalactosamine; GlcNAc = 2,N-acetylglucosamine; NANA = N-acetyneuraminic acid.

The lectins display affinities for carbohydrate residues that occur either as single monosaccharides or as segments of residues of simple and complex carbohydrates.

The specific affinity of lectins for carbohydrates has been exploited for their isolation and purification: glucose-binding lectins can be obtained quickly by saccharide-affinity chromatography using Sephadex G–50 and 0.2 M glucose to displace the adsorbed lectins. Alternatively, glycoproteins and oligosaccharides, can be fractionated through the use of solid support bound lectins.

The molecules of all lectins seem to be multimeric, with pea, lentil and broad bean lectins having a dimeric structure with a molecular weight of approximately 25,000. Concanavalin (MW 104,000) has a tetrameric structure and a similar structure has been claimed for kidney bean lectins. All lectins are metalloproteins and each subunit contains Ca^{2+} and Mn^{2+} binding sites which are essential for carbohydrate binding and mitogenic activity. For the concanavalin subunits (approximate MW 25,000) there are both two separate metal-binding sites for Mn^{2+} and Ca^{2+}, and a hydrophobic pocket as well as a separate binding site for carbohydrate residues. Although pea, lentil and broad bean lectins are smaller two-chain molecules, there are extensive homologues of amino acid sequences for metal-binding sites and the hydrophobic cavity for these lectins and the concanavalin subunit.

The red kidney bean lectin contains two different subunits which can combine to form five different non-covalent tetramers with various functions. In animals, lectins have been found in chicken liver and muscle, but their role is obscure.

PEPTIDE SYNTHESIS WITH PROTEINASES

Proteinases, as typical catalysts are capable of increasing the rates of both the hydrolytic and synthetic reactions. Papain has been used to produce a plastein by catalysing the resynthesis of peptide bonds. Experimentally, synthesis of product can be enhanced by increasing either the concentration of free amino acids (a mass action effect), changing the pH value, or by changing the composition of the solvent. For the food ingredient supply industry peptide biosynthesis may prove eventually useful for the synthesis of small peptides which can be used as 'high value' flavour enhancers, sweeteners, emulsifiers or texture-modifying agents or carriers of essential nutrients. To date it is known that biosynthesis of the sweetener aspartame, has benefited from the use of thermolysin, which permits the specific synthesis of an α-aspartyl phenylalanine dipeptide.

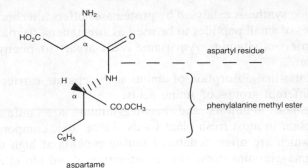

aspartame

KEY FACTS

1. Proteinase enzymes are classified, based on the chemical nature of their active site residues, as serine, cysteine, carboxyl and metalloproteinases.

2. Mammalian proteinases are synthesised as inactive zymogens. Active enzymes are formed by limited proteolysis of the zymogens.

3. The carboxyl proteinases pepsin, chymosin, cathepsins D and E contain two aspartic acid residues in the active site. These enzymes are inhibited by the substrate analogue pepstatin. All cathepsins are proteinases with low pH optima contained within lysozomes.

4. Chymosin destabilises casein micelles by catalysing the hydrolysis of a Phe_{105}–Met_{106} bond of κ-casein. When 85 per cent of κ-casein has been hydrolysed at the Phe–Met bond the casein micelles coagulate.

5. Trypsin catalyses only the hydrolysis of peptide bonds on the C-terminal side of Lys and Arg residues.

6. The serine proteinases contain a pocket for the substrate side chain residues adjacent to susceptible bonds. The hydroxyl group of a serine residue catalyses hydrolysis. Serine proteinases are inhibited by DFP.

7. Metalloproteinases contain Zn^{2+} or Mn^{2+} in the active site of the enzymes. The carboxypeptidases are endopeptidases which remove single amino acids sequentially from the C-terminii of proteins.

8. The sequential action in mammals of trypsin, chymotrypsin and carboxypeptidases rapidly liberates the essential amino acids, Lys, Phe, Tyr, Trp.

9. True collagenases contain Zn^{2+} and catalyse the hydrolysis of a few peptide bonds in the helical part of collagen. Collagenases enhance the tenderisation of meat.

10. Plant proteinases and many cathepsins are often of the cysteine type. The cysteine proteinase inhibitors of egg albumen are now called cystatins.

11.   Peptide synthesis catalysed by proteinases offers a technology for biosynthesis of small peptides to be used as sweeteners, flavour enhancers or carriers of vitamins. Aspartame is α-L-aspartyl-L-phenylalanine methyl ester.

12.   For intestinal absorption of amino acids separate carrier systems exist for different groups of amino acids.

13.   Proteinase inhibitors and haemagglutinins are antinutritional factors present in most fresh plant foods. These toxic components are proteins, which are often denatured during cooking at high temperatures. Haemagglutinins cause the agglutination of red blood cells.

REFERENCES

Anastasi, A., Brown, M. A., Kembhari, A. A. and others (1983) 'Cystatin, a protein inhibitor of cysteine proteinases', *Biochem. J.*, **211**, 129–38.

Barrett, A. J. (1977) 'Cathepsin D and other carboxyl proteinases', in *Proteinases in Mammalian Cells and Tissues*, (ed. Barrett, A. J.), of Research Monographs in Cell and Tissue Physiology, vol. 2 (ed. Dingle, J. T.). North Holland Publishing Company, Amsterdam.

Bender, A. E. (1983) 'Haemagglutinins (lectins) in beans', *Food Chem.*, **11**, 309–20.

Dalgleish, D. G. (1982) 'Enzymatic coagulation of milk' in *Developments in Dairy Chemistry* 1. *Proteins* (ed. Fox, P. F.). Applied Science Publishers, London.

Flotman, B., Pedersen, V. B., Kauffman, D. and Wybrandt, G. (1979) 'The primary structure of calf chymosin', *J. Biol. Chem.* **254**, 8447–56.

Friedman, M., Grosjean, O. and Zahnley, J. C. (1982) 'Inactivation of soya bean trypsin inhibitors by thiols', *J. Sci. Food Agric.*, **33**, 165–72.

Kirschke, H., Langer, J., Riemann, S., Wiederanders, B., Ansorge, S. and Bohley, P. (1980) 'Lysosomal cysteine proteinases', in *Protein Degradation in Health and Disease*, CIBA Foundation Symposium 75. Excerpta Medica, Amsterdam, Oxford and New York.

Laskowski, M. and. Kato, I. (1980) 'Protein inhibitors of proteinases', *Ann. Rev. Biochem.*, **49**, 593–626.

Mahoney, W. C., Hermodson, M. A., Jones, B., Power, D. D., Corfman, R. S. and Reeck, G. G. (1984) 'Amino acid sequence and secondary structural analysis of the corn inhibitor of trypsin and activated Hageman factor', *J. Biol. Chem.*, **259**, 8412–16.

Makinen, M., Gregg, G. B. and Kang, S. (1985) 'Structure and mechanism of carboxypeptidase A', in *Advances in Inorganic Biochemistry*, vol. 6 (eds. Eichhorn, G. L. and Marzilli, L. G.). Elsevier Science Publishers, New York.

Nachbar, M. S. and Oppenheimer, J. D. (1980) 'Lectins in the United States diet: a survey of lectins in commonly consumed foods and a review of the literature', *Am. J. Clin. Nutr.*, **33**, 2338–45.

Richardson, M. (1981) 'Protein inhibitors of enzymes', *Food Chem.*, **6**, 235–53.

Sgarbieri, V. C. and Whitaker, J. R. (1982) 'Physical, chemical and nutritional properties of common bean (*Phaseolus*) proteins', *Adv. in Food Res.*, **28**, 93–166.

Umezawa, H. and Aoyagi, T. (1977) 'Activities of proteinase inhibitors of microbial origin', in *Proteinases in Mammalian Cells and Tissues*, vol. 2 (ed. Barrett, A. J.), of Research Monographs in Cell and Tissue Physiology (ed. Dingle, J. T.). North Holland Publishing Company, Amsterdam.

ADDITIONAL READING

Finley, J. W., and Schwass, D. E. (1983) 'Xenobiotics in foods and feeds', ACS Symposium series 234. American Chemical Society, Washington DC.

Laskowski, M. and Kato, I. (1980) 'Protein inhibitors of proteinases', *Ann. Rev. Biochem.*, **49**, 593–626.

Liener, I. E. (1980) *Toxic Constituents of Plant Foodstuffs*, 2nd edn. Academic Press, New York.

Neuberger, A. and Jukes, T. H. (1979) 'Biochemistry of nutrition' 1. *International Revue of Biochemistry*, vol. 27. University Park Press, Baltimore.

Sharon, N. (1977) Lectins. *Sci. American*, **236**, no. 6 108–119.

Vonk, H. J. and Western, J. R. H. (1984) *Comparative Biochemistry and Physiology of Enzymatic Digestion*. Academic Press, London.

Walstra, P. and Jenness, R. (1984) *Dairy Chemistry and Physics*. John Wiley and Sons, New York.

CHAPTER 5

Molecular structure and functional properties of food proteins

The protein constituents of foods also provide in addition to nutritive value a desirable textural quality. Meat is the example, *par excellence*, of the influence of the primary structure of proteins on the texture of a food. Meat, as animal muscle, is a fibrous material made up of a carefully aligned assembly of mainly fibrillar proteins interspersed by water and soluble salts and enzymes. Fresh meat contains approximately 75 per cent water with the fibrillar structure representing approximately 70 per cent of the volume of lean meat.

Various functional properties of meat are of concern to the food industry. Toughness in meat is not wanted; highly desirable meat is tender, has a high water-holding capacity and thus retains water to maintain juiciness. In further processed products the desirable separate small chunks of meat must maintain their integral structure through the small but significant binding strength of the individual fibrillar components. In comminuted products such as sausages, burgers and re-formed steaks the texture is also influenced by added fat, water and included air.

MEAT PROTEINS

The myofibrillar structure of meat

Muscle consists of a large number of individual fibres: each fibre is a multinucleated single muscle cell and contains the myoglobin, mitochondria and sarcoplasmic reticulum – the latter being analogous to the endoplasmic reticulum of other animal cells. Red muscles are slow acting, while white muscles are fast acting but are easily fatigued. The colour depends on the oxygen-binding haem protein myoglobin, which in horse muscle is approximately 0.7 per cent weight but can be as high as 5.8 per cent in whales and seals where there is a greater need to

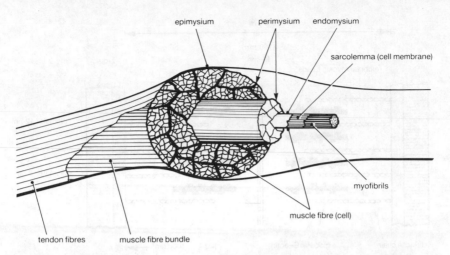

Fig. 5.1 Diagram of the structure of muscle (reproduced with permission
from Winger 1979)

store oxygen. As shown in Fig. 5.1 the fibres (length 3–4 cm) traverse
the whole length of the muscle. Each bundle of fibres is surrounded
by a sheath of connective tissue, the perimysium. Groups of bundles
of fibres are surrounded by the outer connective tissue sheath, the
epimysium.

Each fibre consists of parallel bundles of myofibrils. A fibre with
a diameter of 100 μm could contain up to 10^3 myofibrils each with a
diameter of approximately 1 μm. The main fundamental unit of meat
is the myofibrillar sarcomere which contains the two major muscle
proteins, actin and myosin. These proteins represent approximately 65
per cent of the total dry mass of the sarcomere. The sarcomere consists
of a series of longitudinal filaments of actin and myosin (Fig. 5.2). The
filaments are in register and are therefore seen as banded structures
in longitudinal sections. Myosin constitutes from 50 to 55 per cent of
the myofibrillar protein while actin represents from 15 to 30 per cent.
Six actin filaments surround each thick myosin filament in hexagonal
array.

The myosin molecules, either side of the M-line are packed in a
parallel form. Myosin is a double-headed molecule (Fig. 5.3). The
asymmetric molecule of myosin (MW approximately 500,000) consists
of two heavy chains (MW approximately 200,000) and two pairs of
light chains (MW 15,000 to 27,000). Myosin is a unique protein which
combines both a structural and an enzymatic property. Knowledge of
the molecular structure has been assembled from information gained
for the fragments produced during limited proteolysis with trypsin and
papain. The fibrous end of the molecule has a rod-like tail, starting
with the C-terminals of the polypeptide in the form of a coiled coil of
α-helices composed of heptapeptide repeats. The amino-terminal end

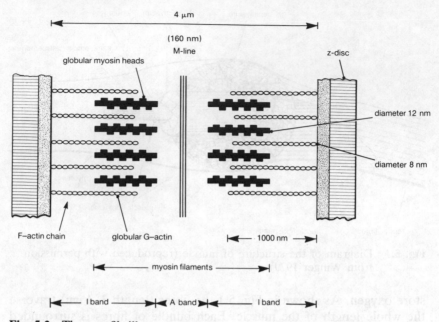

Fig. 5.2   The myofibrillar sarcomere

of the heavy chains is globular and is associated with the two non-covalently bound pairs of light chains in the double-head structures. The enzymatic property of myosin which brings about the hydrolysis of ATP (an ATPase) is associated with the one pair of light chains of myosin which are located in the globular head of the molecule. In the myosin filaments the globular heads of each molecule, are shown as protuberances which occur on the outer surface of the filaments at axial distances of 14.3 nm in a helical manner along the length of the filament. The repeat length of the helical unit in the myosin filament is 43 nm (Fig. 5.4).

An actin filament is four-stranded and consists of two coiled strands of F-actin and two tropomyosin cable-like polymers (Fig. 5.5). The F-actin polymer is made up of chains of spherical G-actin monomers (MW approximately 43,000). Tropomyosin (MW approximately 66,000) is the third major muscle protein composed of two helical subunits and lies within the longitudinal grooves of the coiled F-actin filament. Tropomyosin is a coiled coil α-helix of two subunits. Tropomyosin molecules lie end-to-end in the groove of the actin filaments – one tropomyosin molecule per seven G-actins. At intervals of 38.5 nm each tropomyosin chain is beaded with a trimeric troponin complex (Fig. 5.5).

The troponin complex consists of troponin T (MW 37,000) which binds tropomyosin, troponin I (MW 23,000) which binds to actin, and

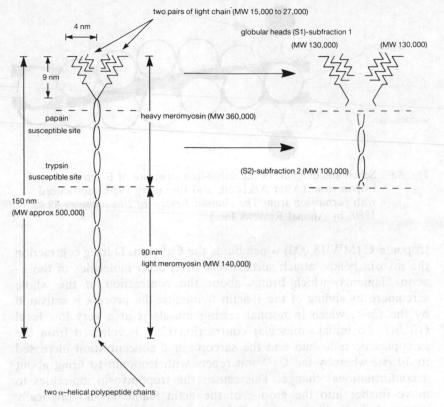

two pairs of light chain (MW 15,000 to 27,000)

globular heads (S1)-subfraction 1

(MW 130,000)   (MW 130,000)

4 nm

9 nm

papain
susceptible site

heavy meromyosin (MW 360,000)

trypsin
susceptible site

(S2)-subfraction 2 (MW 100,000)

150 nm
(MW approx 500,000)

90 nm
light meromyosin (MW 140,000)

two α–helical polypeptide chains

Fig. 5.3 Schematic diagram of a myosin molecule

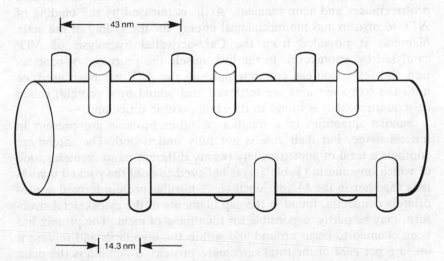

43 nm

14.3 nm

Fig. 5.4 Myosin filament with protruding globular heads in helical array

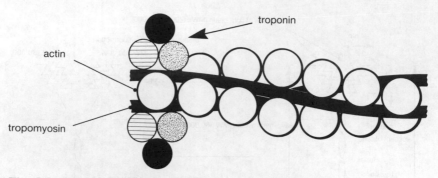

Fig. 5.5 Schematic diagram of the cable-like structure of F-actin and tropomyosin (After Adelstein and Eisenberg 1980, reproduced with permission from *The Annual Review of Biochemistry* **49** © 1980, by Annual Reviews Inc.)

troponin C (MW 18,000) which binds the Ca^{2+} ion. During contraction the myosin heads, attach successively to G-actin molecules of the F-actin filaments, which brings about the contraction of the whole sarcomere by sliding of the F-actin filaments; the process is activated by the Ca^{2+}, which in normal resting muscle is at a very low level (10^{-7}M). To initiate muscular contraction Ca^{2+} is released from the sarcoplasmic reticulum and the sarcoplasmic concentration increased to 10^{-5}M, whereby the Ca^{2+} ion reacts with troponin to bring about a conformational change. This causes the tropomyosin molecules to move further into the groove of the actin filaments and physically expose the actin-binding sites. Ca^{2+} also activates a protein kinase for phosphorylation of Ser-15 of a light myosin chain. Both the phosphorylation of the myosin head and the Ca^{2+}-activated movement of tropomyosin are believed to allow interactions between the myosin protuberances and actin filament. Actin is released by the binding of ATP to myosin and the mechanical energy for the sliding of the actin filaments is provided from the Ca^{2+}-activated hydrolysis of ATP catalysed by actomyosin. In the live muscle the processes of contraction and relaxation can continue until all the ATP has been used, or until the free Ca^{2+} ions are retrieved and bound by a protein, called calsequestrin, that is found in the sarcoplasmic reticulum.

Smaller quantities of a number of other proteins are present in muscle tissue, but their role is not fully understood. The sarcomere contains a total of approximately twenty different minor proteins, one of which, myomesin (Table 5.1) is believed to hold the packed myosin tails together in the M-line junction. A fibrillar protein termed appropriately connectin, found in the gap filaments of the cytoskeletal structure, may be partly responsible for toughness of meat. The protein has been claimed to occur around and within the myofibrils and represent up to 6 per cent of the total sarcomere protein. α-Actinin is the main protein component of the Z-disc. To date the sliding filament hypoth-

Table 5.1 Myofibrillar sarcomere proteins

Protein	Molecular weight
Myosin	500,000
Actin	43,000
Myomesin	165,000
Connectin	700,000
α-Actinin	200,000
Desmin	55,000
Vimentin	58,000
Synemin	23,000
N_2-line protein	60,000

(Davey 1984).

esis, which now encompasses knowledge of first, the molecular structure of myosin and actin, secondly, the Ca^{2+} activation of troponin, and thirdly, the rotation of myosin heads, affords an elegant theory for the mechanism of muscle contraction, whereby simultaneous pulling forces are transmitted to the tendons in the live animal. The energy is provided by the hydrolysis of ATP.

At the point in time immediately after death of an animal the enzymatic control system of the muscle is clearly still intact. The muscle cells become anaerobic due to the lack of oxygen; the muscular glycogen is hydrolysed to glucose-1-phosphate with consequent loss of ATP, and lactic acid accumulates as a result of anaerobic glycolysis (App. III) to produce a subsequent fall of pH value in the muscle to approximately 5.6. The loss of ATP results in further interaction between actin and myosin and contraction of the sarcomere. In the living muscle ATP normally blocks this extensive interaction between actin and myosin.

Muscular contraction and toughness in meat

The rates of post-mortem glycolysis and the initiation of rigor mortis are highly variable, both between animals and indeed between muscles of the same carcase. Rigor mortis arises from an inextensible binding of actin and myosin. Stress on the animal before death, and both premature or incorrect cutting of the muscles or rapid cooling, all influence the rates of post-mortem changes in meat. A relationship between fall of pH value resulting from anaerobic glycolysis and stiffness of the post-mortem muscle is shown in Fig. 5.6.

Excessive shortening of the muscle fibres can be induced by cutting through the muscle shortly after death, or cooling rapidly to temperatures less than 11 °C. At 2 °C the muscle fibres can shorten by as much

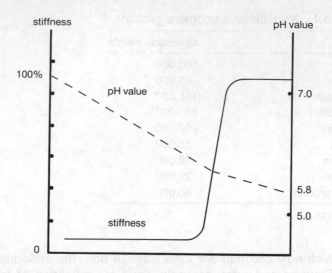

Fig. 5.6 Post-mortem changes in stiffness and pH in beef muscle (after Jeacocke 1984)

as 50 per cent, but this extensive shortening is generally prevented by the attached skeleton. Cold shortening occurs in beef, sheep and turkey meat. Shortening can also occur during the thawing of frozen meat, (thaw rigor), where the meat has been frozen beforc the completion of rigor mortis. For large animals the shortening of muscles that inevitably occurs can be partly overcome by both hanging the carcases to maintain an extension force and by chilling more slowly. However, for small animals, like turkey and chicken, and in some cases for pieces of excised muscle from red meat animals, rapid chilling and freezing is commonly practised soon after death, where the conditions are either created for cold shortening or subsequent thaw rigor shortening. Both the cutting of meat surfaces and cooling to 10 °C or less cause the elevation of levels of Ca+ in the sarcoplasm, whereby muscular contraction is activated with consequent shortening of the length of the sarcomeres. For the shortened sternomandibularis bovine muscle a clear linear relationship between toughness and up to 40 per cent shortening of the fibres has been found (Fig. 5.7). However, during muscle shortening not all sarcomeres decrease in length and shortening is probably related to an increased incidence of shortened sarcomeres (with a length of less than 1.5 μm). As a consequence of shortening, the density of myofibrils per unit area must increase, which explains the observed increase in tensile strength correlated with up to 40 per cent shortening (Fig. 5.7). For shortening beyond 40 per cent, it is proposed that localised regions of extreme shortening develop in the muscle, where an ensuing decrease in tough-

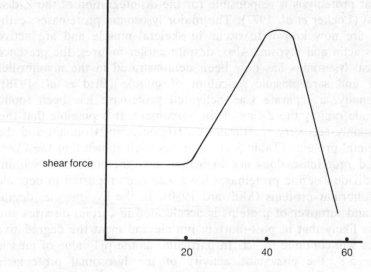

shear force

20   40   60

degree of shortening (%)

Fig. 5.7   Relationship between shortening and shear force in meat (after Davey 1984)

ness is due to a physical disintegration and fracturing of other myofibril regions.

Permanently shortened and tough meat is thought to arise from adverse combinations of myofibrillar shortening and the biochemical changes of post-mortem glycolysis. Permanent toughness arises in cold-shortened muscle, excised muscle and frozen muscle as glycolysis proceeds. The critical temperature–pH combinations are 11 °C before the pH value has fallen below 6.2. Toughness can be avoided by holding the carcases for a brief period at from 35 to 40 °C and ensuring that rigor mortis has taken place before chilling of the carcase below approximately 15 °C. Furthermore, the development of rigor can be brought forward by electrical stimulation which thereby reduces the possibility of shortening during chilling. Such electrically stimulated meat, when de-boned, does not shorten on rapid cooling and freezing. However, the mechanism by which electrical stimulation induces changes in meat is complex and not fully understood, although the increased post-mortem metabolic rate is correlated with tenderness (Fabiansson and Reuterswärd 1985).

Ageing by storage of chilled meat increases tenderness. Slowly the rigor muscle relaxes from its rigid form (the resolution of rigor) and the fibrous structure, after approximately 10 days at 5 °C, starts to break down. Both transverse breakages occur in the myofibrils and the Z-discs also start to disintegrate. The mechanism for the resolution of rigor is not fully understood, but there is now some evidence to indicate that proteolysis is responsible for the disintegration of the Z-disc material (Locker *et al*. 1977). The major lysosomal proteinases, cathepsins, are now known to occur in skeletal muscle and are active towards actin and myosin. Also, despite earlier failures, the presence of typical lysosomes has now been demonstrated in the myofibriller interior and sarcoplasmic reticulum of muscle (Bird *et al*. 1978). Additionally, a separate Ca^{2+}-activated proteinase has been found to degrade rapidly the Z-line of the sarcomere. It is possible that this enzyme only acts very specifically on tropomyosin, troponin and the cytoskeletal proteins (Table 5.1), as it has been shown that the Ca^{2+}-activated proteinase does not hydrolyse myosin, actin or α-actinin. Five individual serine proteinases have also been reported to degrade the myofibrillar proteins (Millward 1980). In the live muscle, degradation and turnover of proteins is accelerated in certain diseases and it seems likely that in post-mortem muscle and meat the degradative enzymes will continue to act. In particular as the pH value of muscle falls to 5.8, the enzymatic activity of the lysosomal proteinases increases and therefore is likely to be significant during the storage of meat. For different muscles there is an overall degree of proportionality between degradation rates and lysosomal proteinase activity.

The tenderness and juiciness of meat is also influenced indirectly by the effect of the intermolecular interactions between different meat proteins on the swelling of meat and its water-holding capacity. The spaces between the myofibrillar proteins in living musculature are mainly filled with water. The spacing itself is influenced by the sarcomere length, the state of post-mortem rigor, the rigidity of the variable skeletal structure of the muscle, the ionic strength and the pH value of the meat. At the isoelectric point of proteins it is well known that the intermolecular electrostatic forces are minimal and indeed Offer and Trinick (1983) have confirmed that the swelling volume of meat decreases by 30 per cent with a lowering of pH values from 9 to 5. The swelling of meat has also been shown to increase at pH values less than 5.0 which are below the isoelectric point of meat proteins. Increasing concentrations of sodium chloride (up to 0.8–1 M) and pyrophosphate (up to 0.3 %) have been used commercially to enhance swelling volume. Pyrophosphate is also thought to mimic the action of ATP and cause the dissociation of actomyosin. The effect of such increases in ionic strength can be explained by both dissolution and extraction of restraining structural components, such as the M-line and Z-disc proteins, and the absorption of ions to increase the electrostatic repulsion between myosin filaments (Offer and Trinick 1983) thereby solubilising myosin.

The tenderness of meat is also finally determined by cooking. Meat cooked to an internal temperature of 60 °C is described as rare, whereas at 80 °C the meat is well cooked and changes to a more granular texture, although the softer fibrillar structure is still an important

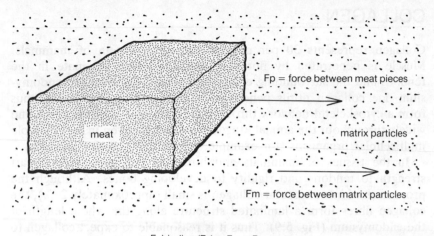

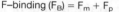

F−binding (F_B) = F_m + F_p

Fig. 5.8 Diagrammatic representation of the binding forces in meat products

and highly desirable characteristic. During the early stages of cooking at temperatures greater than 40 °C, there is an increase in toughness which is associated with a 25 to 40 per cent transverse shrinkage of the muscle fibres. At higher temperatures the heat-induced toughening is partly overcome by both a physical breakdown of the myofibrillar structure, and probably melting and denaturation of the intramuscular collagen.

The myofibrillar proteins also influence the binding properties of pieces of meat. A high binding strength is important, as it enhances the integrity and thus the quality of meat-derived products. The binding strength (F_B) is the force required to separate pieces of meat and includes at least two parameters (Fig. 5.8): these are the forces between the meat particle and the binding matrix (F_p), and the forces required to break the interparticle binding matrix (F_m). The factors which correlate with high values for F_B are enhanced solubility of myofibrillar proteins, the presence of added salts and the temperature of processing. Miller *et al.* (1980) have found a significant correlation between a reduction in total extracted protein and a reduction in binding strength for both beef and pork. Thus the physical treatments such as mechanical agitation and increased ionic strength, which are likely to enhance extraction of meat proteins, increase the values for F_B. As the myofibrillar proteins are denatured at relatively low temperatures (40–50 °C), it seems likely that the released soluble proteins act to enhance F_p by coating the meat particles with a 'sticky' heat-set denatured protein layer. Likewise the heat-setting dispersed soluble proteins dissolved in the matrix will increase the value of F_m.

COLLAGEN

Collagen represents 30 per cent of the total protein of mammals. Muscle is penetrated by fibres of collagen which originate in the tendons and the surrounding epimysium (Fig. 5.1): from the endomysium fine collagen fibrils penetrate between the myofibrils and thus form a cytoskeletal network throughout the muscle. Collagen is found widely throughout the animal kingdom and occurs even in many simple multicellular organisms (for example, jellyfish and marine sponges).

In the tissues of mammals and birds the collagen fibres impart strength to tendons and rigidity to developing bones. Although the proportion of intramuscular collagen is small (approximately 2 %), the collagen fibres form a laminated structure along the whole length of the endomysium (Fig. 5.9). Thus it is reasonable to expect collagen to be a significant contributor to the texture of meat. Furthermore, and most importantly, the unique sequence of amino acids in the collagen molecule dictates the formation of coiled polypeptide chains in tropo-collagen which can then form higher cross-linked polymers of high tensile strength.

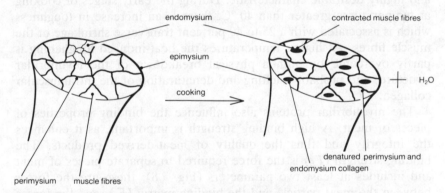

Fig. 5.9   Contraction of collagen and muscle fibres during cooking (after Bailey 1984)

During the cooking of meat at temperatures of up to 80 °C an increase in toughness has been observed. This can be due partly to the large shrinkage that collagen fibres undergo at the denaturation temperature of from 65 to 75 °C. Bailey (1984) has suggested that the shrinkage of collagen compresses the myosin and actin fibres, which then results in both the extrusion of water and an increase in toughness in meat that is related to the increase in density of the fibres (Fig. 5.9). The well known increase in toughness of meat with the age of animal can also be accounted for by the above hypothesis: collagen from older animals is less soluble and more highly cross-linked and thus able to

Table 5.2 Collagen types and molecular composition

Type	Molecular composition	Occurrence
I	$[\alpha 1(I)]_2\alpha 2$	Tendon, bone, skin, cornea muscle epimysium and perimysium
II	$[\alpha 1(II)]_3$	Vitreous humor, hyaline cartilage
III	$[\alpha 1(III)]_3$	Foetal skin, muscle perimysium
IV	$\alpha 1(IV)$ and $\alpha 2$ possibly $(\alpha IV)_3$	Membranes, muscle endomysium
V	$[\alpha IV]_2\alpha 2V$	Human placenta, amniotic membranes, muscle endomysium

impose a greater compression force on both the interstitial fluid and myosin and actin fibres.

There are five types of collagen which vary in their distribution between species and tissues within a single species. Muscle contains types I, III, IV and V (Table 5.2) distributed in the separate morphological parts. Type I is composed of three protein chains, two of which are identical $[\alpha 1(I)]$. The assignment of both arabic and roman numerals to collagens is confusing and it should be noted that it is not intended to imply that there is any close resemblance in structure between the different $\alpha 1$ collagens of types I to V. Similarly $\alpha 2$-chains in the types I, IV and V collagens are not necessarily related. The different types of collagen each contain a collagen molecule composed of three left-handed helical chains supercoiled around each other into a right-handed triple helical cable-like structure of length 290 nm and 1.4 nm diameter (Fig. 5.10). Thus the uncross-linked triple helical tropocollagen molecule (MW 285,000) can be extracted in aqueous solution from immature connective tissue. Type I collagen is the most prevalent and consists of two $\alpha 1$-chains and one $\alpha 2$-chain. The major part of the primary structure and unique sequence of amino acids in all of the type I collagens is surprisingly simple: every third residue is glycine in a triplicate repeating sequence (Gly–X–Y), where X and Y are frequently, but not necessarily, residues of proline or 4-hydroxyproline, respectively (Fig. 5.11). The collagen polypeptide chain (MW approximately 97,000) consists of 1014 residues of amino acids. In the sequence of amino acids the consecutive imino acids confer a helical turn on the collagen polypeptide chains. The hydrogen atoms, on the α-carbon atom of glycine, being of minimal size, do not sterically impede the formation of the triple helix. Glycine is an absolute requirement for packing of the three α-chains. However, the N- and C-terminal ends of the α-chains do not contain the repeating (Gly–X–Y) triplet unit and therefore are not helical. The three α-chains are hydrogen bonded (one H bond per triplet) with each other between the peptide NH and CO groups; the OH groups of hydroxyprolines also stabilise the triple helical structure by hydrogen bonding

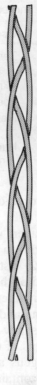

α–chains

Fig. 5.10 Part of the triple helical structure of collagen

with water. Proline and hydroxyproline are conformation-directing imino acids and the helix of individual chains has a pitch of exactly three residues. A similar left-handed helix is formed by L-polyproline in aqueous solution.

An important feature of the non-helical regions of types I, II and III collagens is the presence of a lysine residue at position 9 in the α1-chains (Eyre *et al.* 1984). Similarly lysine is present sixteen residues from the C-terminal end of the α1-chain molecule. The non-triplet N- and C-terminal regions of about fifteen to twenty amino acid residues play a role during the biosynthesis of collagen and also later during the formation of lateral cross-links between collagen molecules.

Following the biosynthesis of separate pro-collagen polypeptides, three parallel α-polypeptide chains are linked laterally through inter-chain disulphide bonds at the C-terminal ends of the molecules prior to the formation of a triple helix (Fig. 5.12). Each α-chain is also stabilised by an intrachain disulphide bond at the N-terminal end of the polypeptide chain. For this purpose the α-chain polypeptides of procollagen contain extension peptides which are probably globular at

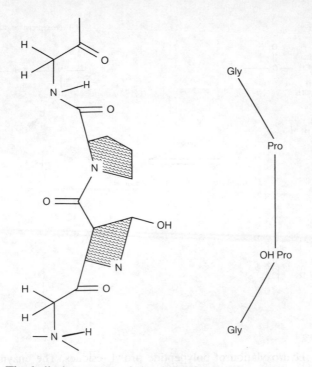

Fig. 5.11 The helical structure of the Gly–Pro–OHPro sequence on collagen-polypeptide chains. The hydrogen atoms of the glycine residues always point in towards the centre of the collagen triple helix. The proline nitrogen atoms and carbonyl groups are available for hydrogen bonding

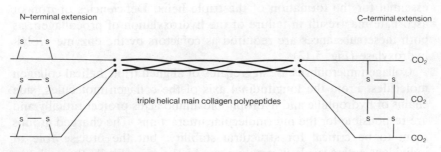

Fig. 5.12 The disulphide-linked extension peptides of procollagen

the N- and C-terminal points. The alignment of the N- and C-terminal regions sets the three chains in register for formation of the triple helical collagen molecule. Subsequently the extension peptides are removed by proteolysis catalysed by procollagen peptidases. The synthesis of procollagen is analogous to the synthesis of the zymogens of proteolytic enzymes. In this instance the biosynthesis of procollagen with its extension peptides seems to prevent the premature formation

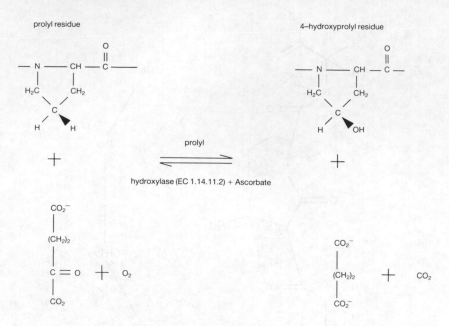

prolyl

Fig. 5.13 Hydroxylation of polypeptide prolyl residues. The enzyme is a
Fe-oxygenase as molecular oxygen is incorporated into the
prolyl residue. Ascorbate acts as reducing agent to maintain Fe²⁺

of collagen fibres in the synthesising cells. Hydroxylation and subsequent glycosylation of procollagen is a post-ribosomal process and is
essential for the formation of the triple helix. Deficiencies of iron or
ascorbate may result in failure of the hydroxylation of procollagen, as
both these substances are required as cofactors by the enzyme prolyl-
hydroxylase (Fig. 5.13).

Collagen microfibrils are aggregates of aligned triple helical collagen
molecules. From the longitudinal axis of the collagen molecules, side
chains of hydrophilic and hydrophobic amino acids project radially and
are responsible for the intermolecular interactions. The charged groups
seem to be critical for structural stability, but the precise role of
individual amino acids is not known. In the microfibrils the collagen
molecules are axially quarter-staggered by 67 nm (1 D) which corresponds to 234 amino acid residues. This staggered arrangement leads
to overlaps of 25 nm and hole zones at 67 nm spacing (Fig. 5.14),
which absorb phosphotungstic acid stains, and give rise to the unique
and characteristic banding pattern observed for collagen fibres in the
electron microscope. As the fibrils of collagen align cross-linking
between the fibrils occurs through the formation of unusual chemical
cross-links found mainly in connective tissue proteins. Hence a strong
collagen matrix is provided at the molecular level, both by linear

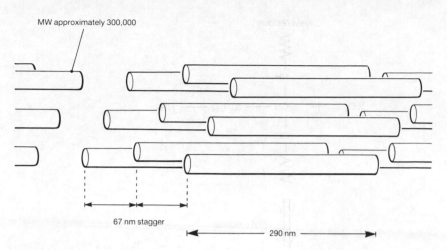

MW approximately 300,000

67 nm stagger

290 nm

Fig. 5.14 Schematic diagram for assembly of layered collagen fibrils in an end-to-tail fashion

twining of the α-chains and the formation of lateral interfibrillar covalent cross-links between the triple helical collagen molecules to provide mechanical strength.

The intermolecular cross-links between the collagen molecules are formed by first, oxidative deamination catalysed by lysyl oxidase (EC 1.4.3.14) of the ε-amino group of a lysyl or hydroxylysyl residues in the non-helical ends of the collagen chains (Fig. 5.15). Secondly, an addition reaction occurs to form a Schiff base between the generated aldehyde group and the free amino groups of other lysine residues (Fig. 5.16). Two pathways of cross-linking are possible. One is based on the lysine-derived aldehydes, and the other on hydroxylysine derived aldehydes. In the α-hydroxyaldimines, –CHOH–CH=N– (Fig. 5.16) spontaneous rearrangements occur to form the more stable ketoamines. The chemical nature of a number of different kinds of cross-links has been determined after their stabilisation by chemical reduction with borohydride. Glycosylated hydroxylysine residues are not oxidised to aldehydes and thus glycosylation may control indirectly the sites for oxidation. In α1-chains there are four sites for cross-linking. Two are located in the telopeptides (the non-helical N- and C-terminal peptides), while the remaining two are found in the helical regions (Fig. 5.17). The quarter-stagger (67 nm) ensures that any aldehyde group in the telopeptide (the N-terminal end of an α-chain) is located alongside an adjacent hydroxylysine-930 N which lies towards the C-terminal part of another collagen molecule. Cross-linking only occurs in insoluble coiled fibre aggregates, and thus insolubility ensures the correct alignment of the lysine residues for the oxidation and head-to-tail condensation reactions.

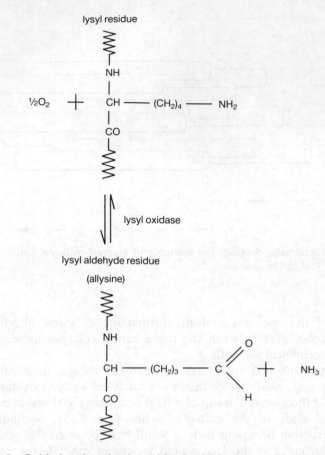

Fig. 5.15 Oxidative deamination of lysyl ε-NH₂ groups. The enzyme is a monooxygenase and contains Cu. It is inhibited by chelating agents and lathrogens from the Leguminosae

Likewise for oxidation of a lysyl residue in the C-terminal end of the molecule (Lys-16C), due to the quarter-stagger arrangement, the enzymatically generated aldehyde group is likely to be adjacent to N-telopeptide lysyl, hydroxylysyl or generated aldehydes in other staggered collagen molecules. Such end-to-end cross-linking results in the formation of rigid three-dimensional collagen fibres of considerable tensile strength. The ketoamino cross-link, unlike the aldimine cross-link is stable at 65 °C and this could account for the shrinkage of collagen during cooking (Bailey 1984). Indirect evidence now suggests that the ketoamino cross-links may act as precursors of pyridinium cross-links between three polypeptides. For formation of a pyridine ring it is proposed that the critical step is an aldol addition reaction between two allysine residues, followed by acid-catalysed nucleophilic

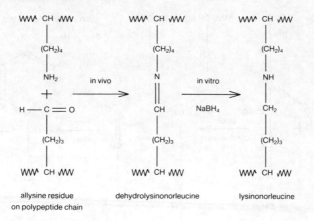

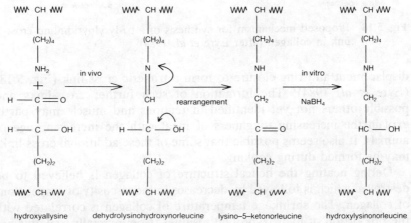

Fig. 5.16 Cross-linking of collagen molecules (Bailey and Etherington 1980)

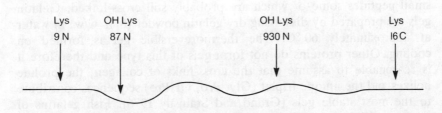

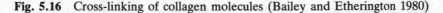

Fig. 5.17 The principal sites for cross-linking in type I, II and III collagens (after Eyre *et al.* 1984)

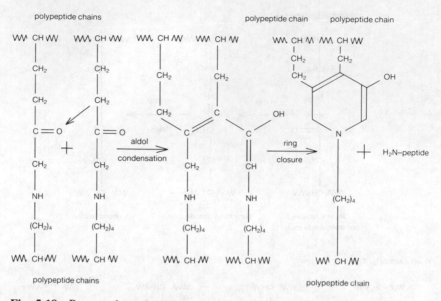

Fig. 5.18 Proposed mechanism for synthesis of a tri-lysylpyridinium cross-link in collagen (after Eyre *et al*. 1984)

displacement and ring closure to form a trimeric cross-link (Fig. 5.18) (Eyre *et al*. 1984). The formation of such further cross-links and possibly others not yet identified in tendons and muscle may partly explain the increasing toughness of meat with the increasing age of animals. It also seems possible that some of these additional cross-links may be formed during cooking.

During heating the helical structure of collagen is believed to be destroyed which is followed by decreases in the viscosity of suspensions of collagen. The shrinkage temperature of collagen is correlated with the proportion of hydroxyproline residues. Commercially, gelatins are obtained by the thermal denaturation and partial hydrolysis with dilute acid or alkali of various types of collagens obtained from bones, cartilage or skin trimmings available from other industries. Thus gelatin is not an homogeneous protein, but a mixture of large and small peptides some of which are probably still cross-linked. Gelatin gels are prepared by dissolving dry gelatin powder (8 % w/w) in water at approximately 60 °C. The thermoreversible gel is formed on cooling. Other proteins do not form gels of this type and therefore it is reasonable to assume that the cross-links of collagen, the proline helixes and the unique triplet (Gly, Pro, OHPro) sequences contribute to the most stable gels (Grand and Stainsby 1976). Fish gelatins of lower pyrollidine content lack the gelling ability of mammalian gelatins. Generally, short segments of the triple helix, joined in a three-dimensional network by segments of single α-chains, probably represent the random polypeptide structure of gelatin. The junction zones may contain a collection of triple helices imitating partially reformed collagen. Thus the physical properties of gelatin, where the association of polypeptide chains is random and not in register, are likely to vary considerably depending on source and hydrolysis conditions. To date a more controlled hydrolysis to produce graded gelatins with a more uniform distribution of molecular size through the use of collagenases has not been achieved.

Collagen-degrading enzymes

There are two classes of mammalian collagen-degrading enzymes. First, both the collagenases and neutral proteinases are active at physiological pH values and thus may be able to catalyse the hydrolysis of collagen fibres in meat. While many neutral proteinases can catalyse the hydrolysis of only the telopeptide region of collagen, collagenases catalyse the hydrolysis of specific peptide bonds in the triple helix region of collagens which is totally resistant to other proteinases. The collagenases seem to catalyse only limited hydrolysis of the separate collagen chains and thus produce large fragments which represent 75 per cent and 25 per cent of the molecule (Harper 1980). Such products of collagenase action are denatured spontaneously at 37 °C and can be degraded further by the action of other neutral proteinases.

Secondly, during the later stages of post-mortem glycolysis where a pH value of 5.8 or less may be achieved, the second group of enzymes, certain lysosomal endo- and exo-proteinases may also be responsible for the degradation of collagen. In particular, it is known that both cathepsins B and N (collagen-degrading cathepsins) will catalyse the hydrolysis of monomeric soluble collagen in the range pH 3 to 6, although both enzymes are inactive above pH 4.5 towards insoluble tissue collagen. Cathepsin B has been shown to catalyse the hydrolysis of the $\alpha1(I)$-chain at Gly-12, Ile-13 and Ser-14 and Val-15, which are located between the cross-links at Lys-9 and the start of the triple helix at residue 16. Thus collagenases and cathepsins may act sequentially. The insoluble nature of collagen, and its dense helical structure, is thought to impede the action of collagen-degrading enzymes. Therefore any tenderisation induced by the endogenous enzymes would clearly be less in older animals, where the cross-linking of collagen is much greater. Both cathepsins B and N are cysteine proteinases, which are inhibited by the microbial proteinase inhibitor, leupeptin (acetyl–Leu–Leu–Arg–CHO). Natural inhibitors of both collagenases and neutral proteinases are likely to be present in muscle and therefore the detection of specific proteinase activity in meat is difficult.

ELASTIN

Animal connective tissues also contain the rubber-like insoluble protein elastin. Tissues where considerable expansion and elasticity are required are rich sources of elastin. These include ligamentum nuchae, visceral pleura, aorta and the parenchyma of lungs. Smaller amounts of elastin are also present in other ligaments and vertebral cartilage. However, elastin is not a major constituent of muscle or other food. Its presence is largely restricted to blood vessels and associated tendons. Also elastin normally exists in an amorphous and relaxed state. Therefore, unlike collagen, it does not exert tensional forces on the muscle fibres.

Consequently the effects of cooking on the small amounts of elastin present in foods would seem to have a negligible effect. However, indirectly elastin has been of particular interest to the meat scientist, because both elastin and collagen are the only known mammalian proteins that contain cross-links derived from lysine. Although similar types of cross-links are believed to be present in eggshell membranes. The identification of the elastin cross-links, as desmosine and isodesmosine (Fig. 5.19) preceded the identification of the cross-links in collagen. However, as in collagen, the initial biochemical reaction for the formation of the cross-links is oxidative deamination of the ϵ-NH$_2$ group of lysyl residues, followed by the subsequent condensation reactions to form pyridinium compounds. Four separate peptide lysyl residues from separate polypeptide chains provide the atomic framework for the pyridinium compounds. Three of these lysyl residues are oxidised to allysine. Elastin also contains very few polar residues but large amounts of non-polar hydrophobic residues. The amount of Gly, Pro and Ala is similar to that of collagen at about 60 molar per cent. However, unlike collagen where the polyproline helix is formed, the proline residues in elastin are thought to be more randomly distributed to form kinks in the polypeptide chains. Studies of the sequence of amino acids in elastin has shown that the molecule contains repeat peptides with sequences of Pro, Gly, Gly, Val residues (Table 5.3). The Pro–Gly dipeptide would produce turns in the polypeptide chain. It has been suggested that the repeat pentapeptide forms spirals, which, together with the helical regions of the molecule, are held together by the pyridinium cross-links to form an elastic polymer

Table 5.3 Repeat amino acid sequences in elastin

Tetrapeptide	Val–Pro–Gly–Gly
Pentapeptide	Ala–Pro–Gly–Val–Gly
Hexapeptide	Ala–Pro–Gly–Val–Gly–Val

(Van Deenen *et al.* 1983).

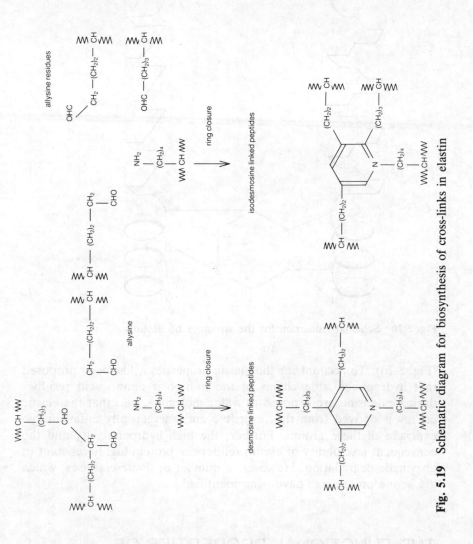

Fig. 5.19 Schematic diagram for biosynthesis of cross-links in elastin

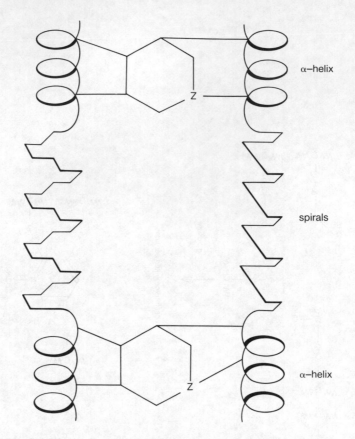

Fig. 5.20 Schematic diagram for the structure of elastin

(Fig. 5.20). To account for the elastic properties it has been proposed that hydrophobic side chains of the non-polar amino acid residues during extension are exposed to water molecules, and that the elastic energy is derived from the reversible and energetically unfavourable exposure of these groups. Further, the high hydrophobicity and the consequent insolubility of elastin render the protein highly resistant to enzymatic degradation. However, a number of tissue elastases, which are serine proteinases have been identified.

THE FUNCTIONAL PROPERTIES OF NON-MEAT ANIMAL PROTEINS

The contribution of milk proteins, egg proteins and seed storage proteins to the texture of whole foods is less obvious than for meat proteins. The proteins are normally non-fibrous and sometimes soluble. The textural properties of some milk and egg-based products such as cheese, egg custards and yoghurt are highly desirable. However, information that relates the structure of egg, milk and plant seed proteins to specific functional properties of foods is still limited, because of the presence in foods of a large number of different proteins and other constituents. Whey proteins, seed proteins including soybean meal and gluten from cereals, have all been used as supplements mainly due to their functional properties. Indeed for the manufacture of new products that incorporate some of these proteins little importance has been attributed to their nutritional value, even when this has been advantageous, as with milk whey proteins. The common terms used widely that describe the functional properties of food ingredients are given in Table 5.4. Although such terminology is empirical, these important physical properties sought by the food industry may be quickly assessed by simple tests for a large number of samples on a routine basis. For example see Tasneem *et al.* (1982).

Table 5.4 The required functional properties of food proteins

solubility, swelling, increased viscosity, gelation, emulsification, foam volume and stability, elasticity, binding properties, extrusion

The swelling and gelation of a protein product is determined by the solubility of the protein, the conformation of the molecule, and the extent of intermolecular interactions at given values of pH and temperature; the gelation property of gelatin obtained by denaturation and limited hydrolysis of collagen is a prime example of the influence of the molecular structure of a protein molecule on a functional property. During the hydrolysis of collagen the protein molecule unfolds but remains joined together by cross-links at specific points to form a three-dimensional framework containing entrapped water. Intermolecular links whether by covalent or non-covalent bonds, as in gelatin and soybean gels, are an essential requirement for gel formation.

Emulsification involves the physical entrapment of droplets in a continuous phase. Emulsions are found in soups, salad dressings, sausages, butter, margarines and ice-cream. The emulsifying capacity for an oil-in-water emulsion is often measured as the volume or weight of oil emulsified per unit weight of protein. Emulsion stability is inversely related to the time for the droplets to coalesce and aggregate which eventually results in phase separation. The molecular mechanism for formation of emulsions between aqueous solutions of proteins and food oils, such as palm oil or soybean oil, must involve diffusion, orientation and unfolding–spreading of the absorbed protein molecules at the oil–water interface. It is obvious that the hydrophobic domains of the proteins will concentrate in the oil phase while the more polar domains of the proteins will associate with water molecules in the aqueous phase. The protein molecules, together with in some instances other simple emulsifiers used as additives, accumulate at the interface to reduce the interfacial tension between the two liquids. An emulsion contains a very large interfacial surface area, which may amount to 1000 cm^2 per cm^3 volume as found in a coarse emulsion like fresh milk. The size of the major constituent protein molecules needs to be adequate to stabilise the emulsion. This is shown by the dramatic effect of proteolysis with pronase on the emulsifying capacity of a protein in Fig. 5.21. Ionic strength, pH value and temperature, affect the structure and properties of proteins and hence their ability to form emulsions. β-Casein, a protein which contains a large proportion of hydrophobic amino acids is surface active and a good emulsifier. The greater surface activity of β-casein results in a rapid absorption of proteins in surface liquid films and an increase in surface pressure. The absorption of proteins in surface films also determines the foaming characteristics and again β-casein gives rise to relatively high-volume foams. Foams are air bubbles with protein skins trapped within a liquid. During the collapse of foams the imbibed liquid drains away.

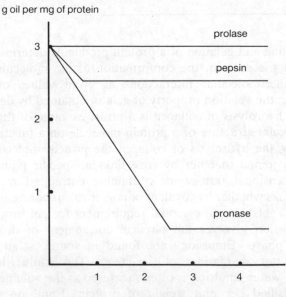

Fig. 5.21 The effect of enzymic hydrolysis on emulsifying capacity (with permission from Kuehler and Stine 1974; reprinted from *Journal of Food Science*, 1974, **39**(2), 380. Copyright © by Institute of Food Technologists)

Typical foam products are angel cake, meringue, soufflé and whipped toppings. Generally, it is thought that protein molecules which unfold and reorientate in the liquid surface film of foams facilitate foam formation. For foam stability the develoment of intermolecular polymer networks in the surface film of the foam is essential. The stabilisation may be provided by other relatively large or aggregated proteins present in complex food systems. A widely used foaming agent in the food industry is egg white, where a mechanically produced foam is stabilised by high molecular weight polymers of ovomucin which seem to form a continuous film to envelop the foam bubble. The need for large protein molecules is shown by the deleterious effect of proteinases on foam stability (Fig. 5.22). For stabilisation of foams and emulsions intermolecular hydrogen bonding, hydrophobic interactions, electrostatic bonding and van der Waals' forces between the various constituents, must be important. However, the complexity of real food systems presently make it extremely difficult to predict the foaming properties of a whole food from knowledge of simpler model systems.

For a full understanding of some of the functional properties, such as gelation and foaming, a detailed knowledge of the molecular structure of proteins may be required. The associative and aggregative properties and tertiary structure of proteins are determined by geneti-

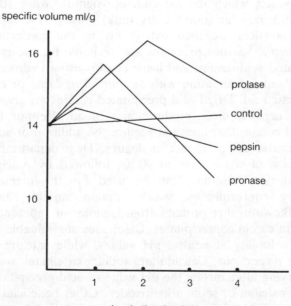

Fig. 5.22   Effect of enzymic hydrolysis on foam volume (with permission from Kuehler and Stine 1974; reprinted from *Journal of Food Science*, 1974 **39**(2), 380. Copyright © by Institute of Food Technologists)

cally controlled biosynthesis of specific amino acid sequences and post-ribosomal modifications. These may include the formation of cross-links between polypeptide chains, or phosphorylation and glycosylation. Knowledge of the amino acid sequences for some milk and egg proteins is available which will aid an understanding of the functional properties of food proteins. For the complex mixture of proteins present in seeds it is becoming clear that many of the proteins are derived from similar precursor proteins. Subsequent proteolysis and oxidation of sulphydryl groups to form disulphide bonds results in modification of the common precursor proteins. For the future, sequencing techniques which are readily available are likely to be increasingly applied to polypeptides derived from plant foods that identify with the desirable functional properties like foaming and emulsification.

Milk caseins

Caseins are the main proteins of milk and represent approximately 80 per cent of the total milk protein. Liquid milk contains approximately 2.7 per cent of caseins. Caseins are defined as those proteins which are precipitated from liquid milk by the addition of acid at pH 4.6. Milk and its products which include cheese, yoghurt, whole dried milk, skimmed milk powder (non-fat dry milk), caseinates, coprecipitates and whey powders are used extensively in the confectionery and baking industry. Various processes are available for the manufacture of precipitated acid caseins and lactic caseins using hydrochloric acid, at pH 4.5, and fermentation with *Streptococcus lactis* or *cremoris* to produce lactic acid. Dried acid precipitated caseins are used for fortification of cereals, meat products and bread. Rennin (chymosin) precipitated casein, that does not require the addition of acid, is used for the manufacture of cheese analogues. Heat denaturation of the whey proteins of whole milk at 90 °C, followed by precipitation in calcium chloride solutions, can be used for the manufacture of casein–whey coprecipitates, which contain variable amounts of calcium. Likewise other proteins from legumes or rapeseed might be used to form casein coprecipitates. Caseinates are valuable because of their high solubility at neutral pH values, while calcium caseinates form stable dispersions. Calcium and sodium caseinates are produced by spray drying after raising the pH value of acid precipitated caseins to 6.7 with calcium or sodium hydroxides. Other beneficial properties are given in Table 5.5, and generally the functional properties of caseinates include the absorption of water, fat binding, whipping and foam stability. Consequently caseinates have been used mainly in comminuted meat products although newer uses have now been found in 'lower energy' margarines, coffee whiteners, whipped confectionery

Table 5.5   The functional properties of caseinate products

Casein product	Functional property
Acid caseinate	Soluble above pH 5.5
Calcium caseinate	White colloidal dispersions
Sodium caseinate	Gels at concentrations above 17 %
Lactic casein	Absorbs less water than acid casein
Rennet casein	Only soluble above pH 9; suspensions above 15 % gel at 25 °C; contains 2.8 % of Ca^{2+}
Casein–whey coprecipitates	High PER values, only soluble at very high pH, or in calcium chelating solutions

toppings and in semi-liquid cheeses. In milk-containing products, the casein micelles largely retain their physical structure and are heat stable. They account for the water-holding capacity in gel and paste-like products such as yoghurt.

In milks there are basically four different types of caseins, α_{s1}-, α_{s2}-, β- and κ-caseins. A range of published values for the amounts of milk proteins present in bovine milk is given in Table 5.6.

Table 5.6   Bovine milk proteins

Proteins	g/100 g of protein	Approximate molecular weight[†]
α_{s1}-Casein	37–58	23,000
α_{s2}-Casein	9.2–12.3	25,000
β-Casein	27.6–33.8	23,900
κ-Casein	9.2–12.3	19,000
β-Lactoglobulin	6.1–12.2	18,300
α-Lactalbumin	3.1–4.6	14,000
Immunoglobulins	1.9–3.1	150,000 to 950,000

(Swaisgood 1982).

Frequently various ratios of the order of 3 : 0.8 : 3 : 1 for amounts of α_{s1}, α_{s2}, β and κ-caseins, respectively, have been quoted for casein preparations. There is genetic variation between breeds of cows, which is expressed by the substitution of some amino acids in the α_{s1} and α_{s2}-caseins. The caseins solubilised in tris-glycine buffers at pH 8.6 can be separated by electrophoresis (Fig. 5.23). The α_{s2} component is not always resolved from α_{s1}-casein depending on the nature of the genetic variants present. The functional properties of proteins are generated from the sequence of amino acids in the casein molecules and in turn from the occurrence and distribution of hydrophilic and hydrophobic domains in the casein subunits. The occurrence of amino acids in all the caseins is similar to that for other globular proteins. However,

Fig. 5.23 Electrophoretic pattern for milk caseins (kindly prepared by Mr
J. Fish). The caseins were obtained from the milk of an
individual cow by precipitation at pH 4.6. The precipitate was
dissolved in tris–glycine buffer (0.033 M tris, 0.078 M glycine, pH
8.8). Electrophoresis was carried out in 7 % polyacrylamide gels
in 0.033 M tris–glycine buffer at pH 8.8 at 1 mA per tube 20 min.
Staining was with 0.1 % naphthalene black 12B in 7 % acetic
acid

small amounts (two residues per mole) of cysteine are only found in
α_{s2}- and κ-caseins. The presence of cysteine allows α_{s2}- and κ-casein to
be purified by affinity chromatography using a thiolated sepharose. For
β- and κ-casein proline is the most frequent amino acid which is likely
to reduce the proportion of α-helical structures in the polypeptide
chains. Post-ribosomal modification of all the caseins resulting in phosphorylation of the hydroxyl groups of serine is an unusual characteristic of caseins. The κ-caseins are also glycoproteins containing
generally from one to three tetrasaccharide or trisaccharide moieties
covalently linked to the hydroxyl groups of Thr-131, -133 and -135.
Microheterogeneity exists between κ-casein molecules because of the

variable occurrence of the oligosaccharide moieties. From the primary structures of the caseins (Swaisgood 1982), it is known that the overall distribution of charged and hydrophobic residues is not random or uniform.

In α_{s1}-casein there are blocks of hydrophobic residues and clusters of negatively charged groups of O-serylphosphates. α_{s1}-Casein contains eight or nine phosphate residues per mole. The α_{s2}-casein is a mixture of four proteins containing either ten, eleven, twelve or thirteen serylphosphate residues per mole. The α_s-caseins are calcium sensitive due to the presence of phosphate groups and precipitate with Ca^{2+} at pH 7.0. α-Helix formation in the polypeptide chains is minimised by the presence of 8.5 per cent proline which is spread throughout the polypeptide chains. Blocks of charged residues are found in α_{s2}-casein (residues 8–12, 56–61) and in β-casein (residues 14–20).

The most hydrophobic component is found in β-casein as a large block of hydrophobic residues (48–209): the polar, hydrophilic and five phosphate residues are contained in the N-terminal region of the polypeptide chain. A typical tertiary structure for such a protein is expected to consist of a tightly folded compact molecule in which the polar groups of amino acids are located on the outer surface and are hydrated. The internal hydrophobic region would contain the apolar groups. Thus β-casein forms aggregates with hydrophobic interiors while the N-terminal hydrophilic parts of the molecules are exposed to solvent.

κ-Casein differs from the other caseins by the presence of only one phosphoseryl residue and the presence of an oligosaccharide moiety. The κ-casein molecule is believed to possess a more stable single disulphide bonded structure with some α-helical and β-sheet regions. The chymosin-susceptible bond is thought to stand out on the surface of the molecule. The C-terminal segment which represents one-third of the κ-casein molecule is strongly anionic and contains the three oligosaccharide residues. The remaining two-thirds of the molecule is highly hydrophobic and corresponds to the *para*-κ-casein product formed after proteolysis catalysed by chymosin at residues 105–106.

Because of the structural similarities for the different caseins, it is relatively easy to understand how both the separate caseins may self-associate and simultaneously interact with each other through hydrophobic and hydrogen bonds. Indeed due to association the monomer of κ-casein has not been isolated at neutral pH values, but is thought to be spherical (radius 9.7 nm). Such interactions between caseins help to explain their insolubility and their interaction with other food proteins. The α- and β-caseins are soluble in neutral and alkaline but not in acid solutions. The binding of Ca^{2+} to the *ortho*-phosphate groups is likely to be particularly important for the formation of casein micelles by reducing the negative charges on the individual molecules.

Casein micelles of from 20 to 600 nm (mean diameter approximately

Table 5.7 A comparison of the frequency of amino acids in the main milk proteins

	α_{s1}-Casein	β-Casein	κ-Casein	β-Lactoglobulin	α-Lactalbumin
			(residues/100 residues)		
Asp	3.5	1.9	2.4	6.8	7.3
Asn	4	2.4	4.1	3.1	9.8
Thr	2.5	4.3	8.3	4.9	5.7
Ser	4	5.3	7.1	4.3	5.7
SerP	4	2.4	0.6	0	0
Glu	12	8.6	7.1	9.9	6.5
Gln	7.5	10	8.3	5.5	4.1
Pro	8.5	16.7	11.8	4.9	1.6
Gly	4.5	2.4	1.2	1.8	4.9
Ala	4.5	2.4	8.8	8.6	2.4
½Cys	0	0	1.2	3.1	6.5
Val	5.5	9.1	6.5	6.2	4.9
Met	2.5	2.9	1.2	2.5	0.8
Ile	5.5	4.8	7.7	6.2	6.5
Leu	8.5	10.5	4.7	13.5	10.6
Tyr	5.0	1.9	5.3	2.5	3.2
Phe	4.0	4.3	2.4	2.5	3.2
Trp	1.0	0.5	0.6	1.2	3.2
Lys	7.0	5.2	5.3	9.3	9.8
His	2.5	2.4	1.8	1.2	2.4
Arg	3.0	1.9	0.6	1.8	0.8
Total number of residues per mole	199	209	169	162	123
MW	23,612	23,980	19,005	18,362	14,174

(Calculated after Swaisgood 1982).

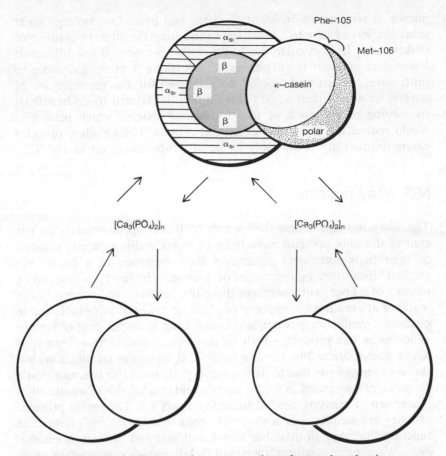

Fig. 5.24 Schematic diagram of a cross section of a casein subunit (diameter 20 nm) with α_{s1} : α_{s2} : β:K-caseins (3 : 0.8 : 3 : 1) and association with other subunits and tricalcium phosphate

120 nm and mean molecular weight 10^8), are thought to exist in milk as voluminous sponge-like structures with the interior of the micelles readily accessible to proteinases. The micelles are generally thought to be composed of subunits 8–20 nm) which associate with each other through tricalcium phosphate of $Ca_3(PO_4)_2$. The micelle contains from 2 to 4 g of water per gram of protein. The K-casein molecules are thought to reside on the surface of the micelles (Fig. 5.24). The subunits are likely to be held together by hydrophobic bonds and through interaction with colloidal calcium phosphate.

As the existence of the casein micelles depends on interactions between four different types of caseins and calcium triphosphate, it is not surprising that the gross composition and structure of the micelles can be changed slightly by temperature, mechanical processing or changes in pH value. Nevertheless, the overall physical structure of the micelle is remarkably resistant to shear and heat. On cooling, slight solubilisation of caseins occurs thus increasing the protein content of milk serum. In particular the hydrophobic β-casein is solubilised at lower than ambient temperatures, thus making it more accessible to proteinases. When such cooled milk is used for the manufacture of cheese, heat-treatment at 60°C for 30 min. is claimed to be beneficial by causing precipitation of the 'solubilised' caseins which otherwise would reduce the yield of cheese curd protein. Unlike whey proteins casein micelles are remarkably stable at temperatures up to 140 °C.

Milk whey proteins

The whey proteins (Table 5.8) which represent approximately 20 per cent of the milk proteins have been of considerable interest, because of their high nutritional value and their existence as a cheap by-product from the manufacture of cheese. However, whole whey consists of 93 per cent water and therefore recovery and concentration methods are required in order to produce an easily transportable stable product. Dried whey powder also contains up to 70 per cent of lactose which gives this product a high dietary energy value. The denatured whole whey obtained by heating to 90 °C is known as lactalbumin, but this is of limited use due to its insolubility. Its main use is a nutritional supplement suspended in soups, cereals and snack foods. Denaturation is assessed by measurement of solubility at pH 4.5. The native proteins of whey are soluble over a wide pH range and have a high degree of functionality; they form stable foams and gels and can act as emulsifiers. Whey protein concentrates and isolates which may contain up to 90 per cent protein may be obtained by ultrafiltration and chromatography. The emulsifying properties of whey, albeit less than caseinates, are less susceptible to changes of pH. For whey protein isolates, gels form at neutral pH values at from 56 to 58 °C. This temperature is close to the gelation temperature (60 °C) of egg white, which has proved to be a most useful but expensive food ingredient. However, whey protein concentrates (5 % w/w) form gels only after heating to

Table 5.8 Whey proteins of bovine milk

Protein	Concentration (g/litre)	Percentage of total whey protein	Approximate molecular weight
β-Lactoglobulin	3.0	54	18,300 (dimer 36,600)
α-Lactalbumin	0.7	21	14,000
Serum albumin	0.3	5	63,000
Immunoglobulins	0.6	10	up to 1 million

(Marshall 1982 and Kinsella 1985).

at least 85 °C and thus gelation of whey is very concentration dependent. A simple and most efficient use of whey proteins can be provided by their retention in the cheese curd. This can be achieved by the use of ultrafiltration to produce a retentate containing all the proteins. Such a product with a high solids content (39 %) has been used for the manufacture of Fetta and Camembert cheeses, which are of higher nutritional value due to the incorporation of whey proteins. The concentrates also produce foams, but the stability of the foam is highly variable due to the lack of stabilising high molecular weight polymers, which occur naturally in competing products like egg albumen.

The individual protein (Table 5.8), α-lactalbumin, has an important biological function and is present in all milks that contain lactose. Galactosyl transferase is the enzyme responsible for the synthesis of lactose. Biosynthesis only takes place when α-lactalbumin acting as a modifier is bound to the transferase enzyme. The molecule of α-lactalbumen is quite heat stable as only 6 per cent is denatured at 70 °C, whereas approximately 32 per cent of β-lactoglobulin, which is the main whey protein, is denatured at 70 °C. The molecule of α-lactalbumin contains four disulphide bonds and is globular. However, little is known about its functional properties, although α-lactalbumin readily associates with β-lactoglobulin through disulphide bonds.

The functional properties of whey, like caseins, are a reflection of the sequence of amino acids and in turn the conformational structure of at least some of the whey proteins. β-Lactoglobulin unlike α_{s1} and β-caseins contains a single sulphydryl group (Cys-119) and two cystine residues (Table 5.7). Therefore both intra- and intermolecular disulphide exchange reactions even with other proteins, like especially κ-casein, in dairy products are easily explained. The native β-lactoglobulin dimer (Table 5.8) dissociates in solution at 60 °C, when Cys-119 becomes more reactive with the increasing exposure of aromatic amino acids to solvent, as measured by difference spectra at 280 nm. Thus the whey proteins are susceptible to denaturation by an unfolding of the tertiary structure and subsequent aggregation through disulphide exchange reactions:

$$\beta\text{-lactoglobulin S-S} + \kappa\text{-casein S-S} \xrightarrow{\text{heat}} \begin{array}{c} \beta\text{-lactoglobulin} \\ | \quad | \\ S \quad S \\ | \quad | \\ S \quad S \\ | \quad | \\ \kappa\text{-casein aggregate} \end{array}$$

Disulphide interchange reactions between α_{s2}-casein and the β-lactoglobulin thiol group might also occur, which would result in the physical attachment of β-lactoglobulin to the caseins in heated milk. Such interchange reactions initiated by small amounts of thiol groups illustrate a general pattern for rheologically related changes in the secondary structure of other proteins, like the wheat glutenins and soybean legumins. The intermolecular interaction for β-lactoglobulin and κ-casein increases the thermostability and retards the aggregation of β-lactoglobulin.

Egg proteins

As a liquid food, the hen's (*Gallus domesticus*) egg is unusual, as it possesses a physically distinct macrostructure: in the fresh whole egg the yolk is held centrally by the chalazae, which are anchored to the thick white gel. The thick egg white gel itself, as shown in Fig. 5.25, is also held firmly in position by its attachment to the inner shell membranes of the egg. For reproduction of the avian species the yolk and albumen provide a source of food for a developing embryo.

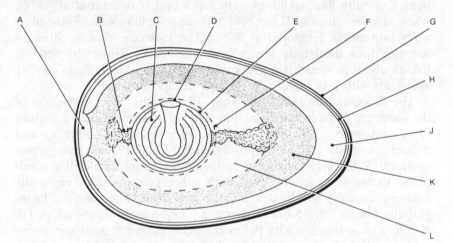

Fig. 5.25   Diagram of the structure of a hen's egg (with permission from Brooks and Hale 1959). A air cell, B chalaza, C yolk, D germinal disc, E vitelline membrane, F mucin, G shell, H shell membrane, J and L thin white, K thick white

For use as human food the organised structure of the egg is important: the central position of the yolk, which is a good medium for microbial growth, ensures for the yolk constituents that contact with the inner shell membranes is prevented. Furthermore, egg white, which is in contact with the shell membranes, is a relatively poor medium for microbial growth, because a substantial number of the egg white proteins possess antimicrobial properties. These include enzyme inhibitors, immunoglobulins, vitamin-binding proteins and the iron-binding protein, now known as ovotransferrin (Table 5.9). Lysozyme is also present in egg white in very substantial amounts; lysozyme itself

Table 5.9 Egg white proteins

Protein	Percentage of total solids	Classification
Ovalbumin	54	Phospho- and glycoprotein
Ovotransferrin	13	Iron-binding glycoprotein
Ovomucoids	11	Trypsin inhibitor glycoproteins
Lysozyme	3.5	Enzyme
Ovomucins	1.5	Glycoproteins
Ovoglycoprotein	0.5	Glycoprotein
Ovoinhibitors	0.1	Protease inhibitor, glycoproteins
Ovomacroglobulin	0.5	Glycoproteins, immunogenic
Other globulins	4.0	
Flavoprotein	0.8	Binds riboflavin, glycoprotein
Avidin	0.05	Binds biotin, glycoprotein

being an enzyme capable of catalysing the hydrolysis of the peptido-glycan component of cell walls of the many microorganisms.

The contents of the hen's egg can be separated easily into egg white (albumen) and yolk. The egg yolk proteins only represent from 15 to 17 per cent of the total yolk, while lipids account for approximately 33 per cent of the total liquid mass: the solids content of egg yolk is approximately 52 per cent. Many of the physical and useful commercial properties of egg yolk and liquid whole egg (albumen and yolk) depend on the high concentration of proteins and lipids. The constituents of the yolk (Table 5.10) act as emulsifying agents; both low and high density lipoproteins are thought to be important for maintaining the open structural network of baked products.

Dried egg products are also used substantially by the food industry. The main criterion used to assess the quality of dried egg products is the ease of reconstitution with water as assessed by measurements of solubility. Egg proteins are easily degraded by enzymes, but little use of this characteristic has been made due to the relatively high cost of eggs.

Table 5.10 Egg yolk proteins

Compounds	Percentage of yolk solids	Classification
Lipovitellin	17–18	Lipoprotein
Lipovitellenin	12–13	Lipoprotein
Livetins	4–5	Globulins
γ-Vitellin	14–15	Phosphoprotein
β-Vitellin	14–15	Phosphoprotein
Vitellenin	8–9	Phosphoprotein
Phosvitin	6	Phosphoprotein

Egg albumen possesses two commercially valuable functional properties, and neither of these can be easily mimicked by other proteins or other food constituents. Ovalbumin which is the major protein of egg white (Table 5.9) is denatured at the relatively low temperature of 60 °C to form at its natural concentration a unique acceptable solid, but soft nutritious food. The properties of the heat-set albumen gel are due to the high proportion of hydrophilic amino acids present in ovalbumin. However, the delicate semisolid gelatinous structure of heat-denatured egg white is disrupted by freezing. Thus it is impossible to store boiled eggs in the frozen state for use in convenience foods. Egg albumen is also very valuable because of its ability to form stable foams. Egg white is an eminent foaming ingredient in confectionery products.

Foam formation, and particularly foam stability, are important for the manufacture of meringues, angel cake, sponge cakes and other confectionery products. The commercially valuable foaming property of egg albumen has been shown to be positively correlated to both the amount of ovomucin, and the interaction of ovomucin with other globulin-type proteins present in egg white. Through the use of separate egg white proteins, obtained by prior fractionation, it has been shown by the application of response surface methodology (Johnson and Zabic 1981a), that the amounts of ovomucin, lysozyme and ovalbumin are positively correlated with angel cake volume. Direct correlations between ovomucin and lysozyme levels with foaming index values have also been observed and the region of optimum response is defined by low levels of lysozyme and high levels of ovomucin. During the baking process ovomucin–lysozyme complexes also offer a protective effect on foam volume, as ovomucin alone merely gives rise to foams which collapse during baking, whereas the addition of small amounts of lysozyme to ovomucin solutions produce a protective effect (Johnson and Zabic 1981b). Egg white from fresh eggs which contain undegraded ovomucins, has a strong positive effect on the volume and stability of the egg white foams.

For a long time it has also been known that ovomucin is important for maintaining the structural integrity of the egg, as shown in Fig. 5.25 where egg white is separated mainly into layers of thin and thick albumen. In fresh eggs the thick albumen layer represents approximately 50 per cent of the total egg white. The gelatinous nature of the thick albumen layer and the integrity of the chalazae are believed to be due to the unique molecular structure of ovomucin glycoproteins. The evidence for the importance of ovomucin resides in the fact that the thick egg white gel fraction contains four times more ovomucin than the thin egg white fractions. The concentration of ovomucin declines with the natural liquefaction of egg white, during the storage of whole shell eggs. Furthermore, fresh eggs which differ in albumen firmness also contain different amounts of ovomucin; those eggs which possess the thickest albumen contain the most ovomucin. During the storage of whole eggs the ovomucins seem to depolymerise by a biochemical mechanism that is still not fully understood. Although, the stability of the albumen gel can be enhanced by small amounts of magnesium ion.

Reduction of the disulphide bonds of ovomucin by mercaptoethanol, in the presence of 8 M urea as a denaturing agent, yields reduced ovomucins. These can be fractionated into two components (α- and β-reduced ovomucins) by preparative ultracentrifugation in density gradients.

Clearly the two α- and β-ovomucins exist, before reduction with thiol reagents, as a complex insoluble and intractable copolymer linked covalently by disulphide bonds. The molecular weight of the reduced α-ovomucin subunit has been calculated to be 210,000, whereas reduced β-ovomucin is an aggregate (MW approximately 720,000) of a smaller subunit (MW approximately 112,000) (Robinson and Monsey 1975). The solubilisation of ovomucin by sodium dodecyl sulphate in the absence of reducing agent only produces large aggregates with sedimentation coefficients of 30S and 35S. Like the other egg white proteins, with the exception of lysozyme, the α- and β-ovomucins are glycoproteins (Table 5.11). β-Ovomucin is unusual, in so far as it contains large quantities of N-acetylgalactosamine, galactose and sialic acid (N-acetylneuraminic acid): these monosaccharides are not present in the other egg white glycoproteins, which contain small amounts of other aldoses, like N-acetylglucosamine and mannose. During the storage of whole eggs the content of β-ovomucin in the thick egg albumen fraction decreases. Therefore it seems likely that the β-ovomucin component is substantially responsible for the gelatinous properties of the thick egg white gel.

Degradative studies on isolated β-ovomucin, using proteolytic enzymes to hydrolyse the peptide moieties, have shown that at least some of the carbohydrate of the β-ovomucin molecule exists as trisaccharide units linked to serine or threonine residues (Fig. 5.26). It is now thought that the β-ovomucin component may be responsible at the molecular level for the gelatinous properties of thick egg white, through either self-association and entanglement, or by electrostatic interaction with lysozyme which is a cationic protein. Unlike some of the other food gels, thick egg white exhibits shear thinning. This thixotropic property suggests that entanglement of polymer chains, rather than the existence of knots and localised junctions, is responsible for the semi-solid nature of the thick albumen gel. However, while it is clear that β-ovomucin is solubilised, and probably degraded, during the natural liquefaction of the thick egg white gel, the mechanism by which the solubilisation occurs remains unknown (Robinson 1987).

Table 5.11 The carbohydrates of egg white glycoproteins

	Glucosamine	Galactosamine
Ovalbumin	1.2	—
Ovotransferrin	1.7	—
Ovomucoids	9.5–17.7	—
α-Ovomucin	5.4	0.5
β-Ovomucins	12.3	8.9
Flavoprotein	8.7	—
Ovoglycoprotein	13.8	—
Ovomacroglobulin	5.5	—
Ovoinhibitors	2.8–5.6	—
Avidin	4.1	—

(From Robinson 1972).

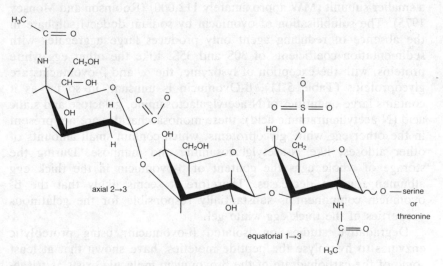

Fig. 5.26 Possible structure of β-ovomucin trisaccharide (by permission of the publishers, Butterworth and Co. (Publishers) Ltd. ©, ed. R. Wells, Robinson 1987)

THE FUNCTIONAL PROPERTIES OF SEED STORAGE PROTEINS

These are of three main types: the water-soluble albumins, the alcohol-soluble prolamins and the salt-soluble globulins. For cereals the prolamins are the main storage protein, whereas the albumins and globulins are of cytoplasmic origin. However, for legumes and many other seeds the salt-soluble globulins are major storage proteins.

Galactose (g/100 g)	Mannose	Sialic acid
—	1.7–2.0	—
—	0.9	—
0.53–4.07	6.4–8.6	0.03–2.23
1.8	4.6	1.0
22.00	0.7	13.8
1.1	3.9	0.86
4.5	9.0	3.0
(0.3)	—	
—	2.1–3.7	0.1–0.3
—	4.6	—

Cereal Proteins

Only the flours of wheat, and to a more limited extent flours of rye, are able to produce a viscoelastic dough which can be baked to produce a high-volume bread loaf. However, all the chemical interactions in wheat dough that occur between the flour proteins, lipids, starch, hemicelluloses, dextrins and enzymes are not understood at a molecular level – as shown by light microscopy wheat flour dough is a continuous matrix. Moreover, it is known that the water-insoluble gluten proteins of wheat, which represent approximately 80 per cent of the total cereal protein, make the major contribution to the rheological properties of bread dough. During the commercial manufacture of the wheat dough, the cereal proteins hydrate and under the influence of sheer stress, produced during mixing, orientate to form a viscoelastic dough. For biscuit manufacture a weak extensible dough with a low degree of elasticity performs best: the wheat flours are often weakened by pre-treatment with metabisulphite to reduce the disulphide bonds of the wheat flour gluten proteins. Likewise cake flours do not require high protein levels, and the characteristic microstructure of such products is provided by the interactions at the molecular level of other ingredients such as egg proteins and fats with the wheat proteins.

For the optimum development of wheat dough for bread manufacture a time-dependent input of mechanical energy is required with prescribed quantities of water, salt and improving agents. During the high-speed mixing used for the manufacture of bread, up to 9.5 kcal of energy per kg of flour are incorporated during a 3-min. period. It is assumed that this energy works the dough into a viscoelastic composite. During the baking of bread the three-dimensional structure of the mechanically developed dough is required to retain carbon dioxide by stretching of the elastic matrix. The carbon dioxide is formed during the fermentation of glucose. After baking, the desirable high volume of the loaf is maintained by a solid, but moist, protein–starch matrix. The rheological properties of the bread dough are correlated with both the total protein content of flour, and the content of insoluble glutenin proteins which form an elastic network within the dough. The overall protein content of the cereal flours should be of the order of 11 per cent. The most 'sticky' and desirable elastic glutens are obtained from wheat flour, whereas rye glutens are the less cohesive. Maize proteins do not possess any viscous or elastic properties.

Wheat gluten is obtained from wheat flour by washing out the wheat starch and cytoplasmic proteins with water. The gluten is a viscoelastic water-insoluble proteinaceous material. Approximately 66 per cent of gluten is water; protein represents approximately 27 per cent and lipid only from 5 to 10 per cent. Wheat gluten represents approximately 80 per cent of the total wheat flour protein. The water-insoluble gluten proteins can be fractionated with 70 per cent ethanol into alcohol-soluble gliadins and insoluble glutenins. The insoluble glutenins are believed to be substantially responsible for the rheological properties of wheat dough: it is believed that the glutenins of high molecular weights mainly determine the tensile strength and elasticity of bread doughs. Thus increasing efforts are being made to understand the amino acid sequences of gluten proteins, and the way in which they interact to form an insoluble, but hydrated, elastic copolymer.

The subdivision of gluten proteins into gliadins and glutenins is mainly historical and arbitrary, but is based on the different solubilities of low and high molecular weight wheat prolamins in organic alcohols like 70 per cent ethanol. The insoluble glutenins (MW $>10^6$), are polydisperse with respect to size and contain both inter- and intrachain disulphide bonds. The gliadins, which are soluble in aqueous alcohol and hence are prolamins, contain the α-, β-, γ-, ω-gliadins and can be separated and identified on the basis of their electrophoretic mobility. Gliadins are monomeric proteins and have molecular weights in the range 35,000 to 75,000. Gliadins contain only intrachain disulphide bonds. The less well defined insoluble glutenins have a similar amino acid composition to gliadins and after reduction of the disulphide bonds are also soluble in organic alcohols. The glutenins can be depolymerised by reduction of the disulphide bonds with mercaptoethanol. The high molecular weight (HMW) reduced subunits (MW 95,000–145,000) are soluble in alcohols, such as aqueous propan-1-ol (50% w/w) at 60°C. Therefore the glutenins can be considered to be just high molecular weight prolamins (Byers *et al*. 1983), which are higher polymers of glutenin subunits rendered insoluble by the presence of interchain disulphide bonds. This new classification for cereal glutenins which is

Table 5.12 Reclassification of cereal prolamins

	Barley	Rye	Wheat
High molecular weight (HMW) prolamins	D-Hordein	HMW secalin	HMW glutenins
Sulphur-poor prolamins	C-Hordein	ω-Secalin	ω-Gliadin
Sulphur-rich prolamins	B-Hordein	γ-Secalin	α-,β- and γ-gliadins and the low MW subunits of glutenins

(After Shewry *et al.* 1984a).

now based on the chemical composition and the known molecular structure of all prolamins is given in Table 5.12.

The wheat flour glutenins with molecular weights of several millions, shown schematically in Fig. 5.27 are believed to form an extensive disulphide-bonded network of polypeptide chains.

By electrophoresis it has been shown that reduced glutenins are composed of approximately fifteen separate subunits. Amino acid analysis of the HMW subunits has shown that glutamine, proline and

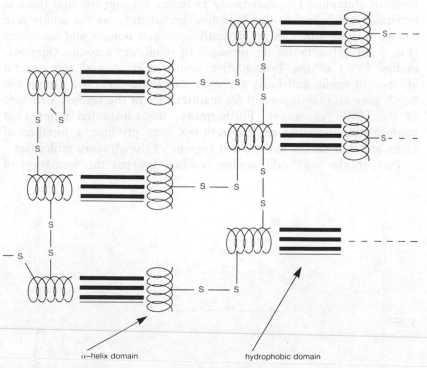

α–helix domain   hydrophobic domain

Fig. 5.27 Schematic diagram of helical, hydrophobic domains and intermolecular disulphide linkages for HMW prolamins of wheat

Table 5.13   The main amino acids (moles %) in some prolamin high molecular weight subunits[†]

Peptide designation	1A,2[‡]	1Bx,7	1Dx,5	1Dy,10
Thr	3.0	3.6	3.0	3.4
Ser	7.0	8.5	6.1	5.9
Glx[§]	39.2	36.8	38.6	33.7
Pro	13.8	12.6	13.5	14.0
Gly	16.0	17.8	17.9	17.7
Ala	2.4	3.2	3.2	3.2
Cys	0.7	0.5	0.6	1.5
Val	1.7	1.5	1.8	2.8
Leu	5.0	3.0	4.7	4.4
Tyr	5.3	7.2	6.0	5.0
Arg	2.2	2.3	1.5	2.2

([†] After Shewry et al. 1984b).

[§] Glx is believed to be 90 per cent glutamine.

[‡] Variety Cheyenne.

glycine represent two-thirds of the total protein (Table 5.13). The high levels of glutamine (approximately 35 moles %) suggests that there is extensive hydrogen bonding between the subunits, as the amide side chains of glutamine can act as both hydrogen donors and acceptors (Fig. 5.28). Also due to the presence of significant amounts (approximately 12%) of the hydrophobic amino acids – and the general absence of acidic and basic amino acids (Table 5.13) – hydrophobic bonds may also be important for maintenance of the tertiary structure of the HMW prolamins. Furthermore, the substantial number of conformation-directing proline residues may produce a number of turns between helical and β-sheet regions of the glutenin molecules.

Polypeptides with odd proline residues prevent the formation of

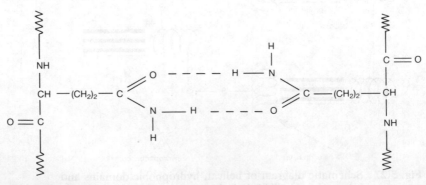

Fig. 5.28 Hydrogen bonding of glutamine residues

Table 5.14 N-Terminal aligned homologous
sequences of high molecular weight prolamin
subunits from cultivars of wheat[†]

Residues	
$1 \rightarrow 5$	Glu–Gly–Glu–Ala–Ser
$7 \rightarrow 11$	Gln–Ile–Gln–Cys_{10}–Glu
$23 \rightarrow 27$	Lys–Ala–Cys_{25}*–Gln–Gln–Val

* The position of the second Cys residue changes slightly for
different varieties due to deletions of amino acids.

([†] From Shewry *et al.* 1984a,b).

α-helices as the ring nitrogen atom forms part of a rigid pyrollidone
ring that prevents free rotation of the peptide bond. Thus proline
residues are frequently found at bends and folds in the peptide chains.
Sequence analysis of some HMW subunits has indicated the presence
at the molecular level of separate protein domains. First there is a high
degree of homology in the N-terminal regions for a number of purified
glutenin subunits, where two important cysteine residues occur at
positions 10 and 25 near to the N-terminus of the polypeptide chains
(Table 5.14). Most of the small number of charged amino acid residues
are believed to be located in the N- and C-terminal regions of the
polypeptide chains of the HMW subunits. This indicates that the
central cores of the subunits may be enriched in hydrophobic amino
acids and thus form hydrophobic domains with regular β-turns
(Fig. 5.27). It is possible that such centralisation of hydrophobic
residues could provide the attractive force required for the elastic
property of gluten (Tatham *et al.* 1985): the coming together of a
number of hydrophobic residues to form central hydrophobic cores in
aggregated subunits during contraction would be energetically favourable. Furthermore, a similar elastic function for hydrophobic amino
acid residues has been postulated for the animal protein elastin (see
p. 206). The presence of covalent disulphide bonds between the α-
helical domains of the HMW subunits is similar to the presence of
cross-links between α-helical regions of elastin. Certainly the
occurrence of the sulphydryl group of cysteine residues at the N-
terminal ends of the molecules provides strong support for the linear
glutenin hypothesis (Ewart 1979).

During the mechanical development of wheat dough it is proposed
that the disulphide bonds rearrange by disulphide interchange reactions to produce more linear elastic polymers. General support for the
overall theory has existed for some time, as large amounts of thiol
reducing agents (e.g. metabisulphite) produce very weak non-elastic
doughs. Furthermore, there is generally a negative correlation between
the baking quality of flour and the content of the natural thiol reducing
agent, glutathione. Also the beneficial effect of flour improvers, such

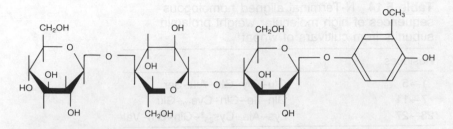

β–D–Glc*p*–(1→4)–β–D–Glc*p*–(1→4)–β–D– Glc*p*–(1→1′)–3′–methoxyhydroquinone

Fig. 5.29 The structure of a wheat flour hydroquinone (Graveland *et al.* 1984)

as bromate and ascorbate, is believed to be due to oxidation of the glutathione sulphydryl group, which otherwise impedes the desirable formation of disulphide bonds. Nevertheless, all the biochemical reactions involved in dough development are not yet understood. It has been suggested (Graveland *et al.* 1984) that a hydroquinone (Fig. 5.29) together with superoxide ion – derived from atmospheric oxygen – could be responsible for reducing disulphide bonds in wheat dough. However, more than a casual relationship needs to be established to prove that the hydroquinone is responsible for initiating disulphide interchange reactions in wheat dough.

The other gluten proteins, traditionally known as gliadins (low molecular weight prolamins), are thought to be responsible for the viscosity of wheat doughs possibly through the formation of microfibrils. The interaction of lipids with other proteins at the molecular level during the development of wheat dough is also not understood.

Electrophoresis of gliadins shows the presence of a large number of different proteins, in the ω-, γ-, β- and α-gliadin fractions. Different characteristic patterns for the gliadins are observed for different cultivars of wheat (Fig. 5.30) and therefore electrophoresis can be used for identification of wheat varieties. The range of molecular weights for rye, barley and wheat prolamins is given in Table 5.15. This classification of all prolamins based on the composition and molecular structure subdivides the gliadins into sulphur-rich and sulphur-poor proteins. However, like the HMW subunits, the gliadins are very

Table 5.15 A comparison of the molecular weights of prolamins†

	Rye	Barley	Wheat
Sulphur-rich	40–75,000	35–46,000	32–44,000
Sulphur-poor	48–53,000	55–72,000	44–74,000
HMW reduced subunits		105,000	95–136,000

† Determined by electrophoresis (after Miflin *et al.* 1983).

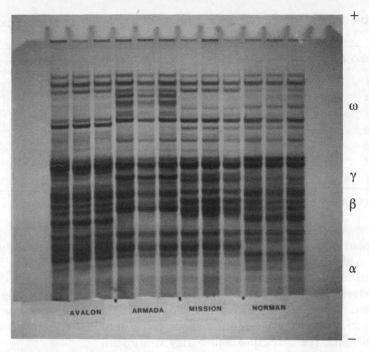

Fig. 5.30 Electrophoretic analysis of gliadin proteins (kindly supplied by
Mrs S. Salmon, Flour Milling and Baking Research Association,
Chorleywood). The proteins of individual wheat grains are
crushed and extracted in 130 μl of 6 % urea. Electrophoresis was
carried out at pH 3.1 in 0.188 M acetic acid–glycine buffer

heterogeneous. The sulphur-rich prolamins (Table 5.15) correspond to
the previously named wheat α- β- and γ-gliadins, barley B-hordein and
rye γ-secalins all of which have a similar amino acid composition
(Table 5.16). However, the sulphur-rich proteins exist as monomers
where the disulphide bonds are of the intramolecular type. The

Table 5.16 The main amino acids (mole %) sulphur-rich prolamins

Amino acid	Rye α-secalin	Barley B-hordein	Wheat gliadins		
			α(A)	β_5	γ_1
Glx	34.8	35.4	38.1	39.6	41.7
Pro	18.4	20.6	14.8	15.8	15.1
Gly	2.4	1.5	2.6	1.9	2.4
Phe	5.3	4.8	3.8	3.7	3.7
Cys	2.5	2.5	2.1	1.8	1.8
Met	1.0	0.6	0.8	1.1	0.9
Lys	0.7	0.5	0.5	0.2	0.1

(Ater Shewry *et al*. 1984a).

Table 5.17   The significant amino acids (mole %) of sulphur-poor prolamins

Amino acid	Rye ω-secalin	Barley C-hordein	Wheat ω-gliadin	
Glx	42.9	41.2	43	53
Pro	30.6	30.6	20	30
Gly	1.4	0.3	0.9	1.4
Phe	7.4	8.8	8.1	8.9
Cys	0	0	0	0
Met	0.1	0.2	0	0.1
Lys	0.3	0.2	0.1	0.3

(After Shewry *et al.* 1984a).

sulphur-poor proteins correspond to the previously well known group of ω-gliadins, barley C-hordein and rye ω-secalins (Table 5.17). Glutamine and proline account for approximately 70 per cent of the residues, cystine is absent, and so ω-gliadins do not form disulphide-linked polymers. Sequence homologies which establish a common ancestral origin have been found for the N-terminal regions of wheat ω-gliadins, rye ω-secalins and barley C-hordein.

In conclusion it must be said that the apparent diversity of the wheat proteins is being resolved through the reclassification of all cereal storage proteins as prolamins. The albumins and globulins are classified as cytoplasmic proteins. For all cereal prolamins, which have previously been given trivial names according to the species from which they have been isolated, it now seems that there are usually two major components of different average molecular weight. Although the genetics of hexaploid wheats with forty-two paired chromosomes contained in three genomes (A, B, D) – each with seven pairs of chromosomes – is complicated, it is thought that the high molecular weight subunits are encoded in small multigene families at single genetic loci on A, B and D chromosomes. With few exceptions all varieties of wheat possess from three to five HMW subunits. The baking properties of wheat flours are probably dependent on the occurrence of specific sequences and spacing of amino acids within the terminal regions of the HMW subunit polypeptide chains. Moonen *et al.* (1985) have claimed that two of their identified subunits (10 and 11) contain more cysteine residues and are therefore capable of forming extended disulphide-bonded glutenin networks.

Legume proteins

No special functional property of major commercial importance has been developed for legume proteins which is comparable to the dough-forming characteristics of cereal prolamins. Only the gelation property of soybean protein has been used in canned foods and particularly by the pet food industry. Generally there are only three types of leguminous ingredients available for use in further processed products; these are legume flours, concentrates (70 % protein) and isolates (90 % protein). Such manufactured ingredients are used for nutrient supplementation, the manufacture of extruded products, and in the case of soybean, the formation of thermostable gels. In general the leguminous storage proteins are insoluble and exist as aggregates in aqueous solutions; they are synthesised by plants to provide a compact source of nitrogen and amino acids for germinating seeds.

In the temperate zones legume crops like peas and beans are seasonal. Legume seeds contain between 18 and 42 per cent protein, and are deficient in the essential sulphur-containing amino acids. The soybean has received considerable attention for use as a protein supplement, due to the high yields obtained per unit area, the availability of land in the United States, freedom of the plant from disease, the high protein content (42 %) and the relative absence of toxic compounds in the seed. In addition to Oriental foods, such as tofu and tempeh, soybean proteins are being added world wide to meat products, soups and dairy products. Protein gels, as opposed to polysaccharide gels, are manufactured from either soybean or gelatin. When heated a dispersion (2 % w/v) of soy protein first increases in viscosity to form a progel which then solidifies on cooling. Gels are also induced by either Ca^{2+} ions (tofu gel), alkali or alkali–alcohol solutions. Upon heating soy proteins initially undergo dissociation followed by intermolecular interactions to form the progel. Excessive heat irreversibly degrades the progel proteins and results in the conversion of the progel to a 'metasol', which does not set on cooling.

$$\text{Soy protein dispersion} \xrightarrow{\text{heat } (>80°C)} \text{progel} \underset{\text{heat}}{\overset{\text{cool}}{\rightleftharpoons}} \text{gel}$$

The crude soy protein is a mixture of different proteins. Historically, soybean globulins have been classified in order of their sedimentation coefficients as measured by analytical ultracentrifugation. The 2S component contains the Kunitz and Bowman–Birk inhibitors (Ch. 4) and the 15S component may be aggregates of the 11S component. The most important component for gelation is the 11S globulin. The basis for the classification is shown in Fig. 5.31 and the proportion of each protein fraction is given in Table 5.18.

The 11S protein fraction of soybean, at a minimum concentration of 2.5 per cent (w/w), forms gels of high tensile strength. Calcium-induced tofu gels, made from the 11S protein fraction, are also harder than those gels obtained from the other main protein sedimenting component (the 7S globulin).

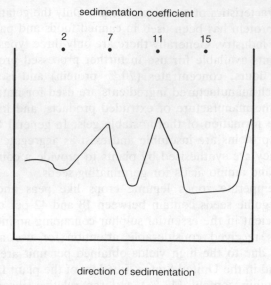

Fig. 5.31 Diagrammatic representation of the ultracentrifugation pattern for water-soluble soybean proteins

Table 5.18 Classification of soybean storage proteins

Sedimentation coefficient	Percentage composition	Protein components	Molecular weights
2S	20	α-Conglycinin Proteinase inhibitors	8000–25,000
7S	35	β-Conglycinin (vicilin) plus enzymes	190,000
11S	30	Glycinin (legumin)	350,000
15S	10	Aggregated legumins	700,000

The seed storage proteins of legumes are located in storage organelles called protein bodies. The storage proteins are of the globulin type, as they are only soluble in aqueous salt solutions or dissociating solvents. Cytoplasmic proteins are the enzymes responsible for catalysis of metabolic reactions and are generally soluble in water or dilute salt solutions. The more insoluble legume storage proteins are characterised by high contents of both glutamine and asparagine. The storage proteins are of two main types: legumins (11S) and vicilins (7S), which traditionally have been classified according to their sedimentation coefficients (Table 5.19). In the case of soybeans, 90 per cent of the seed protein consists of salt-soluble globulins, whereas

Table 5.19   The empirical properties of legumes storage proteins

	Legumins	Vicilins
Sedimentation coefficient	11S	7S
Water solubility	Slightly soluble	More soluble
Sulphur amino acids	Present	Small or absent
Carbohydrate	Absent	Present

Vicia faba, Pisum sativum and *Phaseolus vulgaris* contain only 10 to 20 per cent of globulins. Glycinin and conglycinin are the common names for the soybean 11S legumins and 7S vicilins, respectively, as shown in Table 5.18. The distribution of legumins and vicilins between species is also highly variable; the broad bean (*Vicia faba*) is enriched with legumins, while the great Northern bean (*Phaseolus vulgaris*) contains mainly vicilins (7S); the storage proteins of wrinkled peas may contain up to 66 per cent of vicilins. The soybean storage proteins show a minimum solubility at pH 4.0 to 5.0 (Fig. 5.32) as the two principal storage proteins have their isoelectric points in this pH range. Concentrates and isolates can be obtained by precipitation at the isoelectric point. The legumins can be obtained either after cooling aqueous extracts to 4 °C by calcium precipitation or by gel filtration. A considerable amount of knowledge for the molecular structure of glycinins (Nakamura *et al.* 1984, Peng *et al.* 1984) and other legumins from peas (Gatehouse *et al.* 1984) is now available. Such information permits comparisons and generalisations to be made for the amino acid sequences, subunit and quaternary structures of legumins and vicilins

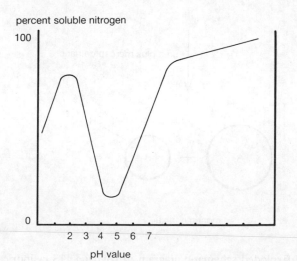

Fig. 5.32   The water solubility of soybean proteins as a function of pH value

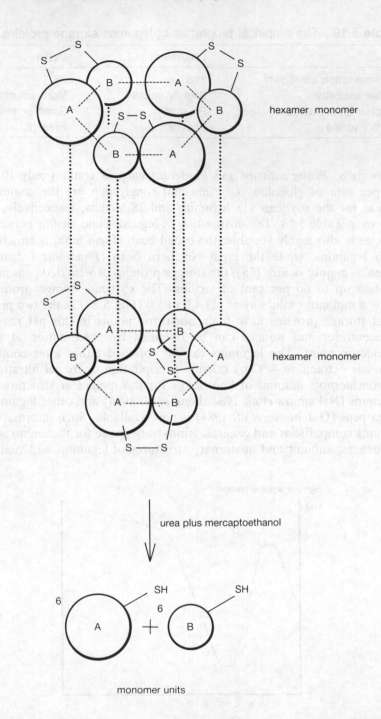

Fig. 5.33 Exploded schematic diagram of soybean 11S cylindrical aggregate of six acidic and six basic monomer units (after Pernollet and Mossé 1983)

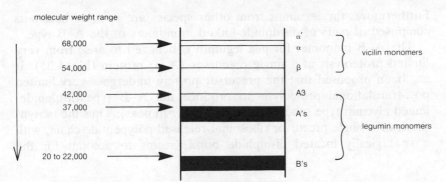

molecular weight range

68,000	α'
	α } vicilin monomers
54,000	β
42,000	A3
37,000	A's } legumin monomers
20 to 22,000	B's

Fig. 5.34 Diagram of sodium dodecylsulphate gel electrophoresis of soybean protein monomers after reduction (after Staswick *et al.* 1983)

for various legume species. All the legumins described to date are oligomers of distinct protein dimeric subunits composed of an acidic and a basic monomer held together by a disulphide bond (A–S–S–B). The legumins are not glycoproteins. The vicilins are also dimers or trimers, but do not contain disulphide bonds. All the vicilins from different species seem to be glycoproteins.

For soybean, the glycinin 11S component (Fig. 5.33) is thought to be composed of two identical hexagonal subunits which form a hollow oblate cylinder with dimensions of $110 \times 110 \times 75$ Å (Peng *et al.* 1984). Each hexagon ring is believed to contain the three smaller intermediary subunits (A–S–S–B type) composed of three pairs of various acidic (MW 34,000 to 38,000)) and basic (MW 7000 to 20,000) proteins. Thus each 11S globulin aggregate (approximate MW 350,000) is a hexamer which consists of six intermediary subunits (6AB) and hence twelve monomeric proteins – six acidic (6A) and six basic (6B) proteins. The different types of legumin acidic (AI to IV) and basic monomers (BI to IV) can be separated by electrophoresis after reduction of the disulphide bond (Fig. 5.34). For the overall hexagonal layered structures of glycinin it is not known whether all the hexagon units possess an identical subunit composition. Sequence analysis for amino acids has shown for the four acidic subunits the occurrence of common sequences in each subunit. The acidic monomer units are characterised by their high contents of glutamic acid and proline, whereas the basic monomer units contain more leucine, tyrosine, valine and phenylalanine. Structural comparisons with legumins isolated from other legume species have also established some sequence homologies. These are particularly apparent for the basic subunits where residues 22 to 29 are identical (Pernollet and Mossé 1983):

Species	Sequence
Soybean	Asp_{22}–Leu–Tyr–Asn–Pro–Gln–Ala–Gly_{29}
Broadbean	
Pea	

Furthermore, the legumins from other species are possibly hexamers composed of pairs of disulphide-linked monomers of the A–B type.

The A–B monomer for pea legumin is believed to arise from very limited proteolysis of a single precursor (A,B) protein (Fig. 5.35). It has been proposed that the precursor protein undergoes very limited post-translational proteolysis to produce the A–B type disulphide-linked glycinin type subunit (α- and β-dimer in peas). Thus the biosynthesis of a single precursor ribosomal released polypeptide chain, with a strategically located disulphide bond, seems to account for the

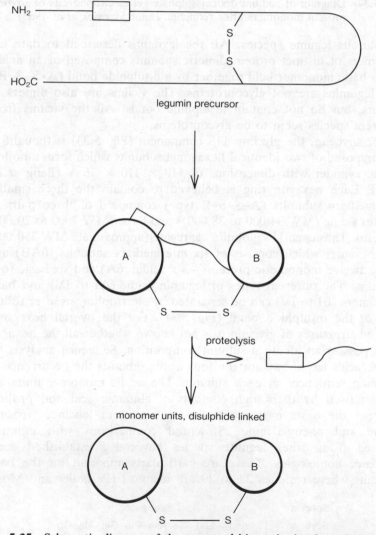

Fig. 5.35 Schematic diagram of the proposed biosynthesis of pea legumin subunits (after Gatehouse *et al.* 1984)

formation of the disulphide linked A–B pairs in legumins.

The major 7S vicilin protein (β-conglycinin) of soybean contains 6 per cent carbohydrate, and is believed to be composed of three subunits. The subunits are compactly folded glycoproteins with significant hydrophobic regions. The subunits are noncovalently linked, as the 7S vicilin dissociates in 6 M urea and reassociates on dialysis to produce a number of trimeric molecules (Lee and Lopez 1984). The vicilins contain negligible amounts of the sulphur amino acids and therefore disulphide bonds are not responsible for the formation of the vicilin trimer. From sequencing of cloned complimentary DNA (cDNA) for pea vicilin (MW approximately 150,000), the amino acid sequence of a precursor protein (MW approximately 50,000) has been predicted (Gatehouse et al. 1984). For pea vicilins it has been proposed that the molecules (MW approximately 50,000) of precursor protein after secretion undergo glycosylation, and some very limited proteolysis before subsequent assembly into a trimeric 7S vicilin component (Fig. 5.36). For the vicilin of pea (*Pisum sativum*) Gatehouse et al. (1983) have shown that proteolytic cleavage of the precursor protein is located in the polar regions of the protein

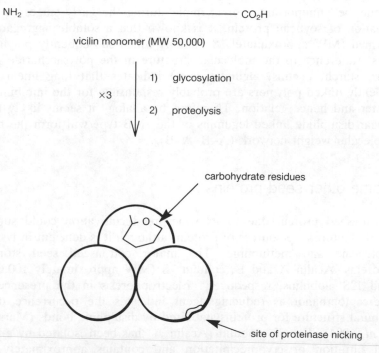

Fig. 5.36   Schematic diagram of the proposed biosynthesis of pea vicilin (after Gatehouse et al. 1984)

molecule. A number of different precursors of pea vicilin give rise to diverse vicilin species, which contain slightly different amino acid sequences which in turn determine the sites of post-translational proteolysis. It seems that the precursors must be specified by a number of vicilin genes which differ in their coding sequences. Smaller protein fragments (MW approximately 33,000, 19,000, 13,500) which are immunologically similar to vicilins are thought to be formed by further proteolytic degradation of the vicilin precursor during the storage of leguminous seeds. For *Vicia faba* seeds it has been shown that the proteinase inhibitor, leupeptin, inhibits the degradation of the bean vicilin (Scholz *et al*. 1983). Thus changes in the subunit composition of vicilins during storage and germination of legume seeds can be explained by proteolysis, and it seems likely that the type of precursor protein (MW approximately 50,000) and trimeric structure (MW approximately 150,000) is common to most legume seed vicilins.

The association of monomers for both the legumins and vicilins and the formation of packed hexagonal and trigonal aggregates, respectively, clearly permits maximum packing of these storage proteins in the seed protein bodies in order to meet the later needs of the germinating seed. However, for the utilisation of legumes as human food, in solution or dispersion, such packing at the molecular level seems be unimportant. For example during the early stages of the gelation of soybean protein, it is known that a soluble aggregate is formed (MW approximately 8 million) which subsequently polymerises. Reference to the molecular structure of the polysaccharide gels (viz. starch, pectins, alginates, etc.) indicates that long linear covalently linked polymers are probably responsible for the imbibing of water and hence gelation. Therefore by analogy it seems likely that linear disulphide linked legumins of the A–B type will form the high molecular weight network $(A–B–A–B)_n$.

Some other seed proteins

Cottonseed protein due to its widespread cultivation could supply limited alternative sources of protein, although it is deficient in lysine, isoleucine and methionine. The major cottonseed seed storage proteins, Acalin A and B, contain 7S (MW approximately 100,000) and 12S globulins, respectively. Electrophoresis in the presence of mercaptoethanol as reducing agent indicates the occurrence of a subunit structure for proteins stabilised by disulphide bonds (Marshall *et al*. 1984). The 7S globulin (Acalin A) has been isolated by either gel filtration or cryoprecipitation and contains approximately six separate polypeptide chains. It is thought that disulphide bonds form covalent links between monomers that aggregate to form the 7S globulin. Proteolysis during storage and isolation of the cottonseed proteins may be responsible for the occurrence of low molecular weight peptides in cottonseeds. However, a clear pattern for the subunit structure for the 7S and 12S cottonseed globulins has not yet emerged.

Although sunflower (*Helianthus annuus*) is a major source of vegetable oil, knowledge of the textural and structural properties of sunflower seed proteins is small when compared with the leguminous seeds. However, high molecular weight globulins (MW approximately 300,000), which represent from 70 to 80 per cent of the sunflower seed protein, with sedimentation coefficients of 11S, have been detected. These are believed (Dalgalarrondo *et al.* 1984) to consist of smaller acidic and basic subunits linked covalently by disulphide bonds to form intermediary subunits of the A–B type. The subunits can be separated by chromatography and electrophoresis in the presence of either mercaptoethanol or dithiothreitol as reducing agents. Based on electrophoresis, the intermediary subunits are predominantly of the A–B type with molecular weights ranging from 23,000 to 42,000. Thus the sunflower globulin subunits are similar in size to those subunits described for pea and bean globulins. Sesame (*Sesamum indicum*) is an oil seed plant of the Pedaliaceae family. An α-globulin which represents approximately 70 per cent of the total seed protein sediments with a sedimentation coefficient of 13S. The protein is oligomeric and is composed of six dimeric units (MW approximately 50,000). As for the soybean 11S globulin, the dimeric unit is of the A–B type linked by a disulphide bond. Likewise sesame proteins form gels on heating. Also it seems that linseed (*Linum usitatissimum*) storage proteins contain a 12S globulin which consists of six subunits.

KEY FACTS

1.   Meat consists of longitudinal filaments composed of mainly linear actin and myosin molecules.

2.   During muscular contraction, glycogen and ATP are hydrolysed and tropomyosin moves further into the groove between actin filaments: binding sites on the F-actin molecules are exposed for increased interaction with the myosin globular heads.

3.   In meat excessive shortening of muscle fibres can be initiated by either stress on the animal before death, or incorrect cutting of the muscle fibres and rapid cooling to less than 11 °C. Released intracellular Ca^{2+} triggers the hydrolysis of ATP and glycogen.

4.   Proteolysis catalysed by cathepsins and a Ca^{2+}-activated proteinase seem to be partly responsible for the processes of tenderisation during the 'ageing' of chilled meat.

5.   The swelling and juiciness of meat is influenced by protein–protein

interactions. Pyrophosphate and sodium chloride used commercially enhance the swelling volume of meat by reducing protein–protein interactions. The adhesive and binding properties of cooked meats are thought to be due to the heat denaturation of solubilised proteins which coat meat particles.

6.   During the cooking of meat, collagen shrinks and imposes a transverse squeezing force on the hydrated myofibrillar proteins.

7.   In the collagen chains the unique triplet amino acid sequence Gly–X–Y is necessary for helix formation. X and Y are conformation-directing imino acids.

8.   A strong collagen matrix is provided at the molecular level by both linear twining of polypeptide chains to form a triple helix and intermolecular cross-links between lysyl and lysyl aldehyde residues. Both aldimine and ketoamine cross-links occur.

9.   Elastin contains cross-links composed of pyridinium compounds. Pentapeptide sequences containing conformational-directing proline residues form spirals. The elastic properties are due to the reversible energetically unfavourable exposure of hydrophobic regions of the elastin molecule to water molecules during extension.

10.   For the formation of food gels, as with gelatin or soybean proteins intermolecular links are required.

11.   Casein micelles are suspended aggregates of α_s, β and κ-caseins. κ-Casein resides on the surface of the micelle.

12.   Alcohol-soluble prolamins, often given trivial names, are the main storage proteins of cereals.

13.   Disulphide bonds, and cysteine residues play an important part through disulphide interchange reactions in the rheological properties of egg albumen, wheat gluten and soybean proteins. The disposition of disulphides and hydrophobic domains in wheat glutenins determines the molecular structure and elasticity of wheat dough.

14.   For leguminous seeds, the major storage proteins are salt-soluble multimeric globulins – legumins and vicilins. Legumins are aggregates of a dimeric protein composed of acidic and basic monomer units joined together by a disulphide bond.

REFERENCES

Adelstein, R. S. and Eisenberg, E. (1980) 'Regulation and kinetics of the actin–myosin–ATP interaction', *Ann. Rev. Biochem.*, **49**, 921–56.

Bailey, A. J. (1984) 'Chemistry of intramolecular collagen', in Special Publication no. 47, *Recent Advances in the Chemistry of Meat* (ed. Bailey, A. J.). Royal Society of Chemistry, London.

Bailey, A. J. and Etherington, D. J. (1980), 'Metabolism of collagen and elastin, comprehensive biochemistry', in *Protein Metabolism*, vol. 19B, part

1 (eds. Florkin, M., Neuberger, A. and Van Deenen, L. L. M.). Elsevier, Amsterdam.

Bird, J. W. C., Spanier, A. M. and Schwartz, W. N. (1978) 'Cathepsins B and D: proteolytic activity and ultrastructural localisation in skeletal muscle'., in *Protein Turnover and Lysosomal Function* (eds Segal, H. L. and Doyle, D. J.). Academic Press, New York

Brooks, J. and Hale, H. P. (1959) 'The mechanical properties of the thick egg white of the hen's egg', *Biochim. Biophys. Acta*, **32**, 237–50.

Byers, M., Miflin, B. J. and Smith, S. J. (1983) 'A quantitative comparison of the extraction of protein fractions from wheat grain by different solvents and of the polypeptide and amino acid composition of the alcohol-soluble proteins', *J. Sci. Food Agric.*, **34**, 447–62.

Dalgalarrondo, M., Raymond, J, and Azanza, J. (1984) 'Sunflower seed proteins: characterisation and subunit composition of the globulin fraction', *J. Exp. Bot.*, **35**, 1618–28.

Davey, L. (1984). 'The structure of muscle and its properties as meat', in Special Publication no. 47, *Recent Advances in the Chemistry of Meat* (ed. Bailey, A. J.). Royal Society of Chemistry, London.

Ewart, J. A. D. (1979) 'Glutenin structure', *J. Sci. Food Agric.*, **30**, 482–92.

Eyre, D. R., Paz, M. A. and Gallop, P. M. (1984) 'Cross-linking in collagen and elastin', *Ann. Rev. Biochem.*, **53**, 717–48.

Fabiansson, S. and Reutersward, A. L. (1985) 'Low voltage electrical stimulation and post-mortem energy metabolism in beef', *Meat Sci.*, **12**, 205–23.

Gatehouse, J. A., Lycett, G. W., Delauney, A. J., Croy, R. R. D. and Boulter, D. (1983) 'Sequence specificity of the post-translational proteolytic cleavage of vicilin, a seed storage protein of pea (*Pisum sativum* L.)', *Biochem. J.*, **212**, 427–32.

Gatehouse, J. A., Croy, R. R. D. and Boulter, D. (1984) 'The synthesis and structure of pea storage proteins', *CRC Crit. Revs. Plant Sci.*, **1**, 287–314.

Grand, R. J. A. and Stainsby, G. (1976) 'N-Terminal imino-acids and gelatin gelation', in *Photographic Gelatin*, vol. 2 (ed. Cox, R. G.). Academic Press, London.

Graveland, A., Bosveld, P., Lichtendonk, W. J. and Moonen, J. H. E. (1984) 'Isolation and characterisation of (3-methoxy-4-hydroxyphenyl)-β-cellotrioside from wheat flour; a substance involved in the reduction of disulphide-linked glutenin aggregates', *J. Cer. Sci.*, **2**, 65–72.

Harper, E. (1980) 'Collagenases', *Ann. Rev. Biochem.*, **49**, 1063–78.

Jeacocke, R. E. (1984) 'The control of post-mortem metabolism and the onset of *rigor mortis*', in Special Publication no. 47, *Recent Advances in the Chemistry of Meat* (ed. Bailey, A. J.). Royal Society of Chemistry, London.

Johnson, T. M. and Zabic, M.E. (1981a) 'Egg albumen proteins and interactions in an Angel food cake system', *J. Food Sci.*, **46**, 1231–6.

Johnson, T. M. and Zabic, M. E. (1981b) 'Ultrastructural examination of egg albumen protein foams', *J. Food Sci.*, **46**, 1237–40

Kinsella, J. E. (1985) 'Milk Proteins: physicochemical and functional properties', in *CRC Crit. Revs. Food Sci. Nutr.*, **21**, 197–262.

Kuehler, C. A. and Stine, C. M. (1974) 'Effect of enzymatic hydrolysis on some functional properties of whey protein', *J. Food Sci.*, **39**, 379–82.

Lee, J. W. and Lopez, A (1984) 'Modification of plant proteins by immobilised proteases', *CRC Crit. Revs. Food Sci. Nutr.*, **21**, 289–322.

Locker, R. H., Daines, G. J., Caŕse, W. A. and Left, N. G. (1977) 'Meat tenderness and the gap filament', *Meat Sci.*, **1**, 87–104.

Marshall, K. R. (1982) 'Industrial isolation of milk proteins: whey proteins', in *Developments in Dairy Chemistry* 1. *Proteins* (ed. Fox, P. F.). Applied Science Publishers, London.

Marshall, H. F., Shirer, M. A. and Cherry, J. P. (1984) 'Characterisation of glandless cottonseed storage proteins by sodium dodocyl sulphate–polyacrylamide gel electrophoresis', *Cereal Chem.*, **61**, 166–9.

Miflin, B. J., Field, J. M. and Shewry, P. R. (1983) 'Cereal storage proteins and their effect on technological properties', in *Annual Proceedings of the Phytochemical Society of Europe*, no. 20 *Seed Proteins* (eds. Daussant, J., Mossé, J. and Vaughan, J). Academic Press I., London

Miller, A. J., Ackerman, S. A. and Palumbo, S. A. (1980) 'Effects of frozen storage on functionality of meat for processing', *J. Food Sci.*, **45**, 1466–71.

Millward, D. J. (1980) 'Protein degradation in muscle and liver', in *Comprehensive Biochemistry, Protein Metabolism*, vol. 19B, part I (eds. Florkin, M., Neuberger, A. and Van Deenen, L. L. M.). Elsevier, Amsterdam.

Moonen, J. H. E., Scheepstra, A. and Graveland, A. (1985) 'Biochemical properties of some high molecular weight subunits of wheat glutenin', *J. Cer. Sci.*, **3**, 17–27.

Nakamura, T., Utsumi, S., Kitamura, K. Harada, K. and Mori, T. (1984) 'Cultivar differences in gelling characteristics of soyabean glycinin', *J. Agric. Food Chem.*, **32**, 647–51.

Offer, G. and Trinick, J. (1983) 'On the mechanism of water holding in meat: The swelling and shrinking of myofibrils', *Meat Sci.*, **8**, 245–81.

Peng, I. G., Quass, D. W., Dayton, W. R. and Allen, C. E. (1984) 'The physicochemical and functional properties of soybean 11S globulin – a review', *Cereal Chem.*, **61**, 480–90.

Pernollet, J-C. and Mossé, J. (1983) 'Structure and location of legume and cereal seed storage proteins', in *Seed Proteins* (eds. Daussant, J., Mossé, J. and Vaughan, J.). Academic Press, London.

Robinson, D. S. (1972) 'Egg white glycoproteins and the physical properties of egg white', in *Egg Formation and Production* (eds. Freeman, B. M. and Lake, P. E.), Poultry Science Symposium no. 8. British Poultry Science, Edinburgh.

Robinson, D. S. (1987) 'The chemical basis of albumen quality', in *Egg Quality – Current Problems and Recent Advances*. Butterworths, London.

Robinson, D. S. and Monsey, J. B. (1975) 'The composition and proposed subunit structure of egg white β-ovomucin: the isolation of an unreduced soluble ovomucin', *Biochem. J.*, **147**, 55–62.

Scholz, G., Manteuffel, R., Müntz, K. and Rudolph, A. (1983) 'Low-molecular-weight polypeptides of vicilin from *Vicia faba* L. are products of proteolytic breakdown', *Eur. J. Biochem.*, **132**, 103–7.

Shewry, P. R., Miflin, B. J. and Kasarda, D. D. (1984a) 'The structural and evolutionary relationship of the prolamin storage proteins of barley, rye, wheat', *Phil. Trans. R. Soc., Lond B.*, **304**, 297–308.

Shewry, P. R., Field, J. M. and others. (1984b) 'The purification and N-terminal amino acid sequence analysis of the high molecular weight gluten polypeptides of wheat', *Biochim. Biophys. Acta*, **788**, 23–34.

Staswick, P. E., Broué, P. and Nielsen, N. C. (1983) 'Glycinin composition of several perennial species related to soyabean', *Plant Physiol.*, **72**, 1114–18.

Swaisgood, H. E. (1982) 'Chemistry of milk protein', in *Developments in Dairy Chemistry* 1. Proteins (ed. Fox, P. F.). Applied Science Publishers, London.

Tasneem, R., Ramamani, S. and Subramanian, N. (1982) 'Functional properties of guar seed (*Cyamopsis tetragonoloba*) meal detoxified by different methods', *J. Food Sci.*, **47**, 1323–8.

Tatham, A. S., Miflin, B. J. and Shewry, P. R. (1985) 'The beta-turn conformation in wheat gluten proteins: relationship to gluten elasticity', *Cereal Chem.*, **62**, 405–12.

Van Deenen, L. L. M., Urry, D. W., Venkatachalam, C. M., Long, M. M. and Prasad, K. U. (1983) 'Dynamic β-spirals and a liberational entropy mechanism of elasticity', in *Conformations and Biology* (eds. Scrinvasan, R. and Sarma, R. M.). Adenine Press, New York.

Winger, R J. (1979) 'The assessment of meat texture', *Food Technol. N.Z.*, **14**(3), 15–25.

ADDITIONAL READING

Altschul, A. M. and Wilcke, H. L. (1985) *New Protein Foods*, vol. 5. Academic Press, London.

Bailey, A. J. and Etherington, D. J. (1980) 'Metabolism of collagen and elastin, comprehensive Biochemistry', in *Protein Metabolism*, vol. 19B, part 1. (eds. Florkin, M., Neuberger, A. and Van Deenen, L. L. M.). Elsevier, Amsterdam.

Bailey, A. J. (1984) Special Publication no. 47, *Recent Advances in the Chemistry of Meat*. Royal Society of Chemistry, London.

Cherry, J. P. (1982). *Food Protein Deterioration. Mechanisms and Functionality.*, ACS Symp. ser. 206, American Chemical, Society, Washington DC.

Daussant, J., Mossé, J. and Vaughan, J. (1983), *Ann. Proc. Phytochem. Soc. Europe* no. 20. *Seed Proteins*. Academic Press, London.

Gatehouse, J. A., Croy, R. R. D. and Boulter, D. (1984) 'The synthesis and structure of pea storage proteins', *CRC Crit. Revs. Plant Sci.*, **1**, 287–314.

Ledward, D. A. (1986) 'Gelation of gelatin', in *Functional Properties of Food Macromolecules* (eds Mitchell, J. R. and Ledward, D. A.). Elsevier Applied Science Publishers. London.

NRC/NAS (1980). National Research Council Committee on Dietary Allowances. *Recommended Dietary Allowances*, 9th edn. National Academy of Sciences Press, Washington DC.

Parry, D. A. D. and Creamer, L. K. (1979) *Fibrous Proteins: Scientific, Industrial and Medical Aspects*, vol. 1. Academic Press, London.

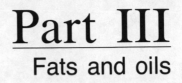

Part III
Fats and oils

CHAPTER 6

Lipids

INTRODUCTION

Fats are used extensively by the food industry for the manufacture of margarine, lard, cream-like products, confectionery products and fried foods.

For animals dietary fats and oils perform a variety of functions. Weight for weight fats offer over twice as much energy (9 kcal per g) as carbohydrates (4 kcal per g). In the SI system the energy values are protein (16 kJ), carbohydrate (17 kJ) and fat (38 kJ) per gram. Fats are the richest sources of energy on a weight basis and most adults eat up to 150 g of fat per day. Unfortunately an excessive energy intake results in fat being laid down as a 'long-term' reserve with the concomitant increase in weight, as glycogen is utilised as the prime source of metabolic energy. Based on the FAO/WHO/UNU (1985) recommendation for energy intake and using a value of 9.0 kcal per g of digestible energy from fat, the calculated amounts of dietary fat intake for 40 per cent of the energy requirement are shown in Table 6.1. As well as being a readily available source of high energy, fats and oils have essential food uses: they provide the dietary essential fatty acids which man cannot synthesise; fats and oils are carriers for vitamins A, D, E and K; they are partly responsible for the structure of cell membranes; fats and oils increase the softness and creaming properties during the manufacture of cakes, bread and pastry; they also affect the flavour of foods.

The terms fats and oils have been used synonymously, as both substances possess the same basic chemical structure. Oils are fats which melt below room temperature. Thus most vegetable seed fats, being liquid at room temperature, are oils. The physical nature of a fat is determined by the types of fatty acids present. Coconut oil and palm kernel oils, which are rich in lauric and myristic acids have lower melting points (approximately 25–28 °C) and are relatively hard solid fats at a temperature between 13 and 18 °C. The main requirement in

Table 6.1   Estimated energy and fat requirements per day

Occupation	Work level	Energy requirement[†] (kcal)	Projected fat intake[‡] (g)
Male office clerk (65 kg)	Light activity	2580	115
Subsistence farmer (58 kg)	Moderate activity	2780	124
Male heavy worker (65 kg)	Heavy activity	3490	155
Retired male (60 kg)	Very light activity	1960	87
Housewife (55 kg)	Light activity	1990	88
Female in developing country	Light activity	2235	99

([†] FAO/WHO/UNU 1985).

[†] To provide 40 per cent of the required daily dietary energy (9 kcal ≡ 1 g of dietary fat).

the food industry is for fat which is solid and firm to withstand mechanical handling and melt just below human body temperature.
The triglycerides are non-polar lipids and are major constituents of plant and animal fats. In plants the triglycerides (triacylglycerols) are found mainly in oil droplets (spherosomes). In cereals the oil droplets are concentrated in the subaleurone layers and are easily extracted with alkanes. The fat content for a number of cereals is given in Table 6.2. In animals, fats are found mainly in the adipose tissue but also in cell membranes and dietary fats supply the essential polyunsaturated fatty acids which are precursors of prostaglandins. In whole milk the small amount of fat exists as a stable oil-in-water emulsion, whereas butter and margarine which contain water droplets suspended in an oil phase are water-in-oil emulsions. For animals, dietary fats also serve as carriers of fat-soluble vitamins.

NOMENCLATURE

The numbering of the carbon atoms in the alkane chain is normally from the carboxyl group. However, the terms n-3, n-6 and n-9 are used to describe polyunsaturated fatty acids and identify families in which the last double bond in the chain is 3, 6 or 9 carbon atoms, respectively, from the terminal methyl group. The polyunsaturated fatty acids may contain from two to six methylene-interrupted double

Table 6.2 The lipid content of cereals

Cereal	Lipid content (approximate %)
Oats	7
Oatmeal	6.2
Maize	4.5
Pearl millet	5.4
Brown rice	2.3
Wheat	1.9
Barley	2.1
Sorghum	3.4
Crude sorghum flour	2.5
Wheat starch[†]	1.1
Wheat germ	10
Barley starch[†]	1.0
Oat starch[†]	1.3
Maize meal	3.9
Maize flour	2.6

([†] Pomeranz and Chung 1983).

bonds. The suffixes *c-* and *t-* denote the geometric configuration of *cis-* and *trans-*.

The naturally occurring fatty acids are mainly saturated or unsaturated straight chain monocarboxylic acids with even numbers of carbon atoms. Although in some fish such as mullet, triglycerides that contain odd numbered fatty acids (C-15 and C-17) are found. The C-14, C-16, C-18 chain length fatty acids account for more than 90 per cent of the fatty acids of seed oils and animal fat depots. The stereospecific distribution in triglycerides of fatty acids shows saturated fatty acids esterified to the primary alcohol groups of glycerol with the more unsaturated fatty acids esterified to the secondary alcohol group at position 2. In biochemical reactions the two primary alcohol groups of glycerol are not identical and therefore it is necessary to adopt a stereospecific numbering (sn) system. The plane projection with the sn convention is shown in the diagram.

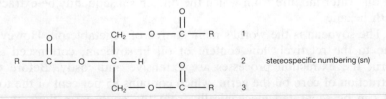

The sterochemistry of various glycerol derivatives is described in the coupled numbering of the carbon atoms which are substituted. Polar lipids include diacyl derivatives of sn-glycerol-3-phosphoryl choline and sn-glycerol-3-phosphoryl ethanolamine (phospholipids) where one hydroxyl group is esterified with phosphoric acid.

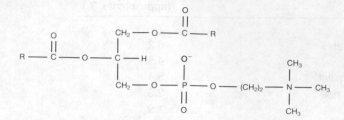

Polar lipids are found in membranes and organelles; the milk fat globule membrane contains 60 per cent of the milk phospholipid. The monoacyl derivatives of sn-glycerol-3-phosphate (the lysophospholipids) are found associated with cereal starch grains. Ether lipids, where an alkoxyl group is attached to the C-1 of the glycerol moiety occur in marine oils and small amounts of cyclopropenoid fatty acids occur in cottonseed oil. Ricinoleic acid, which is a 12-hydroxy acid of oleic acid is a major fatty acid present in the triglycerides of castor oil, but other hydroxy derivatives are less common. Small amounts of keto, epoxy, furanoid and ether fatty acids have been found in more obscure seed oils and fish livers. Cerebrosides (monoglycosyl ceramides) which occur throughout the animal and plant kingdoms do not contain glycerol but are sphingolipids consisting of fatty acids combined as amides of sphingosine, an amino alcohol with a long mono-ene hydrocarbon chain.

EXTRACTION AND REFINING

Several hundred varieties of plants produce oil-bearing seeds, but only a few (Table 6.3) are used commercially and mainly by the food industry.

The oils can be recovered from flaked and dehulled seeds by mechanical crushing or solvent extraction with hexane. From fruit pulps of olives or palm, oils can be recovered by pressing to obtain an oil–water mixture from which the oil can subsequently be extracted with hexane.

The soybean is the world's main source of vegetable oil. However, due to the relatively low content of oil in soybean, cottonseed and corn, the extraction processes are extensive and costly. Before the extraction of corn oil the germ, which contains 85 per cent of the total oil can be separated mechanically from the endosperm flour by dry milling, or from starch by flotation during wet milling. Extracted crude corn oil contains approximately 95 per cent of neutral triglycerides. Peanut, cottonseed, sunflower, coconut and palm oil are used world

Table 6.3 Average oil content of commercially used sources

Sources	Oil content (%)
Castor bean (*Ricinus communis* L)	45
Coconut copra (*Cocos nucifera*)	66
Cottonseed (*Gossypium* species)	19
Linseed (*Linum usitatissimum*)	35
Maize (*Zea mays* L)	5
Olive (*Olea europaea* L)	27
Palm kernel (*Elaesis guineenis*)	47
Peanut (*Arachis hypogaea* L)	45
Rapeseed (*Brassica* species)	42
Safflower (*Carthamus tinctorius*)	30
Sesame (*Sesamum indicum* L)	50
Soybean (*Glycine max* L)	19
Sunflower (*Helianthus annuus* L)	40
Wheat germ (*Triticum aestivum*)	10
Maize germ (*Zea mays* L)	40

wide in varying quantities and diversely, for the manufacture of margarine, cooking oils and salad oils. Olive oil is regarded as the finest vegetable oil, which is in high demand for salad dressings and as a preservative. Sesame oil is used similarly in China, India, African countries and Mexico. Rapeseed oil has been used as a table oil and for cooking purposes. Small quantities of wheat germ oil are specialist products, due to the higher content of vitamin E and octacosanol $CH_3(CH_2)_{26}CH_2OH$. Unlike maize germ, the wheat germ only contains up to 10 per cent oil, and therefore solvent extraction is normally used to increase the yield. The unprocessed wheat germ oil contains small amounts of phospholipids, coloured compounds, fatty acids (less than 6 %) and non-sponifiable matter (less than 8 %). Inedible and less-refined oils from olive kernels, sunflower and castor seed are used in soaps, lubricants or paints. Linseed, which can be grown in cooler European climates, has been used as a drying oil in paints, as it oxidises in air to form an elastic film.

THE OCCURRENCE OF SATURATED AND UNSATURATED FATTY ACIDS

In oils the liquid state is generally due to the presence in the triglyceride molecule of shorter chain length (C-12 and C-14) and unsatu-

Table 6.4 The occurrence of the more common fatty acids in plants

Systematic name	Common name	Symbol	(%)
Dodecanoic	Lauric	12 : 0	4
Tetradecanoic	Myristic	14 : 0	2
Hexadecanoic	Palmitic	16 : 0	11
Octadecanoic	Stearic	18 : 0	4
Octadec-9c-enoic	Oleic	18 : 1	34
Octadec-9c-dienoic	Linoleic	18 : 2	34
Octadec-9c-trienoic	α-Linolenic	18 : 3	5
Docos-13c-enoic	Erucic	22 : 1	3

rated fatty acids. Normally there is a small dominant group of certain fatty acids found in the triglycerides (Table 6.4). Branched-chain fatty acids, acetylenic and substituted fatty acids are rare and only occur in a few species. The different types of glycerides (e.g. saturated, unsaturated, tri-, di and monoglycerides) for a large number of samples can

Table 6.5 The approximate[†] percentage fatty acid composition of plant oil triglycerides

Common name	Fatty acid	Coconut	Cottonseed	Maize	Olive	Palm	Peanut
Caproic	C6 : 0	<1.0	—	—	—	—	—
Caprylic	C6 : 0	7.0	—	—	—	—	—
Capric	C10 : 0	7.0	—	—	—	—	—
Lauric	C12 : 0	48[‡]	—	—	—	<1.0	—
Myristic	C14 : 0	17	1.0	—	—	3	—
Palmitic	C16 : 0	9.0	25	12	13	43	8
Stearic	C18 : 0	2.1	3	2.2	2.5	4	3
Oleic	C18 : 1 (9c)	5.7	18	27	73	40	56
Linoleic	C18 : 2 (9c)	2.6	51	57	8.5	8	26
α-Linolenic	C18 : 3 (6c) <1.0	—	<1.5	<2.0	<1.5	<1.5	—
Arachidic	C20 : 0	—	<1.0	<1.0	<0.5	<1.0	3
Behenic	C22 : 0	—	—	—	—	—	2
Erucic	C22 : 1 (13c)	—	—	—	<0.5	—	—

† The values are taken from various sources (including Egan *et al.* 1981 and Minifie 1982).
‡ Underlined figures are the major components.

be quickly separated and assessed by thin layer chromatography.

The proportion of fatty acids in triglycerides from different sources varies and therefore the proportion of individual fatty acids within an oil provides an important means of identification (Table 6.5). For example, coconut oil is unusual in that 50 per cent of the triglyceride fatty acid is the shorter chain length dodecanoic acid (lauric acid, C12 : 0); for cottonseed, soybean, sunflower and sesame oil, up to 50 per cent of the triglyceride fatty acid is the polyunsaturated fatty acid, linoleic acid, which contains two double bonds. Animal fats can be distinguished by their small amount of polyunsaturated fatty acids and their larger amount of the saturated palmitic and stearic acids (C16 : 0 and C18 : 0). The chemical structures for the more important saturated, monoenoic and methylene-interrupted polyunsaturated acids (Fig. 6.1) are given in Tables 6.6, 6.7 and 6.8.

For analysis of fatty acids as volatile methyl esters, generally a relatively simple gas chromatographic system is sufficient to obtain a profile for the triglyceride fatty acids. For quantitative estimation the odd carbon numbered fatty acids (C15 : 0 or C17 : 0) should be used as internal standards. The *trans*-isomers of unsaturated fatty acids,

Palm kernel	Canadian rapeseed low 22 : 1	European rapeseed high 22 : 1	Safflower	Sesame	Soybean	Sunflower
<0.5	—	—	—	—	—	—
4	—	—	—	—	—	—
5	—	—	—	—	—	—
47	—	—	—	—	—	—
16	—	—	1.0	0.5	0.5	0.5
9	4	4	6	9	11	6
2	2	1	5	5	4	3
18	64	14	25	42	22	23
1	—	15	62	42	53	64
—	9	9	<1.0	<1.0	8	<1.0
—	2	1	<1.0	<1.0	<1.0	<1.0
—	—	—	—	<1.0	—	—
—	<5	46	—	—	—	0.5

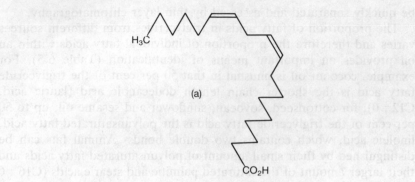

(a)

linoleic acid (C18: n6)

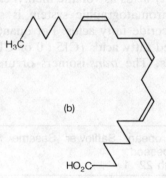

(b)

γ–linolenic acid (C18:3, n6)

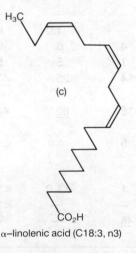

(c)

α–linolenic acid (C18:3, n3)

Fig. 6.1 Schematic diagrams for *cis* di- and trienoic fatty acids

which may arise during hydrogenation in the manufacture of margarines may be determined by infrared absorption at 970 cm^{-1}. For the saturated fatty acids the most common chain lengths are C-16, C-18, C-20 and C-22, although milk fats contain a series of even-numbered fatty acids from C-4 (2 %) to C-20. The fatty acids of shorter chain lengths generally, like the number of double bonds, lower the melting point of the derived triglycerides.

Table 6.6 Common saturated fatty acids found in lipids

Common name	Systematic name	Symbol[†]	MP (°C)	Source
Butyric	Butanoic	4 : 0	−8	Cow's milk
Caproic	Hexanoic	6 : 0	−3.4	Cow's milk
Caprylic	Octanoic	8 : 0	16.3	Milk cocoa fat
Capric	Decanoic	10 : 0	31.3	Milk, palm oils
Lauric	Dodecanoic	12 : 0	43.5	Milk, palm
Myristic	Tetradecanoic	14 : 0	54.4	Milk, coconut
Palmitic	Hexadecanoic	16 : 0	62.9	All fats
Stearic	Octadecanoic	18 : 0	69.9	Milk, meats, pork fat, most seed oils
Arachidic	Eicosanoic	20 : 0	75.4	Peanut oil
Behenic	Docosanoic	22 : 0	79.6	Peanut and rapeseed oils
Lignoceric	Tetracosanoic	24 : 0	84.2	Peanut and rapeseed oils

† Indicates the number of carbon atoms; the number of double bonds for saturated fatty acids is zero (0).

Table 6.7 Some *cis*-monenoic acids found in lipids

Common name	Systematic name	Symbol[†]	MP (°C)	Source
Myristoleic	Tetradec-9-enoic	14 : 1	−4	Fish oils
Palmitoleic	Hexadec-9-enoic	16 : 1	0.5	Fish oils, milk
Oleic	Octadec-9-enoic	18 : 1	16	Major fatty acids of plants and animals
Cetoleic	decos-11-enoic	22 : 1	—	Herring and other fish oils
Erucic	Decos-13-enoic	22 : 1	34	Rapeseed oil
Ricinoleic	Octadec-12-hydroxy-9-enoic	18 : 1	5.5	Castor bean and peanut oils

† Indicates the number of carbon atoms, 1 for the number of double bonds.

LH = 06.

Table 6.8 Some polyenoic acids with two or more double bonds

Common name	Systematic name	Symbol[†]
Linoleic	Octadeca-9c,12c-dienoic	18 : 2 n-6
α-Linolenic	Octadeca-9c,12c,15c-trienoic	18 : 3 n-3
γ-Linolenic	Octadeca-6c,9c,12c-trienoic	18 : 3 n-6
Arachidonic[‡§]	Eicosa-5c,8c,11c-trienoic	20 : 4 n-6
Eicosapentaenoic[§]	Eicosa-5c,8c,11c,14c,17c-pentaenoic	20 : 5 n-3
	Docosahexaenoic	22 : 6 n-3

[†] The family number n, indicates the position of a double bond from the (CH_3) end of the molecule.

The n-6 polyenoic acids, and probably α-linolenic (n-3), are essential dietary requirements for growth of animals. Animals can convert the acids to higher members of the n-families.

[‡] The first number refers to the position of the double bond from the CO_2H end of the molecule.

[§] Precursors of prostaglandins.

For the monenoic acids, oleic (octadec-9-*cis*-enoic) acid is the most widely distributed and substantial amounts are found in animal fats as well as seed oils (Table 6.5). Oleic acid is the major fatty acid of olive oil triglycerides and other monenoic acids are found in fish oils and rapeseed triglycerides (Table 6.7). These monenoic acids are formed from the corresponding saturated fatty acids through the catalytic action of desaturases: oleic acid is derived from stearic acid by the action of a (Δ9) desaturase, acyl CoA desaturase (EC 1.14.99.5). Erucic acid (docos-13-*cis*-enoic acid C22 : 1, n-9) can be a major component (30–50 %) of the fatty acids of rapeseed oil triglycerides, although cultivars producing oils with low levels of erucic acid are now available. Up to 10 per cent eicos-11-*cis*-enoic acid (C20 : 1, n-9) may also be present in oils from *Brassica* species.

The polyunsaturated fatty acids (Table 6.9) contain more than one double bond, and like the monenoic acids generally only occur naturally in the *cis*-configuration. Generally the polyunsaturated fatty acids contain from two to six double bonds that are separated by single methylene groups. The hydrocarbon chain is bent due to the *cis*-configuration at the double bonds (Fig. 6.1). The truly dietary essential fatty acids are restricted to linoleic and α-linolenic acids (Fig. 6.1), although some other polyunsaturated fatty acids are essential metabolites. It has become established practice to refer to the position in the carbon chain of only the first double bond, as the positions of the others must follow along the methylene-interrupted chain. Thus the polyunsaturated fatty acids are classified into n-3, n-6 and n-9 families (Table 6.8), as animals only elongate and desaturate the hydrocarbon chain at the carboxyl terminal end of the molecule. For cottonseed, maize, safflower, soybean and sunflower oils more than half of the

Table 6.9 The occurrence of C20 : 3, C20 : 4 and C20 : 5 polyunsaturated fatty acids (g/100 g of food)†

Common name Symbol	Eicosatrienoic C20 : 3	Eicosatetraenoic C20 : 4	Eicosapentaenoic acids	
			C20 : 5	Total C-20 acids
Raw foodstuff				
Halibut	0.0	0.14	0.17	0.31
Herring	0.0	0.10	1.17	1.27
Mackerel	0.0	0.28	1.07	1.35
Pilchards	0.04	0.03	1.04	1.10
Salmon	0.15	0.05	0.89	1.09
Sardines	0.0	0.0	0.71	0.71
Crab	0.0	0.02	0.78	0.89‡
Lobster	0.0	0.01	0.51	0.58‡

(† Paul and Southgate 1978).

‡ Includes a small amount of C20 : 2 dienoic acid.

total fatty acid present in the triglycerides is linoleic acid. The membrane lipid triglycerides of animal cells in muscle and liver contain significant amounts of linoleic acid and arachidonic acid (C20 : 4 n-6). α-Linolenic acid (C18 : 3 n-3) is only present in small amounts in most seed oil triglycerides with the exception of linseed. However, C18 : 3, n-6 (γ-linolenic acid) is the main fatty acid of the triglycerides in green leaves, phytoplankton and hence some aquatic mammals (e.g. whales and seals). The isomeric trienoic acid (α-linolenic acid (C18 : 3, n-3) occurs in the triglycerides of the evening primrose oil for which medicinal value has been claimed. Some of the higher homologues containing up to five double bonds occur naturally in the triglycerides of pelagic fish (Table 6.9) which therefore offer a direct dietary source of these highly unsaturated long-chain fatty acids. The C-20 and C-22 fatty acids may represent from 25 to 30 per cent of the total fatty acids present in fish oil triglycerides, whereas in vegetable oils the concentrations of these acids is frequently less than 1 per cent. Generally in triglycerides most of the naturally occurring polyunsaturated fatty acids belong to the n-3 family, where the polyenoic acid is attached to the central hydroxyl group of the glycerol moiety.

It is now known that the higher homologues of each family (for example the n-6 family) of polyunsaturated fatty acids can be synthesised in animals by chain elongation and desaturation from lower members of the same series (Fig. 6.2). However, animals, unlike plants, are unable to insert double bonds at n-3 and n-6 positions. The efficiency of such multistage synthesis is unknown and the activities of various required enzymes may decline with age and disease. However, the higher homologues are essential metabolites even though they are not essential dietary nutrients.

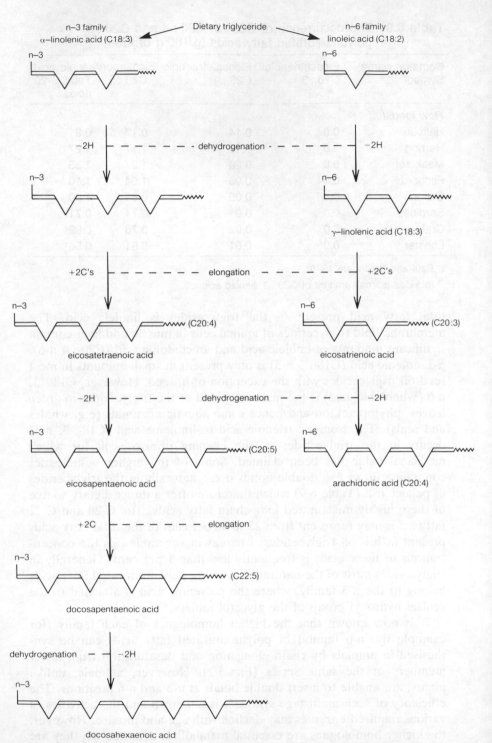

Fig. 6.2 Biosynthesis of higher unsaturated fatty acids in mammals

For each n-family (n-3, n-6 or occasionally n-9) the process of elongation by a two carbon unit and desaturation to form new double bonds occurs to form the C-20 and C-22 polyunsaturated fatty acids (Fig. 6.2). Desaturation to form the new double bond, catalysed by specific desaturase enzymes, always takes place in the carbon chain between carboxyl group and the nearest pre-existing double bond. Each newly introduced double bond is of the *cis*-configuration and is separated from the nearest pre-existing double bond, only by a methylene group. Thus the methylene-interrupted positioning of the double bonds is maintained in the higher homologues.

It has been claimed that the biosynthesis of n-9 acids is suppressed by the presence of n-6 and n-3 acids (Gurr 1984), and thus the relative proportions of the different polyunsaturated fatty acids in the diet may be important. Dietary requirements for the highly unsaturated C 20 acids are being actively investigated (Chen *et al.* 1985). The higher homologues are precursors of some of the physiologically important prostaglandins (Fig. 6.10 and 6.11) thromboxanes and leucotrienes, which are hormones and compounds associated with inflammatory responses. Also in mammals the relative amount of C22 : 6 (n-3) acid in nervous tissue is particularly high.

The variable distribution of fatty acids within triglyceride molecules means that in any one oil or fat large numbers of different triglycerides occur. However, in coconut and palm kernel oil, triglycerides enriched

Table 6.10 The average fat content of animal products

Food	Fat (% in the dry matter)
Cow's milk[†]	3.6
Cream	18
Double cream	48
Clotted cream	55
Whipping cream	35
Yoghurt	1.0
Buttermilk	1.6
Full milk powder	26
Skimmed milk powder	1.0
Full condensed milk	9.5
Skimmed condensed milk	0.2
Butter	82
Cheeses, e.g. Cheddar, Stilton, etc.	45–50
Low fat cheeses, e.g. Edam	40
Ice-cream	5–15
Suet	83–6

([†] Egan *et al.* 1981).

with lauric (C12 : 0) and myristic (C14 : 0) acids predominate and account for a quite sharp melting point at 25 °C. For palm oil, the triglyceride containing three residues of palmitic acid (tripalmitin) represents 10 per cent of the total triglycerides. Fractionation of groups of triglycerides from oils can be carried out by partially solidifying liquid oils by cooling followed by collection of the fat crystals, which for coconut and palm kernel oils have been used for coating confectionery products. Through the use of lipases, many of which first remove the 1,3-positional fatty acids from triglycerides, it is possible to determine by gas chromatography the nature of the fatty acid on the central C-2 hydroxyl group of the glycerol molecule.

FOOD USES

After extraction, oils are refined, bleached and winterised. Refining includes treatment with alkali or steam distillation to remove free fatty acids. Phospholipids can be removed by extraction with water (commonly known as degumming), from which crude lecithin is often obtained. For removal of colour, bleaching is normally carried out by absorption of coloured pigments on to complex silicates (bleaching earths). As well as coloured pigments, undesirable sulphur compounds, metal ions, aldehydes, ketones and peroxides are absorbed during the bleaching process which therefore also results in the removal of odours. Both refining and bleaching can be carried out on the dissolved oil at the solvent-extraction stage in an integrated operation. Further deodorisation can be achieved by steam distillation at reduced pressure. Winterisation is the process for removal, by refrigeration, of high molecular weight triglycerides present in natural and hydrogenated oils which may solidify in food products such as salad oils and liquid shortenings as used in the bread industry.

Together plant seed oils and animal fats can also account for a variable and possibly large proportion of fat intake in developed countries, as fatty tissues of animals may contain from 60 to 90 per cent fat. The crude fat content of foods can be determined quickly by use of the established extractive methods (Egan *et al.* 1981). The approximate content of the total fat present in a number of animal foods is given in Table 6.10. Recovery (rendering) of the fatty tissues of animals to produce tallows from cattle, and lard from pork fat, is carried out by steam or dry heat to melt the fat.

Suet, which contains microscopic particles of fat, each held within a membrane, can be shredded because of its membranous structure. It is obtained from the fatty tissue situated near the loins and kidneys of the sheep or ox. Artificial or prepared suets are manufactured by extrusion of fat and coating of the fibres with wheat flour or rice to prevent coagulation.

Cream is obtained from milk by mechanical separation and butter is obtained by churning cream to separate the excess water. Approximately 16 per cent of water dispersed as droplets in a continuous phase of fat is present in butter. Ice-cream, which is a mixture of milk, fat, sugars, emulsifiers and stabilisers, contains from 5 to 15 per cent fat and dairy ice-cream must contain no fat other than that derived from milk. Other ice-creams may contain vegetable oils in place of milk fat. Normal margarine is a water-in-fat emulsion, which must contain 80 per cent fat, as manufactured from blends of palm, peanut, coconut, sunflower, cottonseed and soybean oils. The proportional use of the different oils varies in different parts of the world and in the United States cottonseed and soybean oils are the main raw materials. Margarines are products which are easy to spread over a wide range of temperatures: characteristics, such as flavour and long-term storage properties, can be controlled very effectively by careful refining of the ingredient oils. Margarines will also coat flour particles easily and therefore are used in the manufacture of short pastry products. Shortenings are simply blends of fats or oils which react with the gluten proteins to soften confectionery products. They need to have a soft texture, be free from foaming and have a low rancidity which excludes the use of coconut and palm oils. The aqueous phase (20 % for normal margarines) can be obtained from fat-free milk cultures of bacteria, or from solutions of protein concentrates, to provide the desirable flavour. However, in order to reduce bacterial growth, particularly in low-fat margarines (fat content 40–50 %), the water droplets must be small and this is achieved by the use of emulsifiers. Annatto and β-carotene are the commonly used colouring agents, which together with vitamins, lecithin and mono- and diglycerides are soluble in the fat phase. The melting characteristics are controlled by hydrogenation, interesterification and fractionation of the ingredient oils.

In one product in particular, namely chocolate, the precise composition and occurrence of triglycerides as the main fat ingredient is extremely important. Cocoa butter is the fat (48 %) of the cocoa bean which exhibits a quite sharp melting point (35 °C) just below body temperature. Softening also occurs at approximately 30 to 32 °C. At room temperature cocoa butter solidifies in a stable crystalline form and does not undergo oxidative rancidity (see p. 286); it is these properties that in turn are related to the chemical composition of the triglycerides which make cocoa butter unique for the manufacture of chocolate products. Only one other natural fat, Illipe butter obtained from seeds of *Shorea*, resembles cocoa butter. However, the melting point is slightly higher at from 37 to 38 °C, which thus imparts slightly different properties to chocolate. Nevertheless, Illipe butter, coconut oil, palm

kernel oil and hydrogenated oils have all been used as partial substi-
tutes for cocoa butter, but their extensive use is restricted by regulations. The United Kingdom provisions apply to chocolate products
and restrict the use of vegetable fats not derived from cocoa beans to
a maximum of 5 per cent (Egan *et al.* 1981). In the United Kingdom
plain chocolate must also contain a minimum of 18 per cent cocoa
butter. However, in Continental Europe cocoa butter is the main fat
component of plain chocolate. The composition of the important cocoa
butter triglycerides is given in Table 6.11.

Table 6.11 The composition of cocoa butter[†]

Symmetry (sus)[‡]		Saturated triglyceride	(%) 3
18 : 0,18 : 1,18 : 0	(SOS)	Oleodistearin	22
16 : 0,18 : 1,18 : 0	(POS)	Oleopalmitostearin	57
16 : 0,18 : 1,16 : 0	(POP)	Oleodipalmitin	4
		Fatty acids	
		Palmitic	24
		Stearic	35
		Oleic	38
		Linoleic	2

([†] Minifie 1982).

[‡] sus = saturated–unsaturated–saturated fatty acids order in a triglyceride.

Each of the above triglycerides possess a certain melting point but
when present in chocolate can solidify in any one of four polymorphic
forms possessing different melting points: α (21–4 °C), β' (27–9 °C)
and β (34–5 °C). The triglyceride molecules possess a tuning fork type
structure with the fatty acid esterified at sn-position 2 projecting in the
opposite direction (Fig. 6.3). In chocolate the type of crystal structure
and melting point is determined by the way the molecules pack
together and hence the types and positions of the fatty acids within the
triglyceride molecules. The β-form of packing is the most stable with
the highest packing density and obviously occurs with triglycerides
which have fatty acids of similar chain length occupying similar
positions within the triglyceride molecules. The type of crystallisation
depends on the rate of cooling, the presence of minor constituents
which can seed the crystals, and the temperature at which the product
is held. For chocolate and other mixed fats the least stable α-form is
obtained on rapid cooling and the most stable β-form by slow cooling.
This is achieved by tempering, when the chocolate is cooled to initiate
crystallisation and then re-heated to transform the less stable α-form
crystals. For unsaturated triglycerides only those which are symmetrical, as in cocoa butter (Table 6.11) can crystallise in the β-form

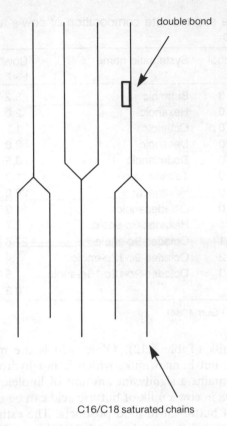

double bond

C16/C18 saturated chains

Fig. 6.3 Three triglycerides packed in the stable β-form

(Fig. 6.3) which gives the closest fit and least freedom of movement for the molecules. The presence of *trans*-unsaturated fatty acids inter- feres with the packing and crystallisation and therefore hydrogenated fats are often incompatible with cocoa butter. Also there may be regions in molecular terms where unsaturated fatty acids come together to give planes of greater fluidity. The white bloom frequently found on the surface of chocolate is believed to be due to the forma- tion during storage – or on melting – of more stable polymorphic β- forms from any less stable α-forms still present at the time of manufacture.

Milk fat

Fat occurs as an oil-in-water emulsion in milk in the form of fat glob- ules (<1 μm). Although fat is the most variable constituent of milk, comparison of the average composition of cow's milk fat against human milk fat shows an unusual occurrence of short chain length fatty

Table 6.12 The approximate composition of cow's and human milk
fats

Common name	Symbol	Systematic name	Cow[†] (%)	Human[‡] (%)
Butyric	C4 : 0	Butanoic	3.2	0
Caproic	6 : 0	Hexanoic	2.0	0
Caprylic	8 : 0	Octanoic	1.2	0
Capric	10 : 0	Decanoic	2.8	1
Lauric	12 : 0	Dodecanoic	3.5	5
Myristic	14 : 0	Tetradecanoic	11.2	7
Palmitic	16 : 0	Hexadecanoic	26.0	27
Stearic	18 : 0	Octadecanoic	11.2	10
Palmitoleic	16 : 1	Hexadec-9c-enoic	2.7	4
Oleic	18 : 1	Octadec-9c-enoic	27.8	35
Linoleic	18 : 2	Octadec-9c-12c-enoic	1.4	7
α-Linolenic	18 : 3	Octadec-9c-12c-15c-enoic	1.5	1
Cholesterol			0.3	—

([†] Egan *et al*. 1981; [‡] Gurr 1984).

acids in cow's milk (Table 6.12). Oleic acid is the major fatty acid
present in milks, but human milk, which is not hydrogenated during
digestion also contains a significant amount of linoleic acid.

The occurrence in cow's milk of butyric acid can be used to estimate
the proportion of butter fat in food products. The estimation can also
be substantiated by analysis of the C-14/C-12 fatty acid ratio, as these
acids are present in milk in a ratio approaching 4 : 1. Thus the adulteration of butter or dairy ice-cream can be detected by analysis of the
fatty acids. Confirmation of dairy ice-cream is obtained by the absence
of sitosterol – cholesterol being the main sterol of milk fat. The longer
chain length saturated fatty acids of cow's milk are randomly distributed in the sn-1 and -3 positions in triglycerides, while human milk
contains the saturated fatty acid (palmitic acid) esterified to the C-2
hydroxyl group of glycerol.

The emulsified fat globules in milk are surrounded by the globule
membrane which consists of glycoproteins, polar lipids, sterols and a
number of enzymes including xanthine oxidase. Unfortunately,
because of the fragility of the membrane disruption of its structure can
easily occur during the pumping and cooling of milk. The existence of
the fat globule membrane is particularly important as it separates the
lipids from the casein proteins and colloidal tricalcium phosphate.
Disruption of the membrane can result in rapid lipolysis catalysed by
either milk lipoprotein lipases or contaminating microbial lipases. Also
absorption of lipid into casein micelles can occur which reduces coagulation by rennin during cheese manufacture. Owing to the chemical

composition of milk fat, which contains predominantly saturated fatty acids (Table 6.12) partial crystallisation of some of the triglycerides and precipitation of immunoglobins on to the fat globule membrane occurs during cooling.

However, for the manufacture of skimmed milk, cream, butter and ice-cream a disruption of the membrane and a breaking of the emulsion is beneficial. The fat content of ice-cream is approximately 10 per cent with the additional fat being provided by either separate additions of milk fat (as for dairy ice-cream) or vegetable oil. During this process homogenisation causes the number of globules and the surface area : fat volume ratio to increase while the size of fat globules decreases. This results in absorption of caseins, whey proteins and surface-active additives on to the exposed surfaces of the fat globule, and during the manufacture of ice-cream the formation of an intricate complex structure of air cells, ice crystals, fat globules and casein micelles. Owing to first, the natural biological variation in milk fat content and composition, together with the commercial use of liquid oils and stabilisers, ice-cream, and also refrigerated cream, can be expected to contain a mixture of crystalline and non-crystalline triglycerides in various polymorphic forms with different melting points. However, due to the complexity of the mixture, the precise distribution and form of all the triglycerides is likely to remain unknown in the forseeable future.

For bread manufacture the importance of monoacyl glycerides as crumb softeners has been known for a long time, but now the importance of both the total lipid and the type of lipid present has been highlighted by the use of rapid high energy mixing processes. Although the amounts of cereal lipids are small, loaf volume shows a peculiar relationship (Fig. 6.4) to total lipid content which differs for various flours (MacRitchie 1983). Furthermore, extractable lipid also decreases during mixing and dough development and is probably related to the presence in gluten of lipid-binding proteins. One of these, termed ligolin (Frazier et al. 1981), is of low molecular weight and possesses a quite different chemical composition from previously identified wheat proteins.

CHEMICAL AND BIOCHEMICAL CHANGES IN FATS AND OILS

For the various uses in margarine, chocolate-type coatings, ice-cream and other confectionery products, the low melting point natural liquid oils are unsuitable. Small quantities of palm oil may form eutectic mixtures when added to cocoa butter and cause bloom on the surface

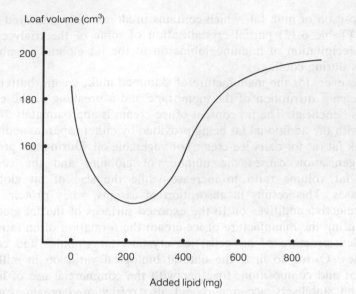

Fig. 6.4 Relationship between bread volume and fat content (with permission from MacRritchie and Gras 1973)

of chocolate products; on the other hand coconut oil may be too hard at ambient temperatures, but yet melt at 21 °C. Also the high degree of unsaturation in plant oils can give rise to oxidative rancidity. However, the properties of oils can be modified by fractionation in suitable solvents, such as acetone, to yield homogeneous mixtures of triglycerides as found in 'Coberine' from palm oil. Coberine has a composition almost identical to cocoa butter and therefore does not form eutectic mixtures.

More profound chemical changes can be achieved by simply hydrogenating vegetable oils to reduce the content of polyunsaturated fatty acids. Generally, hydrogenation is not taken to completion, but to intermediate stages, such that the semi-hardened oils can be prepared with various characteristics. A nickel catalyst is normally used where the nickel atoms spaced 2.5 Å apart correlate closely with a double bond length of 2.7 Å. However, the hydrogenation process is complicated by the migration of double bonds, different rates of hydrogenation for polyunsaturated fatty acids and the structure of the triglycerides. One unfortunate reaction is the formation of *trans*-unsaturated isomers (Fig. 6.5) which have higher melting points than the corresponding *cis*-isomers (Table 6.13). To achieve specific commercial products the pre-treatment of the oil, preparation of the catalyst and the temperature for hydrogenation are carefully controlled, but even so margarines containing hydrogenated vegetable oils have been reported to contain up to 40 per cent *trans*-unsaturated

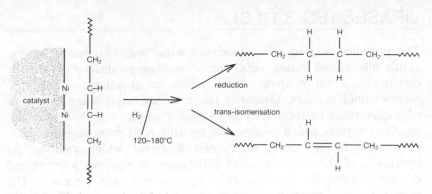

Fig. 6.5 Hydrogenation of triglyceride *cis*-unsaturated fatty acids

Table 6.13 The melting points of some C-18 monenoic acid isomers

Common name	Systematic name	MP (°C)
Oleic	Octadeca-9*c*-enoic	16
Elaidic	Octadeca-9*t*-enoic	42
Petroselenic	Octadeca-6*c*-enoic	30
Petroselaidic	Octadeca-6*t*-enoic	51.9

fatty acids. In other products such as butter biscuits and potato crisps only slightly more than half to two-thirds of the total polyunsaturated fatty acids might exist as true essential fatty acids in the *cis, cis*-methylene-interrupted form (Kochhar and Matsui 1984). The toxicity of *trans*-fatty acids is still being investigated and a complete understanding of their possible effect on cell membrane structure, and their role as inhibitors of desaturases, transferases and prostaglandin synthases is needed.

Triglycerides are also modified by chemical interesterification using sodium metal, sodium methoxide or potassium–sodium alloys as catalysts. This is a process by which the positions of fatty acids on the glyceride are interchanged. At low temperatures (26–38 °C) the interesterification can be directed through the physical removal from the mixture, by crystallisation, of the more saturated triglycerides as they continuously form. At higher temperatures (approximately 80 °C) a more random esterification with palm oil can be carried out. Such a process is useful for changing the low melting point of coconut oils to be used in margarines, which need to be soft in the refrigerator but still solid at room temperature.

LIPASES (EC 3.1.1.3)

The presence of free acids associated with 'soap-like taints' in vegetable oils, cereal grains, milk, cream and egg products is frequently due to the action of lipases. Lipases only act at aqueous–lipid interfaces of lipid micelles. Generally the enzymes catalyse the hydrolysis of triglycerides to form fatty acids and glycerol, but there are also specific enzymes which catalyse the hydrolysis of monoacylglycerides, phospholipids and esters of sterols. Enzymes which catalyse the hydrolysis of the latter group of substances in aqueous solution and do not require the presence of a lipid micelle are esterases. The enzymes occur naturally in plant oils, cereal grains or milk, or are present as a result of microbiological contamination. Lipolysis in fresh milk can be induced by agitation and the addition of often unidentified activators. In milk the natural lipase is a lipoprotein lipase (EC 3.1.1.34) which is absorbed to the casein micelles. The enzyme is activated by cooling or during homogenisation. An activator of the enzyme is present in mammalian blood plasma, and thus contamination in disease states of milk by bovine plasma may also cause lipolysis. In commercial milk samples which have been held at from 6 °C to 10 °C, microbial thermostable lipases synthesised by cold growing psychotrophs (generally pseudomonads) may also catalyse lipolysis even after ultra high temperature (UHT) pasteurisation at 130 °C for 1 or 2 sec. In comminuted meat products, such as minced meats or mechanically recovered meats, the natural animal lipases together with any contaminating microbial lipases – which might be thermostable – can affect the flavour and aroma of the products. Generally, the mode of action of the lipases results in fatty acids being preferentially hydrolysed from sn-1 and -3 positions of triglycerides so as to leave 2-substituted monoacylglycerides (Fig. 6.6). Although subsequent transesterification may occur where the remaining fatty acid moiety migrates to form a 1- or 3-monoacylglyceride, that may then hydrolyse to liberate the transferred fatty acid. However, some microbial and higher plant lipases may also catalyse the hydrolysis of triglycerides in all three positions. The enzymatic activity of lipases can be determined with high sensitivity by measuring the rate of release of ^{14}C-labelled fatty acids from emulsions of glycerol tri[1-^{14}C]oleate. Alternatively,

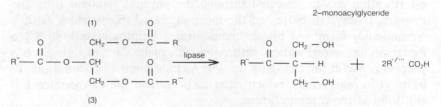

Fig. 6.6 Hydrolysis of a neutral triglyceride by pancreatic lipase

released fatty acids can be determined after extraction into organic solvents by titration or as copper soaps at 440 nm. pH-Stat and acid colorimetric methods of analysis, which measure the acids liberated, are less sensitive for food homogenates due to the buffering capacity of extraneous salts and proteins.

Lipolysis can be divided into three consequential events: formation of lipid micelles, establishment of a water–lipid interface, and absorption of the enzyme prior to the catalysed hydrolysis. The energy for the formation of the lipid micelle arises from the large free-energy change, which occurs with the transfer of alkane moieties from an aqueous to non-aqueous environment. Because of the interfacial nature of lipolysis the velocity of the reaction is proportional to the surface concentrations of the substrate and enzyme in the micelle rather than to their overall concentrations in the suspension. Consequently, the classical relationship between velocity of a reaction and the concentration of substrate in the aqueous phase is not readily found for lipases. The velocity of the reaction is more closely correlated with the available surface area of the lipid micelles. Generally, the enzyme cannot be saturated with substrates due to the finite size of emulsified droplets and thus V_{max} cannot be reached. Therefore only apparent V_{max} and K_m values can be determined. Furthermore, it seems probable that the K_m value may be easily modified by changes in orientation of the active site of the enzyme to the interfacial region of the micelle. A further complication during lipolysis is likely to involve the rearrangement of the micellar constituents as the catalysed reaction proceeds and more polar reaction products accumulate. Thus the localised accumulation of fatty acids from the hydrolysis of triacylglycerides may alter the apparent equilibrium position of the reaction and consequently influence the subsequent hydrolysis of other components like esterified vitamins and sterols.

Plant lipases

Plant seed lipase activity, that cannot generally be detected in ungerminated seeds, increases rapidly after germination. For oil seeds, hydrolysis of lipid – found in lipid bodies (diameter approximately 1 μm – is essential for the mobilisation of the main energy and carbon sources required for embryonic growth. In oil seeds the detected lipase activity has always been associated with either lipid body membranes or the glyoxysomes. However, unbound lipid acyl hydrolases, able to catalyse the hydrolysis of glycolipids, phospholipids and mono- and diacylglycerides, are also present in the cytosol of a number of tubers, leaves and seeds.

The presence of the lipid body membrane-bound lipases in a number of seeds has been demonstrated after ether extraction of the free lipid. Generally the enzymes exhibit maximum enzymatic activity towards either neutral triacylglycerols consisting of short chain fatty acids, or the triglyceride trilinolein. Castor bean membrane-bound acid lipase has been well characterised and shown to require both a thermostable glycoprotein and a tetramer of ricinoleic acid (12-hydroxyoleic acid) as cofactor. The castor bean enzyme catalyses the liberation of short chain fatty acids preferentially from all three sn positions in triglycerides. For soybean, peanut, cucumber and sunflower only glyoxysomal lipases have been detected (Huang 1984). To be effective after germination the glyoxysomal enzymes must contact physically the 'nearby' lipid bodies.

For cereal grains the exact location of lipases is unknown but their presence, even when the lipid content is low (2–7 %), is likely to cause rancid taints in germinating wheat, oats and rice. In wheat a number of acyl hydrolases have been found which probably act on the endosperm glycolipids and monoacylglycerides, but the so-called germ lipase is actually an esterase. For wheat flours, free fatty acids accumulate slowly during long term storage, which may be due to the presence of a natural endosperm enzyme or contamination by the wheat germ lipase or microbial lipases. Greater lipase activity is normally found in the grains of oats and rice, although the enzymes are not well characterised and their location in the grain is uncertain. For oats which have a relatively high fat content (6 %), the lipase has a pH optimum of approximately 7.4. The enzyme is active in low water activity products (a_w, 0.2) even at low temperatures, where the binding of the enzyme to substrate may be increased. Lipase in barley is barely detectable, and in many cereals and oil seeds only appears after germination. Non-specific acyl hydrolases are widespread in cereals and therefore particular use of pure triglycerides (free of monoacylglycerides) is needed when testing for lipase activity. Further difficulties may be caused by the action of acyl hydrolases, which have also been shown to catalyse acyl-transfer reactions. These reactions can give rise to synthesis or deacylation of di- and triglycerides without release of free fatty acids. Such acyl transferase activity has been found in potato tubers.

For microbial lipases, a number of non-specific enzymes have been found which are claimed to release fatty acids from all three positions of the glycerol moiety, although sn-1,3-specificity is still certainly very common among the microbial lipases. Moreover, the lipase of *Geotrichum candidum* preferentially releases fatty acids containing the *cis*-9-double bond as in oleate. The enzyme from *G. candidum* has been extensively investigated by X-ray analysis, but the type of active site has not been identifiied. The enzyme is not inhibited by diisopropylphosphofluoridate (DFP), and a cofactor does not seem to be required. Overall, the mode of action of microbial lipases is very diverse. The existence of numerous lipases with different specificities may accelerate their industrial application.

Milk lipases

Milk from the higher primates – gorillas and man – contains a bile-salt stimulated lipase. A lipoprotein lipase is the only lipase present in the milks of other mammalian species. Immunological cross-reactions and amino acid analysis have demonstrated that the unusual bile-stimulated enzyme (approximate MW 90,000) has a similar composition and structure to a mammalian pancreatic carboxyl ester lipase. In a like manner, the bile-salt stimulated enzyme is non-specific with respect to the fatty acid ester substrates and catalyses the hydrolysis of cholesterol and retinol esters in addition to triacylglycerides. The human milk bile-stimulated lipase is activated by bile salts (0.2–0.5 mM), which means that the enzyme is likely to be readily activated by bile at concentrations of approximately 2 mM present in the lumen of the intestine, while remaining inactive on fresh undigested milk, where the concentration of bile salts is likely to be less than 5 μmole. The enzyme is not hydrolysed by pepsin, and in the presence of bile salts is resistant to proteolysis by serine proteinases. It is estimated that with an enzymatic activity of 6 μmole per min. per cm^3 of milk that all the human milk lipid is quickly hydrolysed following ingestion. Thus the human bile-stimulated lipase has an important physiological role for the new-born infant.

Lipoprotein lipase present in the milk of most mammals is identical to the blood plasma enzyme responsible for hydrolysis of blood lipoproteins and is activated by cofactors. In milks, the enzyme seems to have no function as it is destroyed at low pH values and its enzymatic activity is inhibited by bile salts. The enzyme is a glycoprotein (approximate MW 42,000) which readily aggregates and exists absorbed to casein micelles, although mechanical disruption increases absorption to fat globules. In bovine milk, the lipoprotein lipase is normally inactive, but can be activated by homogenisation, cooling and the presence of activator proteins. This induced lipolysis can result in the condemnation of large quantities of stored bovine milk through very limited catalysed hydrolysis of less than 1 or 2 per cent of the total lipid. The human palate is particularly sensitive to the short and medium chain length volatile fatty acids, which predominate in the milk triacylglycerides. Spontaneous lipolysis in milk, without mechanical disruption, can also occur. Owing to the speed of the reaction, often on the farm premises, the causes of spontaneous lipolysis remain largely unknown, although contamination by activators of lipase enzymes constitutes a likely cause.

The enzyme is active from pH 6.0 to 10.5 and is inhibited by either relatively high concentrations of inorganic salts (>0.3 M), or serine esterase inhibitors. Consequently, the active site is thought to contain an essential serine residue for formation of an intermediate acyl–enzyme complex during the catalytic reaction. The enzyme catalyses the hydrolysis of a wide range of substrates, which include phospholipids and monoacylglycerides. The lipoprotein lipase molecule has a high affinity for heparin and a high isoelectric point (pI 9.0), and therefore the overall charge on the protein is positive at neutral pH values. As only aspartic acid has been found as a N-terminal residue, the monomers of a dimeric form of the enzyme seem to be identical and undergo a very limited and specific cleavage by trypsin. The trypsin-treated 'nicked' enzyme contains a lipid-binding site for the formation of oil–water interfaces, a heparin-binding site, an activator-binding site and the catalytic site. The enzyme can bind fatty acids and detergents, presumably at the lipid-binding site, which may also increase its stability and therefore it is hydrolytic in milk-containing products. Activator proteins are diverse and include a serum apolipoprotein (approximate MW 8800), which is also present in chylomicrons and hen's egg yolk. There is a strong affinity between the activator and milk lipoprotein lipase; the dissociation constant has been reported to be 10^{-6}. For inhibition of lipoprotein lipase, antibodies to the enzyme are specifically effective whereas other proteins, such as serum albumin, may act as non-specific inhibitors by binding to the substrate. Lipoprotein lipase is also particularly sensitive to product inhibition, which is dependent on the presence of Ca^{2+}, or serum albumin to act as fatty acid acceptors and so change the equilibrium position of the reaction.

In milk-containing foods, lipolytic taints are often attributed to either spontaneous or induced lipolysis of milk. In some products lipase taints may arise when raw unpasteurised milk is mixed with other ingredients, such as dry dessert powders or those containing egg yolk, where activators are present. In pasteurised milk, thermostable

Table 6.14 Comparison of the properties of mammalian triglyceride hyrolysing enzymes

Enzyme	Source	MW
Lingual lipase	Human tongue	44,000–48,000
	Rat tongue	45,000
Pregastric esterase	Newborn ruminants tongue	
Pancreatic lipase	Human pancreas	52,000

microbial lipases may be present and their activity may likewise be enhanced by other ingredients.

Lingual and pancreatic lipases

Lingual lipases act preferentially on triacylglycerides containing medium chain length fatty acids. The enzymatic activity of lingual lipases is not stimulated by bile salts. Some of the characteristics of lingual lipases for man and the rat are summarised in Table 6.14, from which it can be seen that the enzyme is particularly stable and active at low pH values and therefore contributes to early digestion of ingested fats.

Although lingual lipase is inactive towards phospholipids, milk fat globules are readily hydrolysed by lingual lipase to produce substantial amounts of monolaurin and free fatty acids. Thus the lingual lipase is unusual in so far as it has a special ability to penetrate the milk fat globule membrane and is not deactivated at the low pH values of the stomach. Therefore commercial production of a similar acid-resistant lipase would be valuable for medicinal use when the secretion of mammalian lipases is impaired.

The control of the lipolytic activity of pancreatic lipase (EC 3.1.1.3) is complex; a pro-cofactor (procolipase) and its activator (trypsin), calcium ions and bile acids are all required to facilitate active lipolysis by pancreatic lipase. The role of calcium ions is not fully understood, although it seems likely that the cation may reduce product inhibition by forming insoluble calcium salts with the liberated fatty acids. It is also possible that the ion influences the activity of the enzyme allosterically (App. VII), as calcium reduces the lag period for the enzymatic activity at low substrate concentration.

The bile acids, are like detergents, where both hydrophobic and hydrophilic moieties act as emulsifiers for fats. They are mainly sodium glycocholate and taurocholate which are synthesised from cholesterol

pH opt.	Optimal substrate
3.5–6	Medium chain length, e.g.
2–6	trioctanoin
4–6.5	Only short chain length, e.g.
	tributyrin
5–9	Long chain length, e.g.
	tripalmitin requires bile salts
	and colipase

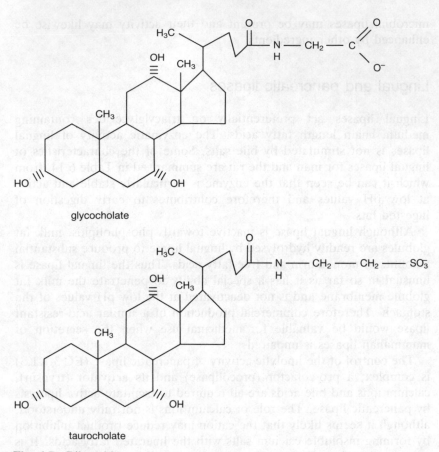

Fig. 6.7 Bile acids

by the liver and are stored in the gall bladder (Fig. 6.7).

Pancreatic lipases have been studied from a number of species and considerable information on the porcine and human enzymes is available (Verger 1984). In pancreatic juice, free of bile salts, the pancreatic lipase exists in a low molecular weight form, which aggregates in the presence of bile, phospholipid and colipase. For ovine, bovine, porcine and human pancreatic lipases the monomeric form of the enzyme has a molecular weight of approximately 48,000. The porcine enzyme has been shown to contain 449 amino acids with six disulphide bonds and two sulphydryl groups. Glycan chains linked to asparagine residues are found in the human and porcine enzymes. However, due to similarities in molecular structure there are immunological cross-reactions between human pancreatic lipase and other mammalian lipases. For human pancreatic lipase two isolipases have been separated with slightly differing isoelectric points.

Sequence analysis of the enzymes has indicated that the distribution of disulphide bonds brings about the formation of small loops of amino acids as found in Bowman–Birk proteinase inhibitors (Ch. 4). The loops contain from six to fourteen amino acid residues. As the lipases constitute a unique class of enzymes that only act at interfaces, the existence of such loops is likely to be very important for essential interactions of the enzyme with cofactor, substrate and bile acids. Investigations of the mode of action of mammalian lipases have shown that k_{cat} and K_m are dependent on an essential histidine residue with a pK value in the range of 5.6 to 6.4. It seems likely that lipases form acyl intermediates with the fatty acids liberated from glycerides similar to the acyl intermediates formed during the hydrolysis of proteins and esters by proteinases. As with the serine proteinases the essential histidine residue could also act as a proton donor and acceptor. It is not yet known whether any of the free sulphydryl groups present in pancreatic lipase are involved in the formation acyl intermediates, as for other hydrolases like papain or β-amylase. However, the pancreatic lipases are not inhibited by oxidation of the sulphydryl groups, nor by the specific active site irreversible serine inhibitors, like diisopropyl-phosphofluoridate. The use of competitive inhibitors which has provided valuable mechanistic information for other enzymes is particularly difficult for lipases, due to the extra complication introduced by the need for interfacial reaction with substrate cofactor and bile salts.

Colipase seems to act as an anchor or linking point for pancreatic lipases in emulsions, as it can competitively remove enzymatic inhibition by bile salts (Verger 1984). The colipase exists in the pancreas as an inactive procolipase, which on secretion into the pancreatic duct and duodenum undergoes proteolysis catalysed by trypsin at both its N- and C-terminii – from which a pentapeptide and possibly decapeptides, respectively, are removed. Colipase is a protein which has been isolated from the pancreas of a number of mammalian species and generally consists of approximately 100 amino acid residues (Borgström and Erlanson-Albertsson 1984). The porcine colipase molecule consists of eighty-four residues and a highly cross-linked core containing five disulphide bonds and hence must, like pancreatic lipase, contain a series of looped regions. One loop containing leucine, valine and three tyrosine residues binds detergents, phospholipids and bile salts and is claimed to be the lipid-binding site. The N-terminal chain is also hydrophobic and contains isoleucine, leucine and valine residues. Although reports of the detailed physicochemical properties of colipase have often been complicated by the variable amount of proteolysis undergone by different preparations, generally it is clear that colipase is absorbed very strongly to interfaces and glass surfaces, even in the presence of bile salts. The binding site of bile salts to colipase, investigated with NMR and neutron scattering, seems to involve a hydrophobic domain on the surface of the molecule which

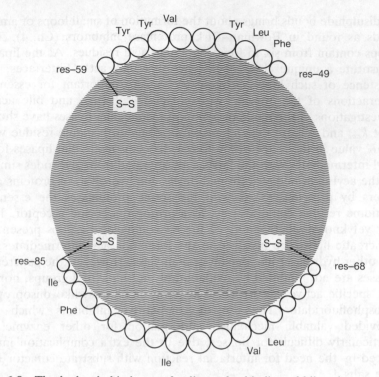

Fig. 6.8 The hydrophobic loops of colipase for binding of bile salts

includes separate looped regions (Fig. 6.8). The calculated dissociation constant in the range of 10^{-6} to 10^{-8}M for the binding of colipase to pancreatic lipase, indicates a high affinity between the enzyme and colipase. The binding between enzyme cofactor is also enhanced by oleic acid, but reduced by bile salts and therefore the main biochemical function of colipase seems to be the restoration of the activity of bile salt-inhibited lipase.

Cholesterol esterase (carboxyl ester lipase EC 3.1.1.13)

This enzyme, which represents 4 per cent of human pancreatic juice protein also catalyses the hydrolysis of other sterol esters. Cholesteryl oleate is a convenient substrate for assay of the enzyme. The enzyme is classified as a lipase because it acts at the interface between lipid and aqueous phases, although there is no requirement for colipase, and indeed the enzyme, unlike pancreatic lipase, can be absorbed on bile salt covered surfaces. The enzyme is also readily absorbed to the surface of siliconised glass beads. At interfaces the presence of bile salts, believed to induce aggregation to a hexamer, enhances the catalysed hydrolysis of long chain fatty acid esters and triacylglycerides

(Rudd and Brockman 1984). The molecular weight of the carboxyl ester lipases from a number of species is reported as from 65,000 to 80,000. As diisopropylphosphofluoridate (DFP) is an irreversible inhibitor of the enzyme, the effects of trypsin and chymotrypsin cannot be easily nullified by the use of DFP during isolation of the enzyme. Thus it is not known whether the enzyme is synthesised as an inactive zymogen, or whether the reported presence of various isoenzymes is due to proteolysis of the lipase.

LIPOXYGENASE (EC 1.13.11.12)

During the storage and commercial milling of dormant seeds, tubers and derived food products, polyunsaturated fatty acids may be oxidised to hydroperoxides by either lipoxygenase-catalysed oxidation, photo-oxidation or chemical autoxidation.

Lipoxygenase has been found in cereals, legumes, potatoes, tomatoes and many other fruits, where it catalyses the oxidation of essential polyunsaturated fatty acids and carotenoids with a consequent loss of nutritional value. Also colour may be lost in products like semolina and pasta. Lipoxygenase-catalysed oxidation, as well as chemical oxidation, may also be indirectly responsible for the formation of rancid off-flavours. On the other hand and particularly in fruits, the required natural flavour substances – often unsaturated aldehydes and ketones – may be formed by further enzymatic degradation of hydroperoxides (see Ch. 9). The bleaching by lipoxygenases of carotenoid pigments in white wheat flour for bread manufacture is also beneficial. Also during dough mixing in air or oxygen, added soybean lipoxygenases, while causing a decrease in the content of polyunsaturated fatty acids, improve the development of bread dough, and bring about a marked increase in the release of bound lipids (Frazier et al. 1973). The beneficial effect of lipoxygenase on dough development, which only occurs if lipid oxidation takes place during mixing in the presence of oxygen, may be due to the coupled oxidation of gluten sulphydryl groups (see Ch. 5). Lipoxygenases, like the oxidative chemicals used as flour improvers, also improve bread loaf volume and retard staling. More recently, lipoxygenases and cyclooxygenase (EC 1.14.99.1) have been discovered in animal tissues, where oxidisation of polyunsaturated fatty acids – like arachidonic acid – to hydroperoxyeicosatetraenoic acids and prostaglandins occurs.

The initial enzymatic reaction catalysed by lipoxygenase only involves the activation of the substrate and the incorporation of oxygen to form hydroperoxides. The enzyme catalyses the peroxidation of the cis,cis-1,4-pentadiene group

$$-CH = CH-CH_2-CH = CH-$$

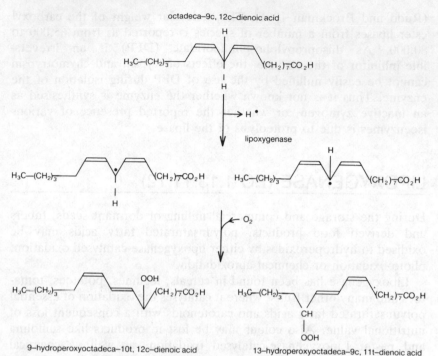

Fig. 6.9 Lipoxygenase catalysed oxidation of α-linoleic acid

of polyunsaturated fatty acids. Oleic acid, with a single double bond is not oxidised by lipoxygenase. A number of isoenzymes have been found which are generally more reactive to fatty acids than triglycerides. The overall reaction results in a direct addition reaction of molecular oxygen to an organic radical and is facilitated by one atom of iron per mole present in lipoxygenase. Activation of the substrate can occur in the absence of oxygen by abstraction of a hydrogen radical (Fig. 6.9) from a reactive methylene group positioned between the two double bonds. Through electron migration the diene radical rearranges to a more stable *trans*-form. Under aerobic conditions activated oxygen (see Ch. 10) reacts to form the peroxide. The reaction is under strict stereochemical control: for linoleic acid it has been claimed that soybean lipoxygenase I isoenzyme abstracts the 11-pro S hydrogen atom and that the 13S-hydroperoxy compound is the predominant product. The free-radical reaction can be propagated by further abstraction of a hydrogen radical from another molecule of substrate with the enzyme controlling the stereospecificity of the reaction. The rate of oxidation can be followed by either measurements of O_2 uptake, increases at 232 nm due to the formation of conjugated diene product, or the formation of products by high performance liquid chromatography. In plant tissues the hydroperoxides may be reduced, isomerised or undergo carbon–carbon cleavage to produce aldehydes through the action of other enzymes (see Ch. 9). The oxidation of carotenoid pigments by lipoxygenase is coupled to enzyme-catalysed oxidation of polyunsaturated fatty acids. Although the hydroperoxide product itself cannot oxidise the pigment, the coupled oxidation by lipoxygenase of an unsaturated fatty acid substrate such as linoleic acid is necessary. Inhibitors of lipoxygenase now include esculetin, nordihydroguaiaretic acid, eicosatetraynoic acid, caffeic acid and diphenyl disulphide.

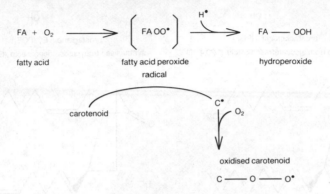

In mammalian tissues various lipoxygenases specific for catalysing the insertion of a hydroperoxide group at different carbon atoms (5-, 8-, 9-, 11-, 12- and 15-lipoxygenases) have been found. Arachidonic acid is normally the main unsaturated fatty acid constituent of cell membrane phospholipids and the metabolically active compounds derived from this and other C-20 fatty acids are now collectively known as eicosanoids. These include the leucotrienes, prostaglandins, thromboxanes and prostacyclins (Fig. 6.10). The leucotrienes contain a triene group and are synthesised by leucocytes; the prostaglandins contain a five-membered carbon ring structure. The series of prosta-glandins A to F represent various levels of oxidation and isomerisation of the cyclopentane ring. The A, B and C series of isomers are formed by dehydration of prostaglandin E series. Prostaglandin D is an isomer

Table 6.15 Physiological action of eicosanoids

Eicosanoid	Physiological action
Prostaglandins	Vasodilation, relaxation of smooth muscle, inhibition of blood platelet aggregation, raise cyclic AMP levels
Thromboxanes	Contract smooth muscle, enhance platelet aggregation
Leucotrienes	Contract smooth muscle, constrict breathing, enhance inflammatory and allergic responses

(After Gale and Egan 1984).

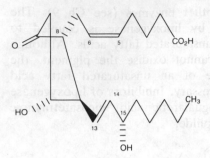

prostaglandin E₂ (PGE₂)

synthesised from eicosatetraenoic acid (C20:4 n6)

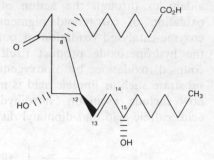

prostaglandin E₁ (PGE₁)

synthesised from eicosatrienoic acid (C20:3 n6)

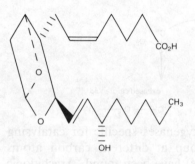

thromboxane A₂ (TXA₂)

synthesised from eicosatetraenoic acid (C20:4 n6)

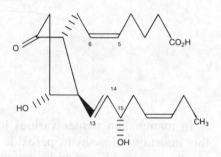

prostaglandin E₃ (PGE₃)

synthesised from eicosapentaenoic acid (C20:5 n3)

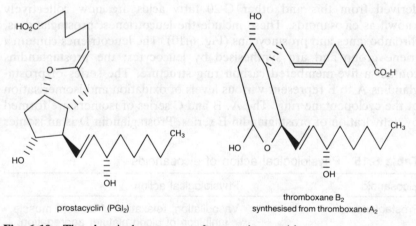

prostacyclin (PGI₂)

thromboxane B₂

synthesised from thromboxane A₂

Fig. 6.10 The chemical structures of some eicosanoids

of prostaglandin E, whereas the prostaglandin F series are formed by reduction of the E series (Fig. 6.11). The thromboxanes contain either an oxetane or pyran ring: prostacyclins are cyclic furan derivatives of prostaglandins (Fig. 6.10).

Some of the important physiological actions of eicosanoids are given in Table 6.15. Surprisingly the different eicosanoids often exert

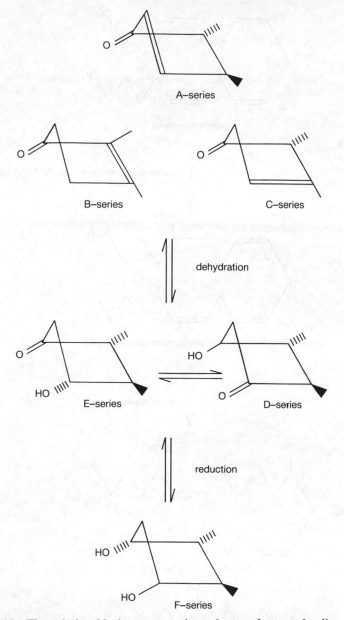

Fig. 6.11 The relationship between various classes of prostaglandin
cyclopentane rings

opposing physiological effects, which indicates that a balanced ratio of
the derived leucotrienes and prostaglandins and thromboxanes is likely
to be desirable for good health.

The leucotrienes are derived from the products formed by the
primary action of mammalian 5-lipoxygenase (Fig. 6.12) on both n-6
and n-3 polyunsaturated fatty acids. Various members of the leuco-

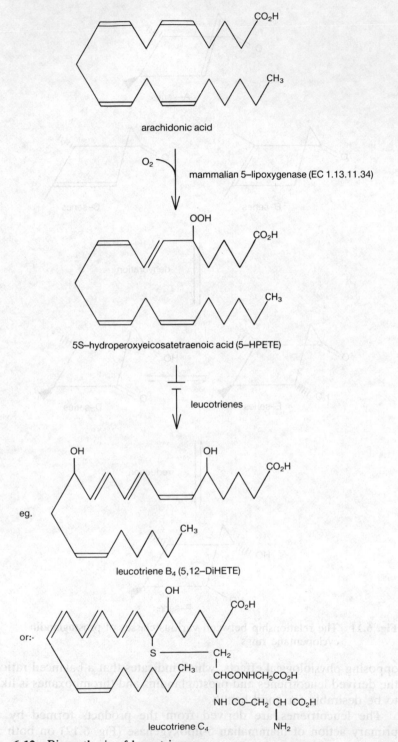

arachidonic acid

O_2

mammalian 5–lipoxygenase (EC 1.13.11.34)

OOH

CO_2H

CH_3

5S–hydroperoxyeicosatetraenoic acid (5–HPETE)

leucotrienes

eg.

OH

OH

CO_2H

CH_3

leucotriene B_4 (5,12–DiHETE)

or:-

OH

CO_2H

S ————— CH_2

CH_3

CHCONHCH_2CO_2H

NH CO–CH_2 CH CO_2H

NH_2

leucotriene C_4

Fig. 6.12 Biosynthesis of leucotrienes

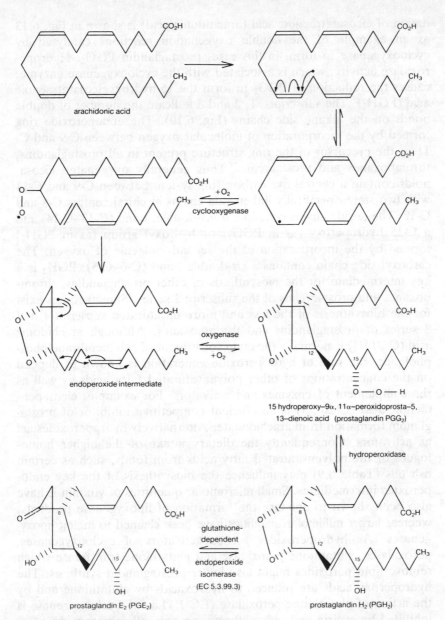

arachidonic acid

+O$_2$
cyclooxygenase

endoperoxide intermediate

oxygenase
+O$_2$

15 hydroperoxy-9α, 11α−peroxidoprosta-5,
13-dienoic acid (prostaglandin PGG$_2$)

hydroperoxidase

glutathione-
dependent
endoperoxide
isomerase
(EC 5.3.99.3)

prostaglandin E$_2$ (PGE$_2$)

prostaglandin H$_2$ (PGH$_2$)

Fig. 6.13 Biosynthesis of prostaglandins

triene family, are also found linked to a sulphur atom of cysteine. During the biosynthesis of leucotrienes from arachidonic acid, 5-hydroperoxyeicosatetraenoic acid (5-HPETE) is the primary product formed by oxygenation of the C-20 polyunsaturated fatty acid.

The prostaglandins, thromboxanes and prostacyclins are derived by oxidation of polyunsaturated fatty acids and transformation of key cyclic endoperoxides (the G and H series, Fig. 6.13). Hydroperoxidation of eicosatetraenoic acid (arachidonic acid) is shown in Fig. 6.13 as an example of the double oxygenation reactions catalysed by cyclooxygenase to form, in this case, prostaglandin PGG_2. Hydroperoxidase activity, which is associated with the cyclooxygenase enzyme, causes the reduction of PGG_2 to form the 15-hydroxyeicosatetraenoic acid (PGH_2). The subscripts, 1, 2 and 3 indicate the number of double bonds on the alkane side chains (Fig. 6.10). The endoperoxide ring formed by the incorporation of molecular oxygen between C-9 and C-11, is the precursor of the ring structure present in all prostaglandins, thromboxanes and prostacyclins. Thus generally oxygenated eicosanoids contain a central five-carbon ring system between C-9 and C-11 with two stereospecifically linked side chains at chiral centres C-8 and C-12. The ω-side chains contain a *trans*-double. bond (C-13–C-14) and a C-15 hydroperoxy (as in PGG_2) or hydroxyl group (as in PGH_2) formed by the incorporation of the second molecule of oxygen. The carboxyl side chain contains a *cis*-double bond (C-6–C-5). PGH_2 is a key intermediate for the biosynthesis of other prostaglandins, thromboxanes and prostacyclins of the subscript 2 series. Similar routes exist for the biosynthesis of the less and more unsaturated subscript 1 and 3 series of prostaglandins and thromboxanes. Although arachidonic acid (C 20 : 4) is normally the main constituent of cell membrane phospholipids, the rate of hydroperoxide generation is known to depend on the concentrations of other polyunsaturated fatty acids as well as the complement of enzymes and activators. For example, eicosapentaenoic acid (C 20 : 5) is an efficient competitive inhibitor of prostaglandin formation from arachidonate. Alternatively hydroperoxides act as activators. Consequently the dietary intake of the higher homologues of the polyunsaturated fatty acids from foods, such as certain fish oils (Table 6.9) may influence the biosynthesis of the key endoperoxide intermediates. Small micromolar quantities of vitamin E have also been shown to enhance the formation of lipoxygenase products, whereas larger millimolar quantities have been claimed to inhibit lipoxygenases. As hydroperoxides act as activators of cyclooxygenases, peroxidases, glutathione peroxidase and glutathione transferase which remove lipid peroxides might also lower prostaglandin synthesis. The hydroperoxy acids are reduced to hydroxacids by glutathione and by the action of glutathione peroxidase (EC 1.11.1.9). Cyclooxygenase is inhibited by aspirin and indomethacin, an anti-inflammatory drug..

Autoxidation can also be responsible for the formation of hydroperoxides. During autoxidation, transition metals act as catalysts and the hydroperoxides formed may be further degraded thermally during cooking to produce alkenes and aldehydes by carbon–carbon and carbon–oxygen bond fission (Frankel 1984). The autoxidation of lipids predominates at low temperature in fish homogenates where a required transition metal exists in denatured haem proteins. The reactions are typically of the free-radical type involving initiation, propagation and termination.

Photo-oxidation occurs in the presence of sensitisers such as chlorophyll or haem pigments, which are easily energised by photons. The higher energy electron of the sensitiser is able to produce singlet oxygen (Ch. 10) that adds directly to double bonds. Autoxidation is inhibited by antioxidants which include propyl gallate, butylated hydroxyanisole and hydroxytoluene. These antioxidants react with the free radicals and thus terminate the propagation reaction. Vitamin E, which is a well known natural antioxidant, acts as a free-radical scavenger. However, the antioxidants are less effective against the lipoxygenase-catalysed oxidations and therefore if relatively thermostable lipoxygenases are present the only effective way to reduce oxidation may require the exclusion of molecular oxygen.

Phospholipids

Phospholipids are acyl derivatives of sn-glycerol-3-phosphate and are classified on the composition of the R phosphate substituent (Table 6.16). Specific phospholipases for each of the positions shown in Fig. 6.14 catalyse the hydrolysis of the acyl and phosphate ester bonds. The action of phospholipase A_2 produces a lysophospholipid whereas the action of phospholipase D produces a diacylglycerophophatide. Both phospholipases C and D can only catalyse the hydrolysis of the separate phosphodiester bonds in intact phospholipids. Phospholipase D can also act as a transferase enzyme and so catalyse the incorporation of methanol or butan-1-ol groups to the phosphate residue during solvent extraction of unheated beans or cereal grains.

Table 6.16 Phospholipids

Chemical structure: 1,2-diacyl-sn-glycerol-3-phosphoryl-R	
Common name	
Phosphatidyl choline	$R=CH_2-CH_2-N(CH_3)_3$
Phosphatidyl ethanolamine	$R=CH_2-CH_2-NH_2$
N-Acylphosphatidyl ethanolamine	$R=CH_2-CH_2-NHCO.R$
Phosphatidyl serine	$R=CH_2-CH-NH_2$
	$\quad\quad\quad\quad\quad\quad\mid$
	$\quad\quad\quad\quad\quad\quad CO_2H$
Phosphatidyl inositol	$R=C_6H_6(OH)_6$

Phospholipids occur mainly in structural components such as cell membranes in animals and plants. In cereal flours the phospholipids are derived from various membranes in the endosperm, aleurone layer and germ tissues of the seed. For milk, approximately 60 per cent of the total phospholipid is found in the fat globule membrane, and in egg yolk phospholipids are mainly associated with the high density lipoprotein granules. Phospholipids, and in particular phosphatidyl

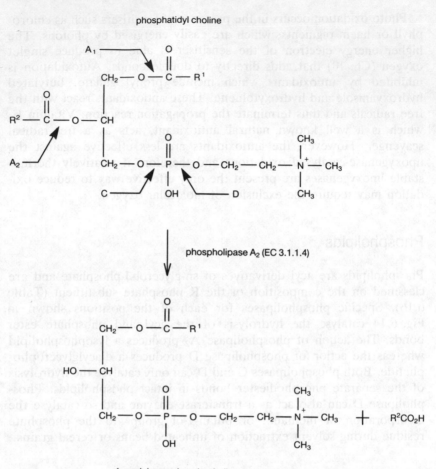

Fig. 6.14   Action of phospholipase A_2. A_1, A_2, C and D represent the sites of hydrolysis catalysed by phospholipases A_1, A_2, C and D (EC 3.1.1.32, EC 3.1.1.4, EC 3.1.4.3 and EC 3.1.4.4, respectively)

choline (lecithin), are used as emulsifiers, in the manufacture of salad creams, chocolate, ice-cream and emulsified meat products. Emulsifiers contain both hydrophilic and hydrophobic groups in the molecule; the hydrophobic fatty acids are soluble within fat globules, whereas the polar phosphate moiety is more soluble in the aqueous phase. For plant oils most phospholipids are removed during refining as 'gums' and in some instances, as for soybean oil, the phospholipids (e.g. lecithin) may be recovered economically.

In cereal starches which contain only small amounts (1 %) of lipid, the unusual monoacylphosphoglyceride has been found to be predominant (Table 6.17). For many years saturated monoacylglycerides have been used as crumb softeners in bread and indeed this property is

Table 6.17 The lipid composition in cereal products

Cereal product	Lysophatidyl choline	Free fatty acids
	(% of total lipids)	
Wheat starch[†]	62.3	11.6
Barley starch[†]	62.4	4.4
Oat starch[†]	51.6	7.7
Wheat flour	9.1	—
Wheat gluten	1.7	—

([†] Pomeranz and Chung 1983.

generally attributed to their ability to form inclusion complexes with amylose (Riisom *et al.* 1984). Inclusion complexes for a model system of amylose and myristate have been shown to be stable up to 65 °C (Bulpin *et al.* 1986). These starch-bound lipids are not easily extracted with petroleum solvents and can only be extracted with polar solvents such as propan-1-ol or with water-saturated butan-1-ol. The included lipid bound with the helical structure of amylose chains (Fig. 6.15) is thought to increase the temperature required for the manufacture of starch pastes and also for starch gelation. Also staling of bread is thought to be retarded by the presence of absorbed lipid which may form a water-impermeable film around partially gelatinised starch grains, and thus act as a barrier against the diffusion of water in the staling process.

Lysophospholipids in other foods can arise from the action of phospholipase A_2 (Fig. 6.14) which catalyses the hydrolysis of the ester bond at the C-2 atom of the phospholipid.

DERIVED LIPID IN FOODS

Glycolipids

Glycolipids contain carbohydrate moieties O-glycosidically linked to glycerol as well as esterified fatty acids. The principal sugar in these glycosyl–glycerides (glycosyldiacylglycerols) is galactose which occurs as monosaccharide (MGDG) and disaccharide (DGDG) units linked glycosidically to the hydroxyl group of C-3 of glycerol (Fig. 6.16). In some instances the primary alcohol group of the carbohydrate is also acylated. In cereals the glycosylglycerides are found exclusively in the endosperm and contain a high amount of α-linolenic acid. The average content of DGDG and MGDG in endosperm is approximately 200 mg and 80 mg per 100 g, respectively, which may represent up to 25 per

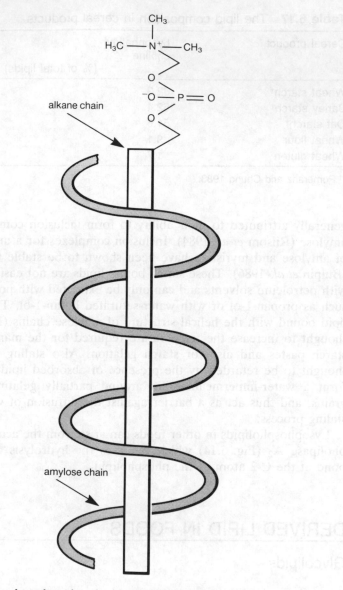

Fig. 6.15 Amylose–lysophosphatidylcholine complex

cent of the total lipid present in wheat flour and wheat gluten. For wheat flour the polar lipids, and in particular the glycolipids, have a marked beneficial effect on bread loaf volume. It has been suggested that increasing the levels of glycolipids by genetic means could be worthwhile.

Other glycolipids found in cereals include the glycosylceramides, where the sugar is attached to an amino alcohol instead of glycerol (Fig. 6.17), but the effect of these on loaf volume is unknown. The

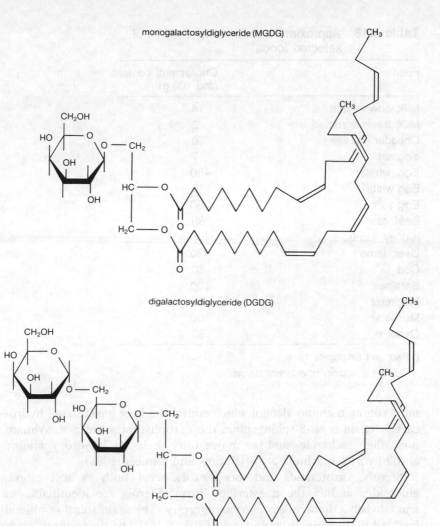

Fig. 6.16 Typical chemical structure of galactosyldiglycerides

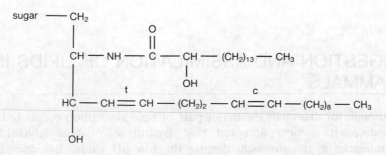

Fig. 6.17 Glycosylcerebroside of hydroxypalmityl-*cis*-8-sphingenine

Table 6.18 Approximate cholesterol content of
selected foods[†]

Food	Cholesterol content (mg/100 g)
Milk, cow's fresh	14
Milk, fresh skimmed	2
Cheddar cheese	70
Yoghurt	7
Egg, whole	450
Egg white	0
Egg yolk	1260
Beef, raw	65
Kidney, lamb	400
Liver, lamb	430
Cod	50
Sardines	100
Mackerel	80
Mussels[‡]	100
Oysters[‡]	50

([†] Paul and Southgate 1978).

[‡] Contain a number of different sterols.

most common amino alcohol which contains a long unsaturated hydrocarbon chain is *cis*-8-sphingenine; the carbohydrates are glucosylman-
nose oligosaccharides and the major fatty acids are 2-hydroxypalmitic
and 2-hydroxyarachidic acids (Fujino and Ohnishi 1983).

Sterols, carotenoids and tocopherols occur both as acyl esters,
glucosides and in the unesterified form. Sterols are identifiable as
trimethylsilylethers by gas chromatography. The main sterol of animal
fats and marine oils is cholesterol (Table 6.18). The phytosterols from
plants include β-sitosterol (which is the most common), stigmasterol,
campesterol and brassicasterol (Fig. 6.18). The presence of these
compounds can be used to identify the source of fats and oils (Table
6.19).

DIGESTION AND ASSIMILATION OF LIPIDS IN MAMMALS

Although for mammals the major part of lipid absorption occurs in the
intestine, it is now accepted that hydrolysis of triacylglycerides
commences in the stomach, despite the low pH value. Evidence for
hydrolysis of dietary fat in the stomach has been obtained by the

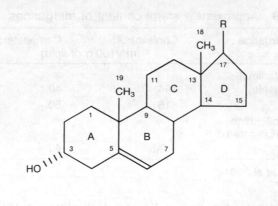

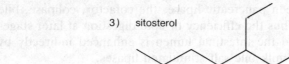

1) cholesterol

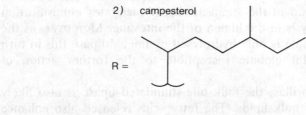

2) campesterol

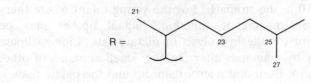

3) sitosterol

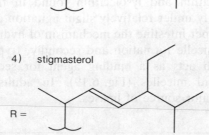

4) stigmasterol

Fig. 6.18 The chemical structures of some common sterols

Table 6.19 Approximate sterol content of margarines

Type of margarine	Cholesterol	Campesterol
	(mg/100 g of lipid)	
Mixed oils (animal, fish/vegetable)	194	40
Vegetable	16	50
Vegetable oils, high in polyunsaturated fats	2.5	40

(From Egan *et al.* 1981).

characterisation of a lingual lipase which differs substantially from pancreatic lipases and esterase. In suckling animals the lingual lipase is particularly important: it is secreted from the von Ebner glands at the base of the tongue, mixed intimately with food and initiates hydrolysis at pH 2.0 to 3.0 in the stomach. For the young infant where there may be insufficient pancreatic function, lingual lipases may be especially important for the hydrolysis of dietary fats. Lingual lipase is secreted rapidly by mammals after feeding: small amounts of other lipases may also arise from oral microorganisms and the palate tissues. Although during a short 15 to 30 min. period only limited hydrolysis occurs to produce mainly diglycerides and free fatty acids, such a preliminary digestion in the stomach clearly facilitates emulsification and further hydrolysis in the lumen of the intestine. Moreover, as the intact milk fat globule is only hydrolysed by lingual lipase this in turn makes the milk fat globule susceptible to the further action of pancreatic lipase.

For man and gorillas, the milk bile-stimulated lipase is also likely to aid digestion of milk lipids. The fatty acids released also enhance the interaction between pancreatic lipase, the cofactor, colipase, bile salts and substrate. Thus the efficiency of lipid digestion at later stages in the duodenum and the intestinal lumen is enhanced indirectly by both lingual and the milk bile salt stimulated lipases.

The chemical mixture of fatty acids, di- and triglycerides, bile salts, phospholipids, lecithin and lysolecithin found in the duodenum is believed to emulsify under relatively slight agitation and shear. In the duodenum and upper intestine the mechanism of hydrolysis is believed to involve first, micelle formation and secondly, trypsin activation of pro-colipase which acts as a binding agent for secreted pancreatic lipase to the lipid micelles (Fig. 6.19). In adults the pancreatic secretion is the major source of lipases.

Fig. 6.19 Schematic diagram for the aggregation of lipid micelles, colipase and lipase

Stigmasterol	β-Sitasterol (mg/100 g of lipid)	Brassicasterol
7.5	52	10
17	140	5
35	165	0

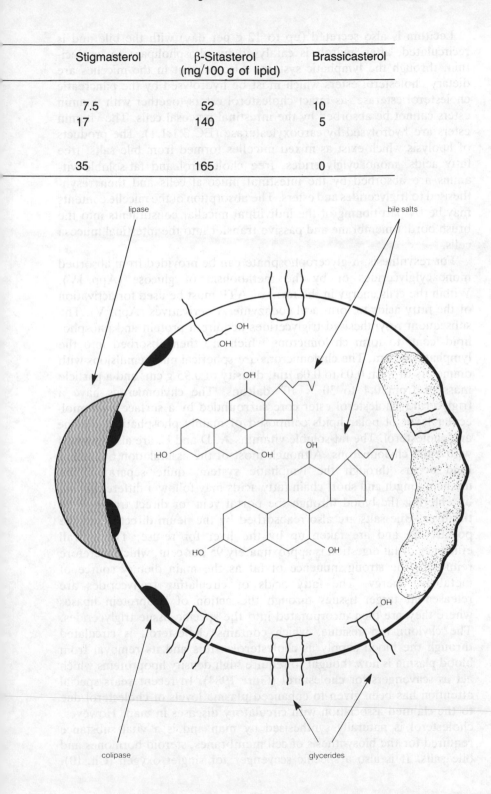

Lecithin is also secreted (up to 12 g per day) with the bile and is recirculated, after hydrolysis catalysed by phospholipase to lysolecithin, through the lymphatic system. Also present in the micelles are dietary cholesterol esters which must be hydrolysed by the pancreatic cholesterol esterase, as intact cholesterol esters together with vitamin esters cannot be absorbed by the intestinal mucosal cells. The vitamin esters are hydrolysed by carboxylesterase (EC 3.1.1.1). The products of lipolysis which exist as mixed micelles formed from bile salts, free fatty acids, monoacylglycerides, free cholesterol and fat-soluble vitamins are absorbed by the intestinal mucosal cells and then resynthesised to triglycerides and esters. The absorption of the micelle contents may be by partitioning of the individual micellar constituents into the brush border membrane and passive transfer into the intestinal mucosa cells.

For resynthesis, α-glycerophosphate can be provided from absorbed monoacylglycerides or by the metabolism of glucose (App. IV). Within the cells energy in the form of ATP must be used for activation of the fatty acids to form acyl coenzyme A derivatives (App. V). The subsequent resynthesised triglycerides acquire a protein and phospholipid 'coat' to form chylomicrons which are then absorbed into the lymphatic system. The chylomicrons are spherical microemulsions with diameters of from 0.03 to 0.06 μm, density of 0.95 g/cm^3 and a particle mass of from 0.4 to 30 $\times$ 10^9 daltons. The chylomicrons have a triglyceride–cholesterol ester core surrounded by a surface monomolecular layer of polar lipids composed of mainly phosphatidyl choline and cholesterol. The fat-soluble vitamins A, D and E, are also imbibed within the chylomicrons. Although most of the assimilation of dietary lipid occurs through the lymphatic system, quite separately the medium length and short chain fatty acids may follow a different route by entering the blood through the portal vein for direct transport to the liver. Bile salts are also reabsorbed by the ileum directly into the portal vein and are taken up by the liver for re-use. The overall efficiency of fat digestion is approximately 95 per cent, which therefore reinforces the strong influence of fat as the main dietary source of metabolic energy. The fatty acids of circulating triglycerides are released at target tissues through the action of lipoprotein lipases where they are then incorporated into the specific tissue triglycerides. The chylomicron residue, which contains cholesterol, is circulated through the blood supply as cholesterol esters and its removal from blood plasma is now thought to require high density lipoproteins which act as scavengers for cholesterol (Gurr 1984). In recent years special attention has been given to enhanced plasma levels of cholesterol due to the claimed association with circulatory diseases in man. However, cholesterol is naturally synthesised by man and is a vital substance required for the biosynthesis of cell membranes, steroid hormones and bile salts. It is also a specific scavenger for singlet oxygen (Ch. 10).

Nevertheless, excess dietary cholesterol may not sufficiently inhibit natural cholesterol biosynthesis and this probably contributes to higher plasma levels. The relationship between dietary cholesterol intake and biosynthesis of cholesterol in man is not fully understood.

Generally, the transport of other lipid-imbibed substances through the lymphatic system may be more significant than previously appreciated, as milk xanthine oxidase entrapped within liposomes in homogenised milk is apparently transported through the lymphatic system to be released unchanged into the blood supply (Ross *et al.* 1980). Therefore other enzymes or macromolecules incorporated into liposomes, accidentally by the food processor, might also pass undetected into the circulatory systems. It has been shown that intact liposomes can release active enzymes on hydrolysis (Ross *et al.* 1980). Also it has been claimed that assimilated xanthine oxidase, as a producer of superoxide anion (Ch. 10) is responsible for the initial development of atherosclerosis in humans (Zikakis *et al.* 1983).

KEY FACTS

1.   Oil seeds contain substantial amounts of neutral triglycerides. Cereals contain only small amounts of oil present mainly in the germ.
2.   Fats provide a readily available source of metabolic energy, (9 kcal per g), fat-soluble vitamins and the dietary essential polyunsaturated fatty acids.
3.   Fats soften the textural properties of foods. The type of crystal structure and melting point is determined by the way the mixture of triglyceride molecules pack.
4.   Oleic and linoleic acids are the predominant fatty acids in plant lipids. Butyric and caproic acids occur mainly in cow's milk. Animal fats contain substantial amounts of palmitic and stearic acids.
5.   Only marine foods contain significant amounts of the higher unsaturated eicosapentaenoic acids (C20 : 5).
6.   Human milk fat differs from cow's milk fat which contains more short chain fatty acids but less linoleic acid.
7.   Milk fat droplets are protected by the fat globule membrane which is composed of phospholipids and glycoproteins.
8.   The melting points and functional properties of fats in foods are modified by chemical hydrogenation and transesterification.
9.   The polyunsaturated fatty acids contain methylene interrupted double bonds and are classified into n-3, n-6 and n-9 families. The polyunsaturated fatty acids are required for the biosynthesis of prostaglandins, leucotrienes and thromboxanes. Linoleic and α-linolenic acids are essential dietary fatty acids, whereas arachidonic acid is an essential metabolite.

10. The actions of natural and microbial lipases in foods are responsible for soap-like taints. Lingual, bile salt stimulated and pancreatic lipases are responsible for the hydrolysis of neutral triglycerides during mammalian digestion.
11. In plant foods, lipoxygenases catalyse the oxidation of polyunsaturated fatty acids to their hydroperoxides.
12. Phospholipids and lysophospholipids act as emulsifiers in foods. Small amounts of lysophospholipids and glycolipids are associated with the endosperm starch of cereals.
13. Hydrolysed lipids, sterols and fat-soluble vitamins are assimilated into the lymphatic system in mammals in the form of chylomicrons.

REFERENCES

Borgström, B. and Erlanson-Albertsson, C. (1984).'Pancreatic colipase', in *Lipases* (eds. Borgström, B. and Brockman, H. L.). Elsevier, Amsterdam.

Bulpin, P. V., Cutler, A. N. and Lips, A. (1986) 'Physical properties of amylose–fatty acid complexes in solution', in *Gums and Stabilisers for the Food Industry* 3 (eds. Phillips, G. O., Wedlock, D. J. and Williams, P. A.). Elsevier Applied Science Publishers, London.

Chen, I. S., Subramaniam, S., Cassidy, M. M., Sheppard, A. J. and Vahouny, G. V. (1985) 'Intestinal absorption and lipoprotein transport of (ω-3)-eicosapentaenoic acid', *J. Nutr.*, **115**, 219–25.

Egan, H., Kirk, R. S. and Sawyer, R. (1981) *Pearson's Chemical Analysis of Foods*, 8th edn. Churchill Livingstone, Longman, London.

FAO/WHO/UNU (1985) 'Energy protein requirements', Report of a Joint FAO/WHO/UNU Expert Consultation World Health Organisation Technical Report series 724. WHO, Geneva.

Frankel, E. N. (1984) 'Recent advances in the chemistry of rancidity of fats', in Special Publication no. 47, *Recent Advances in the Chemistry of Meat* (ed. Bailey, A. J.). Royal Society of Chemistry, London.

Frazier, P. J., Leigh-Dugmore, F. A., Daniels, N. W. R., Russell Eggitt, P. W. and Coppock, J. M. B. (1973) 'The effect of lipoxygenase action on the mechanical development of wheat flour doughs', *J. Sci. Food Agric.*, **24**, 421–36.

Frazier, P. J., Daniels, N. W. and Russell Eggitt, P. W. (1981) 'Lipid–protein interactions during dough development', *J. Sci. Food Agric.*, **31**, 877–97.

Fujino, Y. and Ohnishi, M. (1983) 'Spingolipids in wheat grain', *J. Cer. Sci.*, **1**, 159–68.

Gale, P. H. and Egan, R. W. (1984) 'Prostaglandin endoperoxide synthase-catalysed oxidation reaction', in *Free Radicals in Biology*, vol. VI (ed. Pryor, W. A.). Academic Press, I Orlando, Florida.

Gurr, M. I. (1984) *Role of Fats in Food and Nutrition*. Elsevier Applied Science Publishers, London.

Huang A. H. C. (1984) 'Plant lipases', in *Lipases* (eds. Borgström, B. and Brockman, H. L.). Elsevier, Amsterdam.

Kochhar, S. P. and Matsui, T. (1984) 'Essential fatty acids and *trans* contents of some oils, margarine and other food fats', *Food Chem.*, **13**, 85–101.

MacRitchie, F. (1983) 'The role of lipids in baking', in *Lipids in Cereal Technology* (ed. Barnes, P. J.). Academic Press, London.

MacRitchie, F. and Gras, P. W. (1973) 'The role of flour lipids in baking', *Cereal Chem.*, **50**, 292–302.

Minifie, B. W. (1982) *Chocolate, Cocoa and Confectionery: Science and Technology*, 2nd edn. AVI Publishing Co., Westport, Connecticut.

Paul, A. A. and Southgate, D. A. T. (1978) *McCance and Widdowson's The Composition of Foods*, 4th edn. of MRC Special Report no. 297. HMSO, London and Elsevier, Amsterdam.

Pomeranz, Y. and Chung, O. K. (1983) 'Lipids in cereal products', in *Lipids in Cereal Technology* (ed. Barnes, P. J.). Academic Press, London.

Riisom, T., Krog, N. and Eriksen, J. (1984) 'Amylose complexing capacities of *cis*- and *trans*-unsaturated monoglycerides in relation to their functionality in bread', *J. Cer. Sci.*, **2**, 105–18.

Ross, D. J., Sharnick, S. and Oster, K. A. (1980) 'Liposomes as a proposed vehicle for the persorption of bovine xanthine oxidase', *Proc. Soc. Exp. Biol. Med.*, **163**, 141–5.

Rudd, E. A. and Brockman, H. L. (1984) 'Pancreatic carboxyl ester lipase (cholesterol esterase)', in *Lipases* (eds. Borgström, B. and Brockman, H. L.). Elsevier, Amsterdam.

Verger, R. (1984) 'Pancreatic lipase', in *Lipases* (eds. Borgstrom, B. and Brockman, H. L.). Elsevier, Amsterdam.

Zikakis, J. P., Dressel, M. A., Silver, M. R. (1983) 'Bovine, caprine and human milk xanthine oxidases: isolation, purification and characterisation', in *Instrumental Analysis of Foods, Recent Progress*, vol. 2 (eds. Charalambous, G. and Inglett, G.). Academic Press I, Orlando, Florida.

ADDITIONAL READING

Gale, P. H. and Egan, R. W. (1984) 'Prostaglandin endoperoxide synthase-catalysed oxidation reaction', in *Free Radicals in Biology*, vol. VI (ed. Pryor, W. A.). Academic Press, Orlando, Florida.

Galliard, T. and Chan, H. W.-S. (1980) 'Lipoxygenases', in *The Biochemistry of Plants, a Comprehensive Treatise*, vol. 4, *Lipids: Structure and Function* (ed. Stumpf, P. K.). Academic Press, New York.

Gunstone, F. D. and Norris, F. A. (1983) *Lipids in Foods*. Pergamon Press, Oxford.

Gurr, M. I. (1984) *Role of Fats in Food and Nutrition*. Elsevier Applied Science Publishers, London.

Gurr, M. I. (1984) *The Lipid Handbook*. Chapman and Hall, London.

Gurr, M. I. and James, A. T. (1980) *Lipid Biochemistry: An Introduction*, 3rd edn. Chapman and Hall, London.

Minifie, B. W. (1982) *Chocolate, Cocoa and Confectionery: Science and Technology*, 2nd edn. AVI Publishing Company, Westport, Connecticut.

Rudney, H. and Sexton, R. C. (1986) 'Regulation of cholesterol biosynthesis', *Ann. Rev. Nutr.*, **6**, 245–73.

Walstra, P. and Jenness, R. (1984) *Dairy Chemistry and Physics*. John Wiley and Sons, New York.

Part IV

The chemical elements and vitamins as nutrients

CHAPTER 7

The chemical elements as food components

INTRODUCTION

The distribution of the major elements in the earth's crust is shown in Table 7.1. The eight elements provide more than 98 per cent of the atoms in the earth's crust. Oxygen makes up more than 90 per cent of the total atomic volume occupied by elements. The earth's crust is a packing of oxygen atoms bonded to silicon and the ions of common metals. From these elements, hydrogen, carbon, nitrogen, oxygen and calcium account for more than 90 per cent of the atoms of the human body (Table 7.2). In human tissues which contain 60 per cent water, oxygen and hydrogen represent 63 and 9.3 per cent, respectively. The four most abundant atoms in living organisms, hydrogen, carbon, oxygen and nitrogen have atomic numbers of 1, 6, 7 and 8 and are the smallest and lightest elements which can achieve a stable electronic configuration by adding from one to four electrons to their outer shells to form covalent bonds.

Table 7.1 Average content of the major elements in the earth's crust

Atomic number	Element	% by weight
8	O	46.60
11	Na	2.83
12	Mg	2.09
13	Al	8.13
14	Si	27.72
19	K	2.59
20	Ca	3.63
26	Fe	5.0
	Total:	98.59

(Mason 1966).

Table 7.2   Approximate amounts of the major elements in plants
and adult man

Atomic number	Element symbol	Man	Alfalfa
		(% of dry weight)	
1	H	6.60	5.54
6	C	48.43	45.37
7	N	12.85	3.30
8	O	23.70	41.4
11	Na	0.65	0.16
12	Mg	0.10	0.33
15	P	1.58	0.28
16	S	1.60	0.44
17	Cl	0.45	0.28
19	K	0.55	0.91
20	Ca	3.45	2.31
		99.96	100.32

(From Rankama and Sahama 1964, reproduced with permission, *Geochemistry*
1964, by the University of Chicago).

ELEMENTS AS MACROCONSTITUENTS OF BIOLOGICAL MATERIAL

Of the earth's ninety elements, an increasing number have been
recognised as essential for life. Information of essentiality for trace
elements such as selenium, chromium and molybdenum has been
obtained: discoveries have shown that such elements are vital constituents of enzymes or cofactors. In some instances, a metal ion is only
a constituent of just a few physiologically important enzymes. Nevertheless, in general terms biological selection during evolution has
resulted in the use by living systems of just a small number of certain
elements as essential components of plants, animals and microorganisms.

The major pathway through which the chemical elements pass to
man is through the food chain. Of the twenty-one elements shown
below and definitely established to be essential for living matter, most
are relatively small and only three of these elements have an atomic
number greater than 30. Most of the elements are readily available in
the earth's crust. Their assimilation by plants and animals depends on
their solubility in water and the ease of assimilation and passage across
cell membranes.

Hydrogen	Phosphorus	Chromium	Selenium
Carbon	Sulphur	Manganese	Molybdenum
Oxygen	Chlorine	Iron	Iodine

Nitrogen   Potassium   Cobalt
Sodium   Calcium   Copper
Magnesium   Vanadium   Zinc

In comparison with the earth's crust, carbon, hydrogen, nitrogen, phosphorus, chlorine and sulphur are concentrated in living matter, whereas many of the metals like sodium, magnesium and particularly iron, silicon and aluminium are generally diminished. Clearly despite the abundance of aluminium, a biological role for this element does not exist, although mental illness may be associated with increased levels of aluminium in brain tissues. Certain plants will concentrate some elements: aluminium accumulates in the Lycopodiaceae, silicon in monocotyledons, sodium and chlorine in halophytes, radium in *Lemna spp.* and rubidium in some sea-shore plants.

Nitrogen

Organic nitrogen occurs almost exclusively in the reduced state, where it normally forms three covalent bonds and possesses a lone pair of electrons. It is sufficiently electronegative to form a 'hard' base. This means that it is not readily polarised and as a Lewis base it can donate a pair of electrons to form a coordinate bond. Thus amines, if not protonated, are potential ligands of importance for the hard Lewis acids. Nitrogen serves best as a ligand for metal complexation in heterocyclic rings, such as in the imidazole group of histidine, or as the pyrrole of a porphyrin. More generally, Needham said that nitrogen with its five valence electrons – which is adjacent to carbon in the periodic table – introduces an essential distortion into the symmetry of carbon compounds which provides additional properties of coordination, basicity, charge and redox activity.

Sulphur

Sulphur, like oxygen, is a group VI element but possesses a lower electronegativity than oxygen. Sulphur exists in oxidation states from +2 to +6. As a soft base sulphur ligands form complexes with soft Lewis acids such as Fe^{2+}, Zn^{2+} and Cu^{2+}. Sulphur is involved as a ligand in a number of enzymes and metalloproteins of which the iron–sulphur proteins and copper proteins are the most conspicuous. The sulphydryl group participates in redox reactions and the sulphur atom forms disulphide bonds to give structural stability in proteins. Organic sulphonates may enhance the water solubility of organic compounds as the sulphonic group is ionised at the metabolic pH values. Sulphur can be regarded as an alternative substituent for the more electronegative oxygen, and thus extends the capacity of organic compounds to complex metals, enter into redox reactions and stabilise the structure of proteins by forming covalent disulphide bonds. Such covalent bonds exist as cross-links in proteins which are cleaved by reduction and not hydrolysis.

In both animals and plants sulphur is found mainly in coenzyme A, glutathione and the amino acids, cystine and methionine. In *Brassica spp.* sulphur is found in thioglucosides and in *Allium spp.* as sulphoxides (Ch. 9). Lower plants may contain substantial amounts of organic sulphonates, metalthiolate proteins and iron–molybdenum–sulphur proteins. For animals the sulphur amino acids are essential dietary constituents and are often in short supply. In mammals sulphur is excreted as sulphate(VI) after oxidation of metabolically produced sulphite(IV). The oxidation of sulphite in the liver is catalysed by sulphite oxidase. Reactive species of oxygen may also cause the formation of oxidised sulphur species (Ch. 10).

Phosphorus

The occurrence of phosphorus in foods as inorganic phosphate and organic esters is widespread and consequently deficiencies of phosphorus in animals are rare. Adult man contains approximately 700 g of phosphorus (approximately 1 % of body weight) with more than 80 per cent of the element in the bones. The bones act as a metabolic reserve of phosphorus and calcium as well as a structural component. Animal products are particularly good dietary sources of phosphorus, whereas for cereals and soya-based products the availability of phosphorus is less due to its substantive occurrence also in phytate esters. In all biological materials phosphorus is present in nucleic acids and hence substantial amounts of phosphorus are present in all foods (Table 7.6). In the hen's egg, phosphorus is stored as a covalent ester of serine residues in the protein phosvitin.

In both plants and animals only the fully oxidised state of phosphorus(V) is used for metabolic reactions. At neutral pH values the stable oxyanion exists in the ionised divalent state in equilibrium with substantial amounts of the protonated monovalent anion. Thus, like carbonate, divalent orthophosphate acts as a buffer. The stability of the P–O bond which is not polarised, due to the non-metallic property and lower electronegativity of phosphorus, permits the formation of stable organic esters and anhydrides, like ADP and ATP. These anhydrides are stable in water. The phosphate anhydride stability resides in the strength of the resonating phosphoryl bond which delocalises the electrons. The high energy of the anhydride bonds, as exemplified in ATP, resides as the high energy required to form the P–O–P bonds due to electrostatic repulsion between the three phosphate oxyanion groups. This energy is released on hydrolysis of the O–P covalent bonds. Mixed anhydrides formed with carboxyl groups are also high energy compounds and act as metabolic intermediates (e.g. acetyl phosphate). Phosphate esters, such as glucose-1-phosphate or fructose-1,6-diphosphate are activated intermediates for the catabolism of hexose sugars. Owing to the stability of the covalent P–O bond and the ability of the oxyanion to form stable diesters, the backbone of nucleic acids is composed of phosphate esters.

The oxyanions of phosphorus, like those of sulphur, vanadium and molybdenum, contribute to the electrochemical properties of living material. The main cations are provided by sodium, potassium, calcium and magnesium. These seven ions maintain the electrical neutrality of living tissues and also play a part in maintaining the proper osmotic pressure and volume of fluids.

ELEMENTS AS MICROCONSTITUENTS OF BIOLOGICAL MATERIALS

The trace elements represent a third group of elements used by living organisms. They include the group with periodic table numbers from 23 to 53 in addition to fluorine and boron; boron being essential for plants. The trace elements used by animals and plants are present in only relatively small amounts in the earth's crust (Table 7.3). The known trace elements essential for man are copper, chromium, cobalt, iron, manganese, molybdenum, zinc, selenium and iodine. For all the trace elements, with the exception of iodine, the concentration in man is considerably less than that in the environment.

Although the trace elements are required only in small amounts, nutritionally they are of comparable importance to the vitamins. In many cases the trace elements serve as essential components for many enzymes (Table 7.8), which occupy key positions in metabolism. It is accepted that the extraordinary varied chemistry of the complexes of these metals with organic ligands is the general property that leads to their participation in catalysis by enzymes. The binding of, particularly transition metals, to proteins involves the formation of dative bonds frequently with nitrogen and sulphur atoms; there are many instances where the nitrogens of the imidazole ring of one or more histidine residues serve as ligands. The pyridine-type nitrogen atom of the imidazole ring loses a proton in the presence of a metal cation, which may be at several units of pH less than the intrinsic pK value of the dissociating imidazole residue. Similarly, terminal and ε-amino groups of proteins form dative bonds with metal cations. Coordination, through a lone pair of electrons, can also occur with the oxygen atoms

Table 7.3 Approximate content of nutritionally essential trace elements in the earth's crust and man

Element atomic number		Symbol	Earth's crust[†] (ppm)
5		B[§]	1×10^1
9		F	7×10^2
23		V	1.5×10^2
24		Cr	1×10^2
25		Mn	1×10^3
26	1st series of	Fe	5×10^4
27	transitional elements	Co	2.5×10^1
29		Cu	5.5×10^1
30		Zn	6.5×10^1
34		Se	5×10^{-2}
42		Mo	1.5
54		I[¶]	3×10^{-1}

(† Mason 1966; ‡ Schroeder 1965).

§ Boron is essential for plants.

¶ Iodine is the only trace element which is enriched in a single organ over the environmental concentration.

of both carbonyl groups and phenolic residues. In sulphur-containing ligands, as in cysteine and methionine, vacant d orbitals are also available for bonding. Thus in foods a large number of ligands, as components of proteins and polysaccharides, are potentially available for the substantial binding of the transition elements. Further, it is not always appreciated that some of the trace elements found in foods may be adsorbed and chelated during the processing and manufacture of food products. Thus the values given for the quantities of trace elements in foods are extremely variable. For new food products exposed to metal surfaces during processing, it seems desirable in the future that full spectrographic analyses for mineral elements should be sought. Recently, using inductively coupled plasma emission spectroscopy, average data has been published for the content of iron, copper and zinc in immigrant foods used in Great Britain (Tan *et al.* 1985).

Many of the trace elements are transition metals, which owe their unique properties to their ability to form coordination complexes with ligands. In this way their chemical activity is controlled to allow their use as electron acceptors in biological redox reactions catalysed by metallo-enzymes, where the metal is held deep within the structure of the protein. However, extraneous-bound transition metals may induce uncontrolled oxidative reactions of the sulphydryl, sulphide and amino groups as found in essential amino acids (Ch. 3). Tungsten is also an antagonist to molybdenum (Cohen *et al.* 1973).

Human body‡ (ppm)	(mg/70 kg)
not known	
not known	
3×10^{-1}	20
9×10^{-2}	6
3×10^{-1}	20
5.7×10^{1}	4100
4×10^{-2}	3
1.4	100
3.3×10^{1}	2300
not known	
7×10^{-2}	5
4.3×10^{-1}	30

The transition elements also have important influences on the chemistry of molecular oxygen and its reduced products: both iron and copper may contribute towards the production of toxic species of reduced oxygen. While alternatively iron and copper are contained within enzymes like superoxide dismutase, peroxidase and catalase which provide a defence by destroying superoxide radical and hydrogen peroxide (Ch. 10). Other essential trace elements may include the so-called ultratrace elements (Frieden 1984), lithium, silicon, tin, nickel, arsenic, lead, cadmium, fluorine, bromine, are claimed to be required in less than 50 ng per gram of food. However, except for nickel and silicon, deficiency symptoms in specific animals have not been described for the above elements.

ANALYSIS FOR METAL ELEMENTS

Analyses for inorganic elements in a whole range of foods and living tissues in general have been carried out over a long period and the average values so obtained provide a guide, from which the nutrient value of foods may be estimated. The causes of variation in trace element content are many, with biological variation being of prime importance. The biological variation for food materials of both animal and plant origin is influenced by seasons, age, agricultural practice and exposure in the environment. Furthermore, in recent years methods of chemical analysis for minerals have changed considerably from labour-intensive and time-consuming classical methods to now capital-intensive and highly sensitive instrumental methods. For non-metals, analysis is usually carried out by titration or a colorimetric method as for phosphorus in phosphate. For metals in foods, recent instrumental analysis has been carried out by atomic absorption spectroscopy and inductively coupled plasma emission spectroscopy (Tan *et al.* 1985). A wide range of ion selective electrodes can now also be used for quickly estimating small concentrations of a number of elements and compounds. Analyses of high sensitivity using specialist facilities may include, for potassium gamma-ray counting of ^{40}K which comprises 12×10^{-3} per cent of total potassium. For whole tissues, animals or plants, neutron activation analysis is available. For analysis of surfaces, X-ray fluorescence spectrometry and electron spectroscopy are available. In growing plants and animals the uptake and morphological distribution of elements is partly controlled biologically whereas elements added separately, by intention or otherwise, to foods or other materials, through technological processes, are likely to be adsorbed selectively at surfaces. Consequently surface analysis coupled to analysis of the data by computer could be increasingly used to assess and control the contamination of foodstuffs by mineral elements.

MINERAL NUTRITION

Sodium and potassium occur widely in both plants and animal foods. Additional dietary sources of sodium are from ham, bacon, cured meats (Table 7.4) and monosodium glutamate. Also sodium is frequently added to the human diet in the form of table salt. However, in most foods the concentration of potassium is greater than sodium. The human adult body contains approximately 64 g of Na$^+$ and 180 g of K$^+$. Sodium is the main cation of extracellular fluid, and is only an essential element because it is required mainly to maintain neutrality and the ionic strength of extracellular fluids. In certain halophytic plants sodium is required to maintain turgor pressure in the vacuoles. Such plants may show a favourable growth response to sodium. Owing to the widespread occurrence of Na$^+$ and K$^+$, deficiencies do not normally occur, but a Na$^+$ deficiency can be induced during excessive exercise which results in perspiration, if replacement of sodium from drinking water is not achieved.

Generally, animal cells contain low concentrations of intracellular Na$^+$ and relatively high concentrations of K$^+$ (approximately 100 mM), whereas in blood plasma the concentrations of Na$^+$ and K$^+$ are 140 mM

Table 7.4 Approximate content of sodium and
potassium in selected foods

Food commodity	Na (mg/100 g)	K
Fresh foods		
Brussels sprouts	4	380
Eggs	140	140
Liver	80	310
Milk	50	140
Oranges	3	200
Peas	1	340
Potatoes	7	570
Food products		
Bacon, UK	1480	230
Butter	870	15
Chocolate	120	420
Coffee	40	4000
Margarine	800	5

(From Buss and Robertson 1978).

and 5 mM, respectively. The ionic gradients between extra- and intracellular fluids are maintained by a specific Na^+/K^+ pump mechanism
which uses ATP as the energy source. The specific pump mechanism
has been shown to depend on the presence of a membrane-bound
Na^+/K^+ activated ATPase which is responsible for the pumping out of
Na^+ from intracellular fluids. The energy necessary to pump Na^+ and
K^+ against their concentration gradients is obtained from the hydrolysis of ATP. The uptake of glucose or amino acids by the intestinal
brush border cells is coupled to the simultaneous entry of Na^+. The
rate of entry of Na^+ depends on the Na^+ concentration gradient across
the cell membrane and therefore also depends on the efficiency of the
Na^+/K^+ activated ATPase regulated pump.

The intracellular K^+ clearly neutralises intracellular acids and maintains the cellular osmotic pressure: the ionic strength of intracellular
fluids maintains the conformation of active enzymes, in both animal
and plant cells. The importance of intracellular K^+ as opposed to Na^+
is derived from the larger ionic radius and the smaller hydration energy
of K^+.

Ion	Atomic number	Ionic radius (Å)	Hydration energy (kcal/mole)
Na^+	11	0.95	−72
K^+	19	1.33	−55

Consequently less energy is expended for the replacement of water
molecules in the K^+ hydrated shell by organic ligands. Also for the

Table 7.5 Approximate content of magnesium
in some selected foods

Food commodity	Mg (mg/100 g)
Beef, raw	20
Cheddar cheese	25
Cottage cheese	6
Milk	12
Oatmeal	110
Soya flour	240
Wheat bran	520
White wheat flour	36
Whole egg	12
Wholemeal wheat flour	140
Cockles	51
Cod	23
Oysters	42
Pilchards	39
Plaice	22
Sardines	52
Yeast, dried	230

(Paul and Southgate 1978).

active pumping out of Na^+ from cells advantage is made of the smaller size of the Na^+ ion and the closer approach by negatively charged ligands which can be achieved. The nutritional value of K^+ over Na^+ arises from both the lower polarisation of water and ligands by K^+, and its non-competition for enzyme active sites which specifically require complexing of the divalent and redox metals.

Magnesium is widely found in plant and animal tissues (Table 7.5). Cereal products, potatoes, vegetables and fruits provide most of the human requirement for magnesium. The total human body content of magnesium is approximately 60 g, with 60 per cent of this being located in the skeletal tissues. The level of magnesium in blood plasma is constant at approximately 20 mg per litre. Deficiencies of magnesium are rare but can occur in alcoholics, who have low plasma levels of Mg^{2+}. Also magnesium deficiency, together with deficiencies of other elements, may be associated with kwashiorkor. The magnesium is absorbed in the small intestine but, unlike calcium vitamin D does not aid the absorption of magnesium. The most important properties of Mg^{2+}, as opposed to Ca^{2+}, are the smaller ionic radius (Mg^{2+} 0.65 Å; Ca^{2+} 0.99 Å), its high electrophilic character and hence the high solubility of its salts. Thus Mg^{2+} forms stable complexes with 'hard' electronegative donors, such as the oxygen atoms of the oxyanions. As a highly charged small radius divalent cation, Mg^{2+} can act geometrically as a bridging ion between negatively charged carboxyl and phosphate groups, or electron-donating nitrogen atoms. The polarisation of ligands, caused by ionic bonding with Mg^{2+}, facilitates the attack of substrates by nucleophiles. Mg^{2+}-dependent enzymes are often used for the transfer of phosphate and carboxyl groups; Mg^{2+} also interacts strongly with the nitrogen atoms of pyrolle ligands, as in chlorophyll.

During assimilation and metabolism in animals, the chemical form in which the mineral occurs, as well as quantity, influences uptake and utilisation. Therefore it is important to establish data on the absorption and retention of nutrients for specific foods. No single nutrient acts in isolation as the metabolism of one nutrient is influenced by other nutrients. Rich sources (Table 7.6) of calcium and phosphorous include milk, cheese, leafy vegetables and legumes, but too great an

Table 7.6 Approximate content of calcium and phosphorus in some selected foods

Food commodity	Ca	P
	(mg/100 g)	
Beef, lean	9	180
Cheddar cheese	800	520
Cottage cheese	60	140
Parmesan cheese	1220	770
Whole egg	52	220
Milk	120	95
Cockles	130	200
Cod, raw	16	170
Oysters	190	270
Pilchards, canned	300	350
Plaice	51	180
Sardines, canned	550	520
Wheat bran	110	1200
White wheat flour	15	130
White wheat flour (fortified)	140	130
Wholemeal wheat flour	35	340
Chickpea	120	300
Rhubarb	100	21
Mung bean	160	330
Soybean	200	600
Spinach leaves	600	93
Watercress	220	52
Dried figs	280	92
Yeast	80	1290

(Paul and Southgate 1978; Platt 1962).

intake of phosphorus may block the hydroxylation of 25-hydroxy vitamin D_3 (DeLuca 1980). Sardines and other small fish in which the bones are eaten are also important sources of calcium. In animals, calcium absorption may be hindered by the presence in foods of oxalate and phytate, which can form insoluble complexes with metal salts. In mammals and avian species, vitamin D is required for the efficient absorption of calcium by the intestine, where vitamin D_3 stimulates synthesis of calcium-binding proteins (Ch. 8). The mechanism of entry of calcium into the cell is not known, but intracellular calcium is believed to be bound to the specially synthesised calcium-binding proteins. In man, deficiencies of calcium give rise to both bone loss, as in osteoporosis, and also the failure of muscle fibres to contract because of the weaker activity of calcium-activated ATPases (Ch. 9). The human body contains approximately 1250 g of calcium, of which 99 per cent is found in the bones and teeth. Plasma levels of calcium are maintained at approximately 2.5 mM, through both the absorption of calcium from the intestinal tract and release of calcium from bones; the concentration of calcium and phosphate levels in the plasma is tightly controlled through the interaction of parathyroid hormone, thyrocalcitonin and vitamin D.

In plants, calcium is also accumulated especially in leaves as a complex with phytates, oxalates and organic acids. Ionic interactions between calcium and phospholipids in membranes add to mechanical strength that prevents membrane leakage in both plant and animal cells. Also the hydrophobicity of the membranes may be increased by neutralisation of the negative charges in membranes by Ca^{2+}. However, unlike magnesium, calcium is not associated with the active sites of enzymes. Although Ca^{2+} stabilises the conformational structure of enzymes like α-amylase and Ca^{2+}-activated ATPase by neutralising negatively charged carboxyl groups.

In both animals and plants the concentration of Ca^{2+} in the cytoplasm is low (approximately 10^{-8}M). Ca^{2+} is generally bound to membranes, which act as localised stores of calcium for triggering enzymatic reactions. The low concentrations of cytoplasmic Ca^{2+} are maintained by specific ATPase calcium pumping-out systems, and thus Ca^{2+} is prevented from competing with Mg^{2+} for the active sites of enzymes. The larger ionic radius of calcium results in a lower hydration energy, and hence Ca^{2+} can more readily substitute its water of hydration, $Ca(H_2O)_{6,7 \text{ or } 8}^{2+}$ and react with a variety of ligands. Also due to the larger size of the calcium cation, intermolecular interactions are favoured, where the geometrical demands are less. These properties make it possible for Ca^{2+} to exchange rapidly between hydrated and bound states. Thus calcium induces structural changes in calmodulin, troponin and the sarcoplasmic reticulum proteins of animal muscle; calcium triggers enzymatic reactions like calcium-activated kinases for lipolysis and glycolysis in living and post-mortem tissues (Ch. 9). Also calcium promotes gel formation as with pectic and alginic acids (Ch. 2), although in egg white only Mg^{2+} stabilises the glycoprotein gel, presumably by maintaining a more hydrated cation. The water ligands of magnesium, $Mg(H_2O)_6^{2+}$ are much less mobile.

For trace elements, it is noted that animals or plants cannot live with a deficiency, but also that an excess of an element may be toxic. Indeed large quantities of essential – and sometimes toxic – metals are released from fossil fuel combustion; lead, cadmium, arsenic, antimony, chromium, nickel and beryllium may be released. Consequently, little data is presented here for the very variable quantities of trace elements present in food commodities and thus the latter's contribution to the physiological need for trace elements. Also at the present time, quantitative data for the inorganic composition of foods is unsatisfactory, partly because of the continually changing local and worldwide geographical sources of food ingredients. However, it is generally recognised that certain plant- and animal-derived foods, such as cereal grains and liver, supply much of man's mineral requirements (Table 7.7).

For some elements, like vanadium and molybdenum, there is a lack of data relating to both the human requirement and the chemical form in which the element may best be assimilated. It is also thought that many other elements, often considered to be toxic are required in ultratrace amounts. These include arsenic, silicon, lead, nickel and many other elements found in the higher periods of the periodic tables (Frieden 1984). Specific biochemical functions have not been found for the ultratrace metals except for nickel. In ruminant animals, nickel supplementation enhances urease (EC 3.5.1.5) activity for the release of ammonia which is used by rumen microorganisms for the biosynthesis of amino acids.

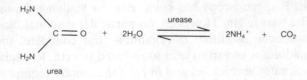

Table 7.7 The main dietary sources of trace elements

Element	Food commodity
Vanadium	Fruits, grains and vegetables
Chromium	Vegetable oils, meat
Manganese	All foods
Iron	Eggs, meat, legumes, leafy vegetables
Cobalt	Meat and milk
Copper	Meat
Zinc	All foods
Selenium	Seafoods, grains and meat
Molybdenum	Legumes, cereals, liver, milk
Iodine	Marine foods, some vegetables

Overall the environment is rich in manganese, iron and silicon, but poor and deficient in the elements selenium, molybdenum and iodine. It seems that evolution has led to the development of highly specific homeostasis in mammals, that prevents an intake of excess of trace elements, such as iron and chromium. These elements are present in large amounts in the environment. The concentration of iron is maintained in the body by mainly controlled absorption of the element from haem, organic complexes and ferritin. Likewise chromium is more readily absorbed as an organic complex (the glucose tolerance factor) as found in baker's yeast. However, severe trace element deficiencies do not seem to occur in industrial countries, though some of the dietary intakes may be marginal. For the possible detection of deficiencies of essential trace elements several methods are in use which include: (a) demonstration of decreased tissue levels; (b) demonstration of increased excretion; and (c) demonstration of decreased levels in blood or occasionally hair.

Vanadium

The oxidation states of vanadium are +5, +4, +3 for the $3d^0$, $3d^1$ and $3d^2$ electronic states, repectively. Vanadium is the lightest of the transitional elements. As for chromium and manganese, vanadium readily forms oxyanions due to the vacant 3d orbitals. At physiological pH values vanadium exists mainly in the +5 oxidation state as vanadate (H_2VO_4 and HVO_4^{2-}). For vanadium (IV), vanadyl species (VO^{2+}) are stabilised and complexed with proteins and other chelating agents, such as citrate and amino acids. For vanadyl species with a single $3d^1$ electron, EPR spectroscopy has been used for studying the binding to proteins like transferrin. However, no particular essential biochemical function has been ascribed to vanadium, but complete absence of dietary vanadium is known to lead to reduced growth, low survival and reproduction rates in chickens and in rats; the dietary requirement may be less than 1 ppm. Vanadium (1–100 μg) is also required for growth of algae. Nevertheless, like other transition metals, vanadium is known to be toxic at concentrations exceeding 1 mg per kg body weight in rabbits and probably in humans.

Vanadium compounds are known to exert biochemical effects, but such observations do not establish a physiological function. Vanadate at pH 6 to 8 inhibits the enzyme-catalysed hydrolysis of phosphates. Vanadate also copurifies with ATP. The ion transporting systems Na^+, K^+-ATPase and Ca^{2+}-ATPase are strongly inhibited (K_i 10^{-6}M) by low concentrations (approximately 4 nM) of vanadate. Other enzymes inhibited by vanadate are phosphorylase kinase (hence the hydrolysis of glycogen by phosphorylase-a is inhibited), acid phosphatases, ribonucleases, phosphoglucomutase and phosphoglycerate mutase

(Chasteen 1983). Vanadate has also been claimed to depress serum cholesterol and triglycerate levels. The biochemical effects and the unknown biological function of vanadium have been reviewed by Boyd and Kustin (1984).

Chromium

For chromium, Cr^{3+} the biological requirement is small. The requirement in man is approximately 20 μg per day. There is no known requirement for chromium in plants. Not surprisingly, many foods are likely to contain variable amounts of chromium, some of which must arise from the widespread use of stainless steel in the food industry in addition to the large scale industrial use of chromium elsewhere. However, most of the chromium may not be readily available for assimilation.

In mammals chromium is claimed to have one specific function as an integral part of a glucose tolerance factor (GTF). This factor potentiates the action of insulin: chromium deficiency is claimed to result in insulin resistance and glucose intolerance. However, inorganic chromium compounds are poorly absorbed in mammals, whereas chromium present as an organic complex in brewer's yeast is readily absorbed. GTF of brewer's yeast is composed of glutamate, glycine, chromium and nicotinate. The complex is chemically labile and it seems likely that it is destroyed during the cooking and processing of foods. To date, biologically active chromium has been estimated by measuring the effect of alcohol extracts of food on the oxidation of glucose by specially prepared chromium-deficient rat adipose tissue. Although GTF has not been fully characterised, it has been reported that a number of synthetic amino acid–complexes will mimic the GTF. Such active chromium complexes contain a pair of nitrogen atoms that are diagonally displaced with respect to the chromium atom as shown in Fig. 7.1. The different complexes adopt geometries in which the distance between the nitrogen atoms is similar.

Manganese

The Mn^{2+} ion is relatively stable with a single electron in each of the 3d orbitals. The oxyanions MnO_4^{2-} and MnO_4^- do not have a known biological function. The Mn^{2+} ion resembles Mg^{2+} which it can replace in many enzymatic reactions. However, in both animal and plant fluids Mg^{2+} is present in large excess and therefore Mn^{2+} is unlikely to substitute for magnesium *in vivo*.

The few known functions of manganese and those of other trace elements are given in Table 7.8. Pyruvate carboxylase (Ch. 8) is a

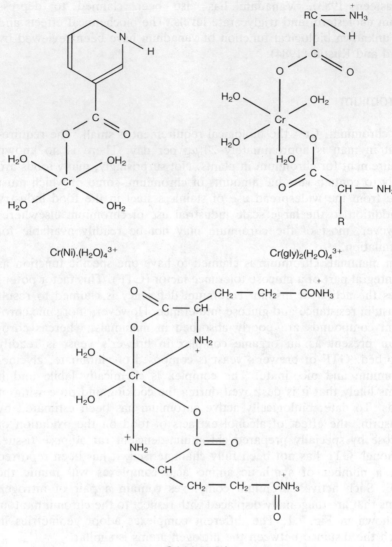

Fig. 7.1 Proposed chemical structure for glucose tolerance factors (after
Cooper *et al.* 1984)

tetrameric enzyme that contains four atoms of manganese. In plants
the redox system of photosystem II requires Mn^{2+}, where it may act
as an electron carrier. Mn^{2+} also has a structural role in phytolectins
where, together with Ca^{2+}, the cation stabilises the conformation of
the protein moiety (Ch. 4). For animals the manganese-dependent
enzymes include superoxide dismutase and the glycosyl transferases
required for the biosynthesis of glycoproteins. It has been suggested

Table 7.8 Some functions of trace elements

Element	Biological function
Boron and vanadium	Required by plants and rats for growth
Arsenic, tin and nickel	Unknown
Chromium	Part of a glucose tolerance factor in man
Manganese	Required for photosynthesis, cofactor for arginase, superoxide dismutase, glycosyl transferases, pyruvate, carboxylase, amino peptidases
Iron	For redox reactions (see Table 7.9)
Cobalt	DNA synthesis
Copper	Contained in: ceruloplasmin (required for synthesis of haemoglobin), cytochrome oxidase, superoxide dismutase, lysyl oxidase, amino oxidase, galactose oxidase, phenolase, ascorbic acid oxidase, plastocyanin
Zinc	Cofactor for: carbonic anhydrase, carboxypeptidase, several dehydrogenases, superoxide dismutase, RNA and DNA polymerases, alkaline phosphatases, phospholipases
Selenium	Cofactor for one enzyme: glutathione peroxidase
Molybdenum	Cofactor for: xanthine oxidase, nitrogenase and sulphite oxidase
Iodine	Part of the thyroxine molecule
Fluorine	Increases the stability of bones and teeth by substituting for hydroxyl groups on hydroxyapatite

that deficiencies of these enzymes may have caused skeletal and inner ear defects in manganese-deficient offspring. The human body requires approximately 20 mg of manganese, although there are very few metallo-enzymes which contain manganese.

Increased intestinal absorption of manganese has been closely linked to non-haem iron absorption in humans and increased incidences of iron deficiency. For instance in miners suffering from manganese poisoning, iron-deficiency anaemia may be responsible for some of the neurological symptoms which are more commonly associated with vitamin B_{12} deficiencies. In addition to manganese, cobalt, nickel and zinc also share the iron absorptive mechanism. The absorption of the toxic heavy metals, lead, cadmium and plutonium is increased for experimentally induced iron deficiencies (Valberg and

Flanagan 1983), which suggests risks to individuals who might be exposed to greater than normal amounts of heavy metals that compete with iron absorption.

Iron

Ionic Fe^{3+} contains five unpaired electrons and is chemically more stable than Fe^{2+}. The solubility at neutral pH values, where Fe^{3+} readily forms insoluble ferric hydroxide, can be maintained by replacement of coordinated water molecules in $Fe(H_2O)_6^{3+}$, with ascorbate or citrate. Hence the chemical composition of foods and the contents of the intestinal tract influence the solubility of iron and its assimilation in animals. Both Fe^{3+} and Fe^{2+} will enter into octahedral complexes depending on the nature of the ligands which also influences the redox potential for the two ions and the catalytic properties of haem-containing enzymes. In haemproteins, four of the coordinate positions of each iron ion are occupied by pyrrole nitrogens (Ch. 9 and 10).

The redox potentials of iron-containing proteins vary and for haem-containing proteins depend on the chemical nature of the substituents in the porphyrin ring, the nature of the linkages of the porphyrin to protein and the axial coordination group of the iron complex. In redox reactions where oxygen or hydrogen peroxide are involved, the axial position coordinates with an oxygen atom. In plants, iron is also mainly associated with the redox enzymes present in chloroplasts, mitochondria and peroxisomes, as plants do not contain the oxygen-transporting pigments, although some non-haem iron is stored as Fe^{3+}-phosphoprotein (phytoferritin) in leaves and is transported in plants as a Fe^{III}–citrate chelate. In eggs, Fe^{3+} is complexed with the phosphate groups of phosvitin. Hence dietary iron exists in two forms, haem and non-haem iron, which during digestion forms two chemically separate pools.

Table 7.9 The biological functions of iron

Occurrence	Biological function
Complexed with porphyrins:	
Haemoglobin	Oxygen transport
Myoglobin	Oxygen transport
Cytochromes	Enzyme-catalysed redox reactions
Peroxidases	Enzyme-catalysed redox reactions
Catalases	Enzyme-catalysed redox reactions
Non-haem iron:	
Lipoxygenases, cyclooxygenases	Activation of diatomic oxygen
Iron–sulphur clusters	Redox reactions

The human body contains approximately from 3 to 4 g of iron, which is vital for many body functions (Table 7.9). In man approximately two-thirds of the total iron is present in haemoglobin and approximately 3 per cent in muscle myoglobin. Minute quantities of iron exist in respiratory enzymes (0.3 %) and plasma. The majority of stored iron is in the form of ferric hydroxide–protein complexes (ferritin) found in the spleen, liver and bones. The ferric hydroxide core is surrounded by aggregated protein composed of small subunits (MW 18,000 to 21,000). Non-haem iron is found in iron–sulphur proteins associated with electron transport and the dioxygenases – lipoxygenases and cyclooxygenases (Ch. 6).

Given the widespread distribution of iron in many foods (Table

Table 7.10 Approximate content of iron in some selected foods

Food commodity	Fe (mg/100 g)
Plant food	
Chickpea	9.0
Cocoa powder	14
Cowpea	5.0
Lentil	7.0
Lima bean	6.0
Locust bean	4.0
Mung bean	9.0
Soybean seed	7.0
Spinach leaves	4.0
Oatmeal	4.1
Wheat bran	12.9
White wheat flour	1.5
White wheat flour, fortified	2.2
Wholemeal wheat flour	4.0
Animal foods	
Beef, lean	1.2
Egg yolk	6.1
Liver	10
Fish	
Cockles	26
Oysters	6
Pilchards	2.6
Sardines	2.9
Other types	
Yeast, dried	20

(Paul and Southgate 1978; Platt 1962).

7.10), it might, at first sight, be thought that iron deficiency in animals should be rare, but this is not so as ionic iron is poorly assimilated. Iron is unusual, in so far as it is required in only trace amounts by living organisms, but yet it is abundant in substantial amounts in the earth's crust (Table 7.3). Consequently many organisms have devised systems where absorption is very effectively restricted; at the same time, because of the essentiality of the element, excretion of iron is also minimal. Therefore the outcome of such protection against excessive intake is to precipitate a deficiency in circumstances where the dietary intake may be marginal. Any loss of blood, due to even minor disorders, can eventually result in marginal cases of anaemia of which there is thought to be a high incidence in human populations. Through the use of radioactive iron (^{55}Fe), it has been shown that haem iron is more readily assimilated. Intestinal mucosal receptors for haem have been identified and after cellular absorption, iron is released from haem by the catalytic action of haem oxygenase (Valberg and Flanagan 1983).

Non-haem iron in the digestive tract becomes single pool iron, the availability of which depends on the composition of the rest of the diet. The intestinal uptake of non-haem iron can be very rapid, when iron reserves are low and special binding sites may be involved. Inhibition of non-haem iron uptake occurs with phytates, present in bran and wholemeal products, and also in the presence of polyphosphates. The absorption of non-haem iron, irrespective of its source, whether it be from eggs, vegetables or iron added as a nutritional supplement to flour, is enhanced by the presence of meat and ascorbic acid. It is possible that such enhancement is due to the reduction of Fe^{3+} to Fe^{2+} which is more soluble at neutral pH values. Iron is also assimilated more efficiently from human milk, and this may be due to specific interactions between human milk glycoferrins and the corresponding receptors in the intestinal cells. Excess dietary iron that enters intestinal mucosal cells is excreted into the lumen as ferritin contained in sloughed cells.

After the intestinal absorption of iron, intracellular synthesis of ferritin occurs where iron atoms are incorporated into the ferritin molecule. For further use in the synthesis of haem proteins iron is believed to be released from ferritin in small quantities and passed to the blood plasma by means of the iron-transferring protein, transferrin. The iron is carried by transferrin in the Fe^{3+} state. Ferritin serves as a reserve in the mucosal cells and is therefore involved in iron storage, whereas mucosal and plasma transferrins provide the vehicle for the transport of Fe^{3+} to tissues. However, because iron delivery from the gastrointestinal tract is controlled and complicated, metabolic deficiencies in the presence of adequate dietary iron might still occur, although it is rare for the transport proteins themselves to be lacking. If such a mechanism for iron absorption involving the uptake of Fe^{2+}

by the mucosal cell, and the transfer of Fe^{3+} to blood plasma occurs, then the overall assimilation of iron may well be regulated primarily by the ratio of ferritin to transferrin biosynthesis and thus be controlled by DNA and messenger RNA synthesis.

Copper

Unlike iron, generally copper-dependent enzymes both react directly with atomic oxygen and cause its reduction to either hydrogen peroxide or water. Such chemical properties make the element both extremely beneficial for catalysing oxidative reactions and extremely toxic. Normal amounts of copper are required by both plants and animals and generally dietary deficiencies in humans do not normally occur. However, a copper deficiency can give rise to anaemia, neurological disease, disorders of connective tissue and depigmentation. A low activity for the copper-dependent enzymes, lysyl oxidase (EC 1.4.3.14) and tyrosinase (EC 1.14.18.1), explains some of the deficiency symptoms, including emphysemia. Cytochrome-c oxidase (EC 1.9.3.1) activity and superoxide dismutase activity (EC 1.15.1.1) may also be reduced in copper-deficient states. The most important metabolic function of copper is undoubtedly its involvement in the cytochrome-c oxidase of the mitochondrial respiratory chain.

During digestion in animals copper, like other reactive metals, is likely to be bound to various ligands which will include small peptides and amino acids. Consequently the absorption of copper may be influenced by the composition of the diet. Furthermore, the presence of other metals, such as zinc, may also affect the uptake of copper by competing for common ligands. Absorption of copper may also be decreased in the presence of phytates provided by some high-fibre diets. Intestinal cells contain the protein metallothionein which as an essential component seems to offer protection against copper toxicity. As a metal-binding protein metallothionein contains up to from 5 to 7 g atoms of metal per molecule with zinc and copper as the predominant bound metals. Metallothionein has no apparent enzymatic function and therefore is an intracellular binding macromolecule for both copper and zinc. Metallothioneins contain approximately 25 to 30 per cent cysteine where the –SH group is presumably responsible for metal binding.

After absorption in animals, most of the copper is stored in the liver and transported in the blood complexed with ceruloplasmin. Ninety per cent of plasma copper is bounded tightly to the ceruloplasmin. The small amount of exchangeable copper in plasma is bound to serum albumin and small peptides like glycyl histadyl glycine. In animals, copper is necessary for haemoglobin synthesis where copper may act as an oxidising agent for the transport of transfer-bound Fe^{3+}.

Normally excess copper is discharged with bile salts, but toxic quantities can be chelated with penicillamine. In man, Wilson's disease is a recessively inherited disorder characterised by a high accumulation of copper in the liver, kidney and brain and by a low plasma level of ceruloplasmin, even though normal amounts of apoceruloplasmin are present in serum of diseased patients. In contrast to Wilson's disease, Menke's disease is characterised by a copper deficiency. This inherited copper deficiency results from the malabsorption of copper, which then accumulates to a large extent in the intestinal mucosal cells.

In plants, copper is present in oxidative enzymes (Table 7.8), where it takes part in redox reactions. The role of copper in reactions catalysed by phenolase, ascorbic acid oxidase and superoxide dismutase is described in Ch. 10. In plants, lignification is dependent on the formation of diphenols and their subsequent oxidation by the copper-dependent phenolases.

Zinc

The special properties of the zinc cation, which permit its incorporation into both the active sites of enzymes and as a protein conformational stabilising cation, are undoubtedly due to the fact that zinc is not strictly a transition element, as the 3d orbitals are completely filled. Consequently zinc tends to form tetrahedral complexes and favours the softer ligands containing nitrogen and sulphur. Unlike the true transition metals zinc does not initiate redox reactions, and hence fulfils the need of a metal able to form dative bonds where redox reactions are unwanted. Consequently zinc does not possess the reactivity and hence the toxicity of the adjacent transition element copper, and unlike copper, zinc is abundant in most plant and animal tissues. Man is estimated to contain from 1.5 to 2 g of zinc. Liver, kidney and muscle are good dietary sources of zinc. The zinc in human milk has a high availability, whereas for cow's milk which contains more caseins that are not readily digested by infants, zinc is less available due to strong binding of the cation by the caseins. The predominant use of cereal proteins by the majority of the world's population is an important cause of zinc deficiency, due to the low availability of zinc in such diets that contain substantial amounts of phytate. Indeed it has been shown that the separate additions of phytic acid and dietary fibre to diets reduces the absorption of zinc. Deficiencies have been reported in Iran, Egypt and other Mediterranean countries.

For humans and rats it is clear that a deficiency of zinc also retards growth, produces hypogonadism in males, poor appetite, mental lethargy, dermatitis and an increased susceptibility to infection with *Candida albicans*. The widespread effect of zinc deficiencies in both plants and animals is explained by the need for zinc as a constituent of a very large number of diverse enzymes. In plants, a zinc deficiency reduces the nucleic acid content which probably accounts for the drastic effects on protein content and chloroplast formation.

Zinc has a vital role in many biochemical reactions; 100 enzymes or more require zinc for catalytic activity. These include dehydrogenases, peptidases, aldolases and many enzymes required for DNA synthesis, which clearly affects a wide range of metabolic functions including the immune response. However, those enzymes which bind zinc very strongly are still fully active in a zinc deficiency state, whereas three enzymes – alkaline phosphatase, carboxypeptidase and thymidine kinase – are particularly sensitive to zinc restriction in experimental animals. A deficiency of zinc can also arise either from bowel disease or be of a genetic origin. Unlike copper, a proportion of zinc at the physiological pH values of the intestinal lumen contents might also exist as the negatively charged zincate anion which may be less readily absorbed.

For the assimilation of zinc, absorption by the intestinal mucosa is influenced by other metals, such as copper and iron which act antagonistically with each other, whereas haem iron has no such effect. Other dietary factors (as for copper absorption) such as protein restriction, influence zinc uptake which suggests that amino acids act as ligands for Zn^{2+}. Zinc in blood plasma is mainly bound to serum albumin, but it does complex with other binding proteins like transferrin and ceruloplasmin. Amino acids with unprotonated amino groups, for example lysine and glutamine, and sulphydryl groups bind zinc. As for copper and other metal cations, intracellular zinc is bound by metallothionein. However, the release of such metal cations varies, with zinc leaving the protein during proteolysis, while cadmium remains bound to degraded polypeptides.

Molybdenum

Approximately 0.1 μg of molybdenum per gram is found in plant tissues, with much higher quantities being present in nodulated roots. Molybdenum is a specific component of the enzyme nitrate reductase, which occurs in symbiotic bacteria and catalyses the fixation of nitrogen. Small amounts of molybdenum are required by animals for enzymes with specific oxidative functions, such as xanthine oxidase (EC 1.1.3.22) and sulphite oxidase (EC 1.8.3.1). In sheep, molybdenum decreases the retention of excess copper: the effect is believed to be due to the formation of a dietary insoluble copper thiomolybdate. Consequently, copper deficiency could also arise from a diet enriched with molybdenum and particularly so as an excessive intake of molybdenum may also enhance the excretion of copper. Higher dietary levels of molybdenum might occur where substantial quantities of sorghum are consumed. Sorghum has been reported to contain higher levels of molybdenum and this may have been caused by environmental factors like mineral mining or volcanic activity in some sorghum-producing areas.

Molybdenum is the only element of the second period of transition elements, that is definitely known to be essential nutritionally. Tungsten acts antagonistically and can induce a sulphite oxidase deficiency (Cohen *et al*. 1973). Molybdenum very readily forms oxyanions, due to the empty d orbitals, with oxidation states of +4, 5 and 6 (MoO_4^{2-}). Consequently the molybdate anion can act as either a one or two electron acceptor ($Mo^{IV} \rightleftharpoons Mo^{V} \rightleftharpoons MO^{VI}$), or donor. Molybdate is the only complex anion known to function in biological redox reactions. Unlike the other transitional elements, molybdate is the anion of a weak acid and therefore can conceivably also act as a redox coupled proton carrier in membranes:

$$e + H_2MoO_4 \rightleftharpoons HMoO_4^- + H^+$$

$$e + HMoO_4^- \rightleftharpoons MoO_4^{2-} + H^+$$

In this way, redox reactions catalysed by molybdenum-containing enzymes may be efficiently coupled to translocation of protons in cell membranes.

Selenium

In the periodic table selenium and sulphur are members of group VI, and thus selenium possesses many of the properties of sulphur but is less electrophilic. Selenium, like sulphur, exists as oxyanions and can substitute for sulphur in both cysteine and methionine. It is thought that the chemical form of selenium may influence its biological activity, as selenomethionine is assimilated better than the selenite anion. The requirement for selenium might be up to 100 μg per day. It is known that deficiencies are associated with certain geographical locations as in New Zealand, Finland and Sweden where the soils contain little selenium.

In animals, selenium is remarkable, in so far as its only known biochemical function is as an essential constituent of glutathione peroxidase (EC 1.11.1.9).

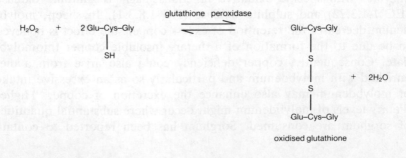

Rats fed a selenium-deficient diet show a large decrease in glutathione peroxidase activity. The enzyme is necessary to maintain low levels of intracellular hydrogen peroxide and organic peroxides. The selenium atom is present in the enzyme in the form of selenocysteine. The enzyme catalyses the reduction of 12-hydroperoxy-5,8,10,14-eicosa-tetraenoic acid to the 12-hydroxy unsaturated fatty acid. This function is complimentary to the action vitamin E, catalase and superoxide dismutase, which are also responsible for the removal of toxic reduced oxygen species. Selenium also reduces the extremely toxic effects of substances such as paraquat which generate superoxide (O_2^-).

Other essential elements not described here are cobalt and iodine. Cobalt is required in the form of vitamin B_{12} (Ch. 8) and iodine is the only trace element present in man in larger concentrations than in the surrounding environment. Assimilation processes are responsible for the concentration of iodine in a specific part of the body, namely the thyroid gland, for the synthesis of thyroxine. This is an iodinated compound synthesised from tyrosine.

RECOMMENDED DAILY AMOUNTS

Recommendations for the estimated daily amounts of individual elements have been made in the United Kingdom, the United States and by FAO/WHO, even though only empirical estimates are available for the bioavailability of elements from foods.

The meaning of the values for recommended daily amounts (RDA) are often misunderstood. The RDA values are the levels of intake of nutrients considered to be adequate to meet the estimated nutritional needs of man. However, whether the diet of the individual consuming less than the RDA for any nutrient is adequate or not depends entirely on that person's requirements. For example, it is not possible to state definitely that because the RDA values are being met by a single person, that either there is no nutritional inadequacy, or that a diet which meets two-thirds of the RDA value is considered to be adequate for an individual. The recommendations by the United Kingdom and FAO/WHO are restricted to calcium and iron. Whereas for the United States recommended range values for calcium, phosphorus, iodine, iron, magnesium and zinc have been suggested (NRC/NAS 1980). The specific recommended daily allowances by FAO/WHO for calcium and iron are summarised in Table 7.11. For the United States the recommended daily amounts for trace elements and electrolytes for selected age groups are summarised in Table 7.12.

In Great Britain, since the Second World War, regulations have been in existence which require white flours to contain minimum quantities of calcium, iron and two B-vitamins, thiamin and niacin. This

Table 7. 1 Summary of the recommended daily allowances for calcium and iron by FAO/WHO[†]

Age, (years)	Ca (mg)	Fe (mg)
under 1	500–600 (600)[‡]	5–10 (6)
7–9	400–500 (600)	5–10 (10)
13–15	600–700 (700)	9–18[§](12)
19 +	400–500 (500)	5–9 (10)

([†] FAO/WHO 1974).

[‡] Approximate UK values from DHSS (1981).

[§] For females from 12+ years of age a range value of 12 to 28 mg per day of Fe is recommended.

requirement arises because minerals and vitamins from the outer layers of the grain are lost during milling for the manufacture of white flour. Calcium carbonate and ferrous sulphate are added to flour; the product must contain 0.65 mg of iron and 235–390 mg of calcium carbonate per 100 g of white flour. Losses of other essential elements can also take place during the refining of sugar and the polishing of rice. In particular, sodium, potassium and a range of trace elements including chromium, zinc, manganese and copper, may be lost during such refining of ingredients. The present legal requirements do not contain provision for the presence of trace elements in processed food ingredients, even though with modern analytical techniques it should be possible now to establish appropriate standards.

In view of the toxicity of many elements, if taken in excessive quantities, it is surprising that range values for RDA data have not been used earlier. The concept of range values emphasises that a healthy organism can maintain desirable tissue concentrations of trace elements over a wide range of dietary intakes. Furthermore, the range value allows for variation in the biological availability of many of the

Table 7.12 Summary of the recommended daily allowances for elements in the United States

	Age (years)	Sodium (mg)	Calcium (mg)	Potassium (mg)	Phosphorus (mg)	Magnesium (mg)
Infants	0.5–1.0	500	540	1100	360	70
Children	4–6	900	800	1550	800	200
Males	15–18	1800	1200	3250	1200	400
	23–50	2200	800	3900	800	350
	51+	2200	800	3900	800	350

(From NRC/NAS 1980).

trace elements, which depends substantially on the chemical form in which the elements occur in foods; iron being a particular example. Also there is antagonism between metals, such that excessive intake of one metal may impair the uptake of another element present in minimal amounts. Furthermore, the organic constituents of a diet also influence the uptake of metals as exemplified with iron, where meat-based foods and vitamin C (present in fruits and vegetables) enhance iron uptake. The use of range values may also emphasise that what may be adequate for one individual may be inadequate for another individual of identical race, sex, age and size.

KEY FACTS

1.   The elements essential for life belong to the lower periods of the periodic table.
2.   H, C, N, O and Ca account for more than 90 per cent of the human body.
3.   Many of the dietary essential trace elements are transition metals.
4.   The transition metals are often required as integral parts of enzymes involved in redox reactions.
5.   Many of the transition elements compete with each other for assimilation from the intestinal contents in mammals.
6.   The content of metals varies widely for different foods. Animal foods act as good dietary sources of iron, zinc and copper.
7.   The RDA values for elements are the amounts considered to be adequate to meet the estimated needs of man. Whole wheat flour is often fortified with iron and calcium to replace these elements which are lost during the milling of wheat grains. Other trace elements, like zinc and copper, that are also lost during milling, are not replaced.

Copper (mg)	Iron (mg)	Zinc (mg)	Manganese (mg)	Iodine (µg)	Selenium (mg)	Molybdenum (mg)
0.85	15	5	0.85	50	0.02–0.06	0.04–0.08
1.7	10	10	1.75	90	0.03–0.12	0.06–0.15
2.5	18	15	3.75	150	0.05–0.2	0.15–0.5
2.5	10	15	3.75	150	0.05–0.2	0.15–0.5
2.5	10	15	3.75	150	0.05–0.2	0.15–0.5

REFERENCES

Boyd, D. W. and Kustin, K. (1984) 'Vanadium: a versatile biochemical effector with an elusive biological role', *Advances in Inorganic Biochemistry*, vol. 6 (eds. Eichhorn, G. L. and Marzilli, L. G.). Elsevier Science Publishing Co., New York.

Buss, D. and Robertson J. (1978) *Manual of Nutrition*. Ministry of Agriculture, Fisheries and Food, HMSO, London.

Chasteen, N. D. (1983) 'The biochemistry of vanadium', in *Copper, Molybdenum and Vanadium in Biological Systems. Structure and Bonding* 53. Springer Verlag, Berlin and Heidelberg.

Cohen, H. J., Drew, R. T. and Johnson, J. L. (1973) 'Molecular basis for the biological function of molybdenum. The relationship between sulphite oxidase and the acute toxicity of bisulphite and SO_2', *Proc. Nat. Acad. Sci.*, **70**, 3655–9.

Cooper, J. A. Blackwell, L. F. and Buckley, P. D. (1984) 'Chromium (III) complexes and their relationship to the glucose tolerance factor Part II. structure and biological activity of amino acid complexes'. *Inorg. Chim. Acta*, **92**, 23–31.

DeLuca, H. F. (1980) 'Some new concepts emanating from a study of the metabolism and function of vitamin D', *Nutr. Rev.*, **38**, 169–82.

DHSS (1981) Department of Health and Social Security. Report on Health and Social Subjects 15. 'Recommended daily amounts of food energy and nutrients for groups of people in the United Kingdom', Report by the Committee on Medical Aspects of Food Policy, 2nd impr. HMSO, London.

FAO/WHO (1974) *The Handbook of Human Nutritional Requirements*. FAO Nutritional Studies no. 28, Rome. WHO Monograph Series no. 61.

Frieden, E. (1984) *Biochemistry of the Essential Ultratrace Elements. Biochemistry of The Elements*, vol. 3 (ed. Frieden, E.). Plenum Press, New York.

Mason, B. H. (1966) *Principles of Geochemistry*, 3rd edn. John Wiley and Sons, New York.

NRC/NAS (1980) National Research Council Committee on Dietary Allowances. *Recommended Dietary Allowances*, 9th edn. National Academy of Sciences Press, Washington DC.

Paul, A. A. and Southgate, D. A. T. (1978) *McCance and Widdowson's The Composition of Foods*, 4th edn. of MRC Special Report no. 297, HMSO, London and Elsevier, Amsterdam.

Platt, B. S. (1962) 'Tables and representative values of foods commonly used in tropical countries', Medical Research Council Special Report series no. 302. HMSO, London.

Rankama, K. and Sahama, T. G. (1964) *Geochemistry,* University of Chicago Press, Chicago.

Schroeder, H. A. (1965) 'The biological trace elements', *J. Chron. Dis.*, **18**, 217–28.

Tan, S. P., Wenlock, R. W. and Buss, D. H. (1985) 'Immigrant foods', second supplement to *McCance and Widdowson's The Composition of Foods*. HMSO, London, and Elsevier/North Holland Biomedical Press, Amsterdam.

Valberg, L. S. and Flanagan, P. R. (1983) 'Intestinal absorption of iron and chemically related metals', in *Biological Aspects of Metals and Metal Related Diseases* (ed. Sarkar, B.). Raven Press, New York.

ADDITIONAL READING

Clarkson, D. T. (1980) 'Mineral nutrition of higher plants', *Ann. Rev. Plant Physiol.*, **31**, 239–98.

Combs, G. F. and Combs, S. B. (1984) 'The nutritional biochemistry of selenium', *Ann. Rev. Nutr.* **4**, 257–80.

Nielsen, F. H. (1984) 'Ultratrace elements in nutrition', *Ann. Rev. Nutr.*, **4**, 21–47.

Sarkar, B. (1983) *Biological Aspects of Metals and Metal Related Diseases.* Raven Press, New York.

Stadtman, T. C. (1980) 'Selenium-dependent enzymes', *Ann. Rev. Biochem.*, **49**, 93–110.

Underwood, E. J. (1977) *Trace Elements in Human and Animal Nutrition*, 4th edn. Academic Press, London.

CHAPTER 8

Vitamins in foods and their biochemical function

INTRODUCTION

For this very diverse group of chemicals, biochemical knowledge is required in order to understand why small amounts of vitamins are so essential for health. Vitamins, which help to regulate biochemical reactions, are – unlike hormones – not synthesised by the human or animal body. Therefore they must be supplied from the diet. Generally the biochemical functions of the water-soluble vitamins that have been known for some time, have been well documented: for the fat-soluble vitamins further information on their more diverse biochemical functions is still being revealed. The accurate analysis of vitamins has proved to be difficult: each vitamin exists in a number of different chemical forms often of varying biological activity, and frequently only microgram quantities are present per 100 g of food. Biological assays, although time-consuming, do measure the biologically available vitamin in complex natural products such as foods, without hydrolysis and extraction. However, now through the application of high performance liquid chromatography, better chromatographic resolution of vitamin derivatives and their isomers is possible. This should enable a fuller evaluation of the biological activity of the various vitamers and their importance in different foods.

The term 'vitamer' is frequently used, and refers to different chemical compounds that can replace a vitamin requirement. Further information is required for the biochemical roles of many vitamers including those of vitamin E, vitamin K and folate in metabolism. Generally it is not known whether during the storage and processing of food, some vitamers are preferentially degraded or even isomerised.

The diseases arising from acute deficiency states have been known for a long time and are given in Table 8.1. However, the minimum amounts of vitamins that are required to prevent the deficiency diseases are not dietary optimums for the maintenance of health. The minimum requirement for many vitamins is often considerably less

Table 8.1 Extreme deficiency symptom

Vitamin A	Light perception, night blindness
Vitamin D	Rickets, osteomalacia
Vitamin E	Oxidation of fats and membrane lipids
Vitamin K	Haemorrhaging
Vitamin C	Scurvy, defence against infections
Vitamin B_1 (thiamin)	Beri-beri, neuritis
Vitamin B_2 (riboflavin)	Tiredness, mouth and tongue lesions
Niacin	Pellagra, skin lesions
Vitamin B_6 group (pyridoxal)	Atrophy of organs, lack of growth, widespread disruption of metabolism
Pantothenic acid	Widespread disruption of metabolism
Biotin	Acidosis, skin rash, neurological problems, anorexia, immunodeficiency
Folic acid	Megaloblastic anaemia
Vitamin B_{12}	Pernicious anaemia (megaloblastic anaemia and neurological damage)

than the amount required to maintain constant plasma levels and certainly saturation of tissues. Water-soluble vitamins, which are widespread in all metabolising cells, are easily excreted and thus deficiencies may occur quickly. On the other hand, fat-soluble vitamins are stored in relatively large quantities in certain organs. For example, vitamin A is stored in the liver and the time period for a deficiency to develop, which is dependent mainly on the levels of the reserves, can be considerable. Also localised deficiencies may occur more rapidly in some tissues, while perhaps the whole body status for a particular vitamin remains satisfactory. However, generally the minimum requirement for each vitamin has been evaluated clinically by observing the onset of known deficiency symptoms, coupled to determinations of the amounts required to correct deficiencies. Obviously blood plasma levels of some individual vitamins, for example pyridoxal phosphate and folic acid, can indicate both the state of health of individuals and the adequacy of the dietary intake. However, for other vitamins, such as vitamin A, the plasma level may be unrelated to a current dietary intake, due to the mobilisation by the liver of large amounts of stored vitamin A. The amounts of water-soluble vitamins excreted in the urine may also indicate the vitamin status of the tissues, although this may be influenced by other metabolic or dietary insufficiencies.

The amounts of vitamins estimated to be present in foods by microbiological assay and classical methods of chemical assay on extracts of foods have been reported extensively by Paul and Southgate (1978). However, for diverse compounds like vitamins, which occur in a very

Table 8.2 Blood enzymes as indicators of vitamin states

Vitamin	Cofactor	Enzyme	Tissue
Thiamin	Thiamin pyrophosphate	Transketolase (EC 2.2.1.1)	Erythrocytes
Riboflavin	Flavin adeninedinucleotide	Glutathione reductase (EC 1.6.4.2)	Erythrocytes
Vitamin B_6	Pyridoxal-5'-phosphate	Glutamic acid transaminases (EC 2.6.1)	Serum
		Alanine transaminase (EC 2.6.1.2)	Erythrocytes

wide range of foodstuffs, such methods of assay are often cumbersome and inaccurate. Many food tables still reveal contradictory values. Now vitamins D, E, folates and the isomers of vitamin A are being quantified more accurately by the use of high performance liquid chromatography in extracts of foods. Nevertheless, for the future greater numbers of analyses for various food products, blood and tissue samples may be required and thus other assays based on the use of vitamin-dependent enzymes may prove useful. For example, a few enzymes are now known to be particularly sensitive to depleted physiological concentrations of vitamins (Table 8.2), and therefore assay of the activity of such enzymes can be used to estimate vitamin-deficiency states.

Deficiency states can also arise from poor assimilation of vitamins. Deficiencies of the dependent apoenzymes and genetic defects in coenzyme synthesis which can give rise to vitamin-related metabolic errors have been highlighted. Sometimes megadoses of vitamins help to overcome such multivarious defects, where the medical conditions are described as vitamin-dependent rather than deficient.

FAT-SOLUBLE VITAMINS

Vitamin A

Retinol is the primary alcohol derivative made up of four isoprene units (Fig. 8.1). It is regarded as the active form of vitamin A, because it is readily oxidised enzymatically to other metabolically active compounds like 11-*cis*-retinal and retinoic acids. It has been known for a long time that *cis*-retinal is required for night vision, and deficiencies cause blindness. More recently it has been discovered that retinoic

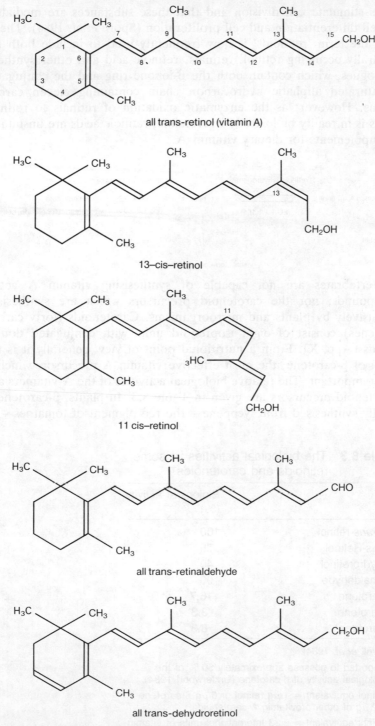

all trans-retinol (vitamin A)

13–cis–retinol

11 cis–retinol

all trans-retinaldehyde

all trans-dehydroretinol

Fig. 8.1 Chemical structures of some retinoids

acids stimulate cell division and that these substances are mediators of cell differentiation and cell proliferation (Sporn *et al.* 1984). Therefore the term 'retinoids' is now frequently used to include both the naturally occurring retinol, retinals, retinoic acid and other synthetic analogues, which contain both the β-ionone ring and the conjugated unsaturated aliphatic hydrocarbon chain containing eleven carbon atoms. However, as the enzymatic oxidation of retinals to retinoic acids is in reality biologically irreversible, retinoic acids are unsuitable as supplements for dietary vitamin A.

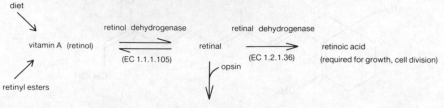

Vertebrates are not capable of synthesising vitamin A active compounds, nor the carotenoid precursors which are synthesised exclusively by plants and microorganisms. Carotenoids (forty carbon terpenes) consist of eight isoprenoid units with conjugated double bonds (App. X). From a nutritional point of view generally it is the level of β-carotene, the most effective vitamin A precursor, which is most important. The relative biological activities of the A-vitamers and carotenoid precursors are given in Table 8.3. In plants, β-carotene is finally synthesised from lycopene – the red pigment of tomatoes – by

Table 8.3 The biological activities of some retinoids and carotenoids[†]

	Biological activity (%)
All *trans*-retinol	100
13-*cis*-Retinol	75
Dehydroretinol	40
Retinaldehyde	90
β-Carotene	16.7
α-Carotene[‡]	8.3
γ-Carotene[‡]	8.3

([†] Sivell *et al.* 1984).

[‡] Reported to possess approximately 50 % of the biological activity of β-carotene (Underwood 1984).

1 retinol equivalent = 1 μg retinol or 6 μg β-carotene or 12 μg of other provitamin A carotenoids.

1 retinol equivalent = 3.33 International units of vitamin A.

cyclisation of the two ends of the molecule to form the β-ionone rings (App. X). In yellow varieties of tomatoes, lycopene is replaced by β-carotene, but due to differences in colour these fruits have not yet been widely accepted. Apocarotenoids are thirty-carbon compounds which contain a shortened hydrocarbon chain. Generally the apocarotenoids have less biological activity than β-carotene. Owing to their unsaturated chemical structure, carotenoids and retinoids are sensitive to oxidation during the storage and processing of foods; they are easily co-oxidised by lipid hydroperoxides in a reaction catalysed by lipoxygenases (see Ch. 10). Also photoisomerisation can occur in sunlight. With high performance liquid chromatography the natural occurring isomers of A-vitamers, and the various carotenoid pigments, can now be quantified separately in extracts of foods. Thus a more meaningful value of total vitamin A activity in foods – in terms of retinol equivalents – is now possible. Values for the retinol equivalents of beef, chicken and other animal foods which are consumed in significant amounts are given in Table 8.4. In human milk, vitamin A is present as retinol and retinyl esters, generally in the form of the palmitate. Small amounts of retinal and dehydroretinal have been found in cod products, salmon and trout.

Table 8.4 Vitamin A active compounds in some important foods[†]

Commodity	All trans-retinol (μg)	13-cis-Retinol (μg)	β-Carotene (μg)	Total retinol equivalents (μg)
Cow's milk	36	2	12	40
Dried milk[‡]	320	40	5	351
Cheese, Cheddar	300	56	126	363
Margarine, polyunsaturated	774	3	143	800
Liver pate,[§] fine	6200	2500	0	8075
Eggs	132	53		190[¶]

([†] Sivell et al. 1984); [‡] Reynolds 1985); [§] Paul and Southgate 1978).
[¶] Included nineteen equivalents from retinaldehyde (21 μg).

Following the digestion of foods, retinol is absorbed by the intestinal mucosal cells. Retinol is liberated from retinyl esters by intestinal esterases (EC 3.1.1.1), and in the presence of human milk possibly by bile salt stimulated lipases. In most vertebrates, perhaps with the exception of carnivores β-carotene is cleaved oxidatively to retinal and then reduced to retinol. The cleavage enzyme is β-carotene 15,15′-dioxygenase (EC 1.13.11.21). The atoms of molecular oxygen are incorporated into the aldehyde products. Although theoretically 1 of β-carotene should yield 2 moles of retinal, the oxidative and subsequent reductive reactions are less than 100 per cent efficient and thus losses of potential vitamin A occur. Consequently for nutritional purposes β-carotene has been generally equated to one-sixth of all *trans*-retinol. After absorption by the intestinal cells retinol is esterified, mainly as the palmitate, and then imbibed in the hydrophobic core of the chylomicrons and transported via the thoracic duct to enter the systemic blood. Although retinol is stored in the liver mainly in the form of retinyl palmitate, it is transported to target tissues as protein-bound retinol after hydrolysis by retinyl esterase. The overall process is shown schematically in Fig. 8.2.

At target tissues intracellular binding proteins for retinol, retinal and retinoic acids together with the enzymes retinol dehydrogenase

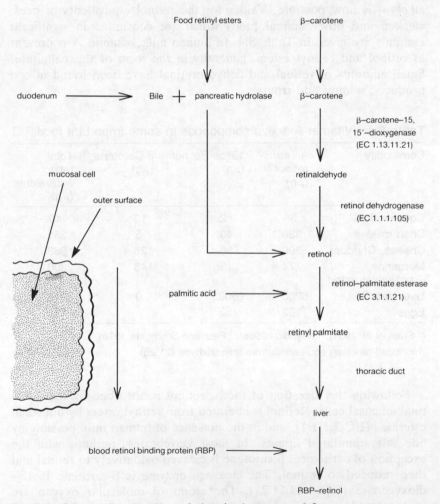

Fig. 8.2 Scheme for digestion of vitamin A esters and β-carotene

and retinal dehydrogenases have been identified. For its role in vision the oxidation of retinol to all *trans*-retinal is catalysed by the NAD-dependent retinol dehydrogenase. After isomerisation catalysed by retinal isomerase (EC 5.2.1.3) the 11-*cis*-retinal combines with the glycoprotein opsin to form rhodopsin. The visual process involves photoexcitation and isomerisation of 11-*cis*-retinal back to all *trans*-retinal. The related structural changes in the rhodopsin molecule, resulting from the *cis–trans*-isomerisation, influence cell membrane permeability in the retina and subsequent excitation of the optic nerve.

Retinoic acid and various hydroxy- and oxo-derivatives are now thought to be involved in controlling epithelial differentiation. Whether isomerisation in the unsaturated aliphatic chains is also an important event for such control processes is unknown. Retinyl phosphates, retinyl α-mannosyl phosphate and retinyl galactosyl phosphate have also been identified. Their physiological role is poorly understood.

Vitamin D

In mammals vitamin D_3 in tissues arises from either the action of ultraviolet light on 7-dehydrocholesterol to form first, previtamin D_3 and secondly, cholecalciferol (Fig. 8.3), or from the intestinal absorption of vitamin D_3 itself. Dietary sources of vitamin D_2 arise from the analogous photoconversion in plants of ergosterol to ergocalciferol (vitamin D_2). The two vitamers and other related metabolites differ only in the structure of the side chain at C-17. In light-skinned humans the maximum level of pre-D_3 is reached in approximately 15 min. of photoexposure, after which the biologically inactive compounds, lumisterol and tachysterol are formed. Pre-D_3 formed by photoexposure is then isomerised thermally (non-enzymatically) in skin tissues to D_3 prior to its transport in blood serum: such a process avoids vitamin D intoxication by excess sunlight.

The D-vitamins and all their metabolites are secosteroids in which the characteristic ring structure of steroids has been broken by cleavage of the 9,10 carbon bond of ring B (Fig. 8.3). The ring cleavage arises from the absorption of ultraviolet light by the diene structure and excitation of the B-ring in 7-dehydrocholesterol and ergosterol. The vitamin D secosteroids possess a stable conjugated *cis*-triene system which exhibits a strong absorption in the ultraviolet spectrum at 265 nm. Owing to the fission of the B-ring in the secosteroids, rapid conformational changes of the A-ring are possible in solution (Fig. 8.4).

It is now well established that vitamin D is hydroxylated enzymatically to form hormonal type compounds. Ingested vitamin D_3, now regarded as a prohormone, is metabolised first, in the liver to form 25-

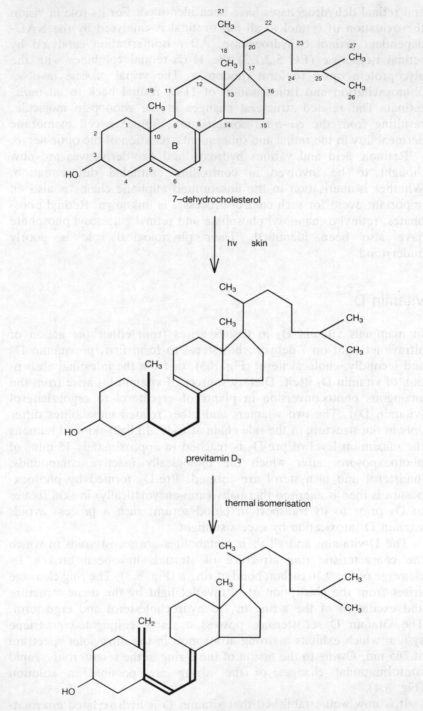

7–dehydrocholesterol

hv   skin

previtamin D$_3$

thermal isomerisation

vitamin D$_3$ (cholecalciferol)

Fig. 8.3   Formation of vitamin D by ultraviolet light

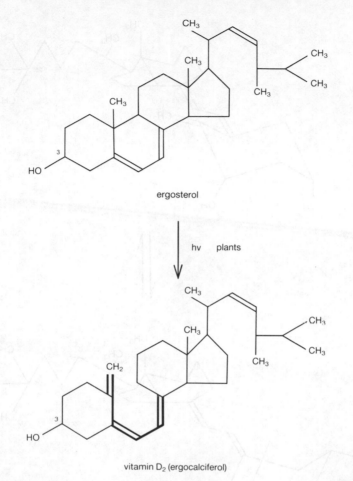

ergosterol

hv   plants

vitamin D₂ (ergocalciferol)

Fig. 8.3   (Cont'd)

hydroxyvitamin D₃ (25-OHD₃), and secondly, in the kidney to form 1,25-dihydroxyvitamin D₃ (1,25-(OH)₂D₃) (Fig. 8.5). The hydroxylation reactions may be catalysed by the mitochondrial cytochrome P-450 type mixed function oxidases (see Ch. 10), which derive their reducing equivalents from NADPH. 25-OHD₃ is the main chemical form of vitamin D circulating in blood plasma and generally the plasma level of 25-OHD₃ is a good indicator of vitamin D status. The 1,25-(OH)₂D₃ is the most important metabolite of vitamin D, as it acts like a steroid hormone by directing the synthesis of calcium-binding proteins. The other dihydroxy derivatives 24,25-(OH)₂D₃ and 1,24,25-(OH)₃D₃ are less active and their physiological roles have not been elucidated. The dihydroxy derivative is bound to 'high-affinity' components in the cytoplasm. These subsequently bind tightly to components in the nucleus to stimulate the synthesis of new messenger RNA required for

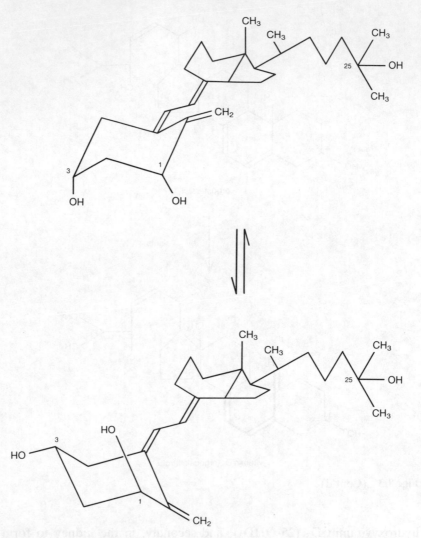

Fig. 8.4 The conformations of 1,25-dihydroxy vitamin D₃ in aqueous
solution. The 1α- and 3β-hydroxy groups of the A-ring interchange
equatorial and axial positions

the synthesis of calcium-binding proteins. Such proteins are important
for transport of calcium through the walls of the small intestine,
calcium transport in blood plasma and for bone formation. 1,25-
$(OH)_2D_3$ also stimulates the production in bone γ-carboxyglutamyl
proteins (osteocalcins). The biosynthesis of the γ-carboxyglutamyl
residue also depends on the presence of vitamin K. This reveals a
remarkable unexpected obscure interaction between two of the four
fat-soluble vitamins. Other tissues are influenced by 1,25-$(OH)_2D_3$,
and it seems that this novel hormone may also influence insulin

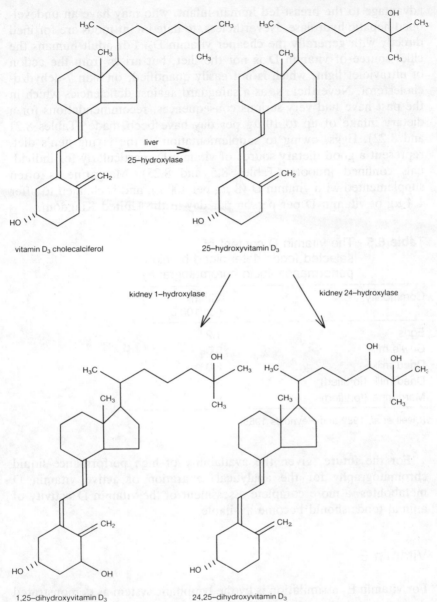

Fig. 8.5 Hydroxylation of vitamin D₃

secretion, cell growth and differentiation.

The amounts of vitamin D present in foods are extremely small. High performance liquid chromatography has now been used to determine more accurately the amounts of vitamin D_2 and D_3 in milk and milk products and eggs. However, in human milk, analysis by HPLC has identified 25-OHD₃ as the main D-vitamer. This may afford an advantage to the breast-fed human infant, who may have an undeveloped hepatic hydrolase. Nevertheless, to date infant foods are fortified directly with generally the cheaper vitamin D_2. For adult humans the chief source of vitamin D is not the diet, but arises from the action of ultraviolet light, which is not easily quantified, on skin 7-dehydrocholesterol. Nevertheless, as a safeguard against deficiencies which in the past have had very serious consequences, recommendations for a dietary intake of up to 10 μg per day have been made (Tables 8.21 and 8.22). Eggs, owing to supplementation of the laying hen's diet, represent a good dietary source of vitamin D, particularly for individuals confined indoors (Tables 8.5 and 8.25). Margarine is often supplemented with vitamin D (8 μg per 100 g), and is claimed to offer 1.4 μg of vitamin D per person per day in the United Kingdom.

Table 8.5 The vitamin D content of selected foods determined by high performance liquid chromatography

Commodity	Vitamin (μg/100 g)
Eggs	1.2
Cow's milk	0.08
Dried milk	2.0
Dried milk (fortified)	5.0
Margarine (fortified)	8

(Sivell *et al.* 1982 and Reynolds 1985).

For the future, given the availability of high performance liquid chromatography for the analytical separation of active vitamin D metabolites, a more complete assessment of the vitamin D activity of animal foods should become available.

Vitamin E

For vitamin E, assimilation is by the lymphatic system as demonstrated during cannulation of the thoracic duct. It is presently assumed that the vitamin is stored in adipose tissue and the liver. The average dietary intake in the United States is estimated to be 7.4 mg per day. However, absorption of vitamin E is inhibited by substances present in some foods such as peas and kidney beans. Also the feeding of nitrite in the diet of rats has been reported to produce a deficiency of vitamin E.

The eight naturally occurring compounds with vitamin E activity are the α, β, γ, and δ-tocopherols and the corresponding tocotrienols

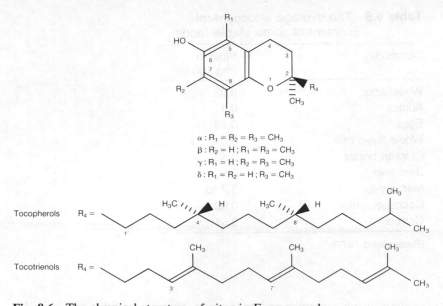

α : R₁ = R₂ = R₃ = CH₃
β : R₂ = H ; R₁ = R₃ = CH₃
γ : R₁ = H ; R₂ = R₃ = CH₃
δ : R₁ = R₂ = H ; R₃ = CH₃

Fig. 8.6 The chemical structure of vitamin E compounds

(a) The tocopherols contain sixteen-carbon saturated isoprenoid units. For the tocopherols there are three centres of asymmetry at C-2, C-4' and C-8' with the R configuration

(b) The tocotrienols contain a triene isoprenoid sixteen-carbon unit. The tocotrienols have the 2R, 3'-*trans*- and 7'-*trans*-configuration

(Fig. 8.6). The individual tocopherols differ by their substituents in the benzene ring. The tocotrienols contain an unsaturated isoprenoid type hydrocarbon chain containing three double bonds. In foods the tocopherols and tocotrienols – due to the long linear hydrocarbon side chains – are likely to be dissolved within the lipid phases and monolayers. The richest sources are vegetables, oils and nuts. α-Tocopherol is the predominant form present in human tissues, although it is not synthesised by mammals. There is a great variability in the content of vitamin E in foods, which is decreased by virtually any kind of storage and processing. Values indicative of the likely α-tocopherol content of some main food ingredients are given in Table 8.6. However, such data must be used with considerable caution due to the highly variable effects of harvesting, storage and processing of foods. Generally, the content of vitamin E in milk is higher in summer seasons, perhaps due mainly to the consumption of fresh grass by cattle. In foods, the losses of vitamin E activity are due to either direct oxidation of E-vitamers by molecular oxygen, or chemical reaction with hydroperoxides. A wide range of values have been found for the content of vitamin E in margarines, due to the use during the manufacture of margarine of many different natural vegetable and seed oils. Biological methods of

Table 8.6 The average α-tocopherol content of some staple foods

Commodity	Vitamin (mg/100 g)
Wheat flour	0.03
Apples	0.31
Eggs	0.46
Whole liquid milk	0.04
Chicken breast	0.42
Beef liver	0.5
Margarines	3.2 to 32
Cabbage, white	0.02
Carrots	9.51

(Bauernfiend 1977).

analysis using animals, and inaccurate chemical methods, are being replaced by high performance liquid chromatography for total evaluation of the tocopherol and tocotrienol content of foods. Values for the tocopherol content of some oils determined recently by HPLC are given in Table 8.7. Because higher dietary intakes of polyunsaturated fats are being frequently advised, the vitamin E requirement both for the satisfactory storage of foods and the physiological needs of man is likely to increase. Therefore such detailed analyses as shown in Table 8.7 are likely to be required for a whole range of foods.

Generally the E-vitamers are the natural fat-soluble antioxidants in foods and living animals. The vitamin is thought to protect cells, and

Table 8.7 The concentration of vitamin E active compounds in seed oils[†]

Commodity	α-Tocopherol	β-tocopherol	γ-Tocopherol
		(mg/100 g)	
Olive oil	17.9	0.2	1.1
Sesame oil	1.0	0.05	51.7
Sunflower oil	78.8	2.5	1.9
Soybean oil	10.7	2.7	74.3
Safflower oil	57.5	1.8	1.6
Maize germ oil	32.4	1.3	74.9

([†] Speek et al. 1985; [‡] calculated using the data of Burton et al. (1983) for antioxidant activity against styrene).

in particular cell membranes, against oxidation by peroxyl radicals:

$$LOO + AH(antioxidant) \rightarrow LOOH + A$$

The primary physiological function in animals seems to be that of an antioxidant. Vitamin E compounds have been claimed to be the major radical scavengers present in human plasma. A number of other chemical and enzymatic reactions involving oxygen and haemoglobin, or xanthine oxidase may also give rise to superoxide anion ($O_2^{\bar{}}$), hydroxyl radical (OH$^{\bullet}$) and hydrogen peroxide. In living tissues polymorphonuclear leucocytes involved in mammalian inflammatory reactions also produce $O_2^{\bar{}}$ and H_2O_2. In some instances various types of anaemia, eye and lung damage have been ameliorated by administration of vitamin E. Owing to its action as a scavenger of free radicals, vitamin E can also be expected to influence lipoxygenase- and cyclooxygenase-catalysed reactions in animal tissues; vitamin E deficiency has been claimed to increase prostaglandin synthesis in blood platelets.

Using model systems containing polystyrene, or ditertiarybutyl ketone for the generation of peroxyl radicals, kinetic studies have shown the E-vitamer, α-tocopherol, to be the most effective antioxidant. Generally, the order of antioxidant activity (Table 8.8) is the same as that claimed for biological activity. The more effective antioxidants are believed to be the molecules where the phenolic O–H bond is weakest. This is thought to result from the stabilisation of the generated unpaired electron of the phenoxyl radical by overlap with the orbital lone pair of electrons of the ethereal oxygen atom. Further information is needed on the biological value of the non-α-tocopherols, because metabolic conversions of the other tocopherols and trienols might occur through methylation and reduction reactions.

δ-Tocopherol	α-Tocotrienol	Approximate total vitamin E‡ activity
(mg/100 g)		(mg α-Tocopherol equivalents)
0.05	0.05	18.2
0.05	0.05	14.9
0.7	0.05	79.0
55.6	0.05	38.1
0.05	0.05	58.0
4.1	2.1	53.0

Table 8.8   Antioxidant activity of tocopherols

	Relative vitamin E activity[†]	Relative antioxidant activity towards[‡]	
		(a) styrene	(b) di-*tert*-butylketone
α-Tocopherol	100	100	100
β-Tocopherol	30	71	
γ-Tocopherol	15	66	27
δ-Tocopherol	3	27	13

([†] As stated by Paul and Southgate 1978; [‡] calculated from Burton *et al.* 1983).

Vitamin K

The K-vitamers are synthesised by plants and beneficially by gut microorganisms in animals; thus the need for vitamin K by mammals is provided by both microbial synthesis and dietary intake. Consequently deficiencies in mammals – which result in low levels of blood clotting factors – are rare and have only been reported in adult man when antibiotics such as neomycin are given to reduce colonic bacteria. The presence of bile and fat are necessary for the absorption of vitamin K from ingested food and deficiencies may also occur when there is biliary obstruction. Vitamin K is incorporated into the chylomicrons, appears in the lymph and is transported to the liver. Recently it has been shown that samples of human milk may contain only very small amounts of vitamin K (1 μg per litre), and thus deficiencies may arise in infants where there is little microbial synthesis. The requirement for infants is estimated to be 5 μg per day (Olson 1984).

The K-vitamers are 2-methylnaphthoquinones substituted in the 3-position (Fig. 8.7) Phylloquinones occur extensively in plants and contain a monounsaturated phytyl side chain. The menaquinones are of microbial origin and contain unsaturated isoprenyl side chains where a suffix indicates the number of isoprene units. The unsubstituted 2-methyl-1,4-naphthoquinone (menadione) is a provitamin which can be converted to menaquinones by animals. Values indicative of the vitamin K content of some of the main staple foods are given in Table 8.9. However, as a number of closely related menaquinones exhibit vitamin K activity, considerable caution is required when determining the vitamin K content of a food by chromatographic analysis. Biological studies of the homologues have shown them to differ in their vitamin K activity. Menaquinone-7, -8 and -9 have been found in human liver which implicates bacterial sources as being important.

In microorganisms, menaquinones are required for electron transport, oxidative phosphorylation and photosynthesis. The biochemical function in mammals of the K-vitamins involves the additional γ-

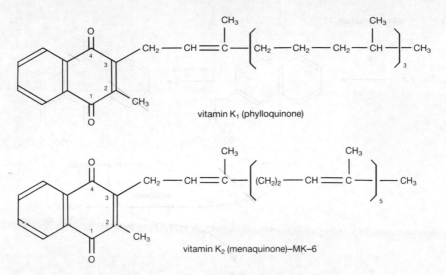

Fig. 8.7 Chemical structure of vitamins K_1 and K_2

Table 8.9 The average vitamin K content of some staple foods

Commodity	Vitamin K (μg/100 g)
Wheat flour	4
Apple sauce	2
Eggs	11
Whole liquid milk	5–17
Ground beef	7
Beef liver	92
Cabbage	125

(Olson 1982).

carboxylation of glutamate residues in a series of proteins, associated with blood clotting and calcifications. The carboxylation reactions are catalysed by vitamin K-dependent carboxylases. The γ-carboxyglutamate residue has been identified by mass spectrometry of peptides obtained from prothrombin and calcifying bone proteins.

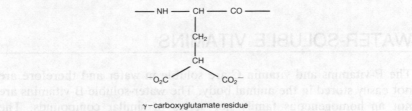

γ–carboxyglutamate residue

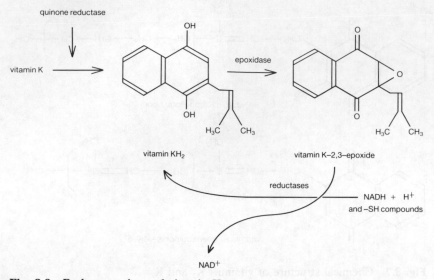

Fig. 8.8   Redox reactions of vitamin K

The γ-carboxyglutamate residue is responsible for the binding of Ca^{2+} to prothrombin, which is necessary for the release of thrombin and subsequent blood clotting. Osteocalcin, a calcifying protein in bone, has also been found to contain γ-carboxyglutamate. Dicoumarol, found in sweet clover, is a vitamin K antagonist and causes fatal bleeding in cattle fed on hay contaminated with clover. The rodent poison warfarin, which also causes fatal bleeding, has a naphthoquinone structure. Studies of the cation of these antagonists has revealed that the reduced vitamin (KH_2) and a 2,3-epoxide are active intermediates in a cyclic vitamin K redox system (Fig. 8.8). The reduced vitamin KH_2 is formed directly through the catalytic action of a NAD(P)H-linked reductase on the quinone (vitamin K). The mechanisms for the γ-hydrogen abstraction from glutamyl residues and the fixation of carbon dioxide are unknown, but are believed to be linked to the epoxidation of the reduced vitamin. Vitamin KH_2 which is necessary for the activity of the vitamin K dependent carboxylases is regenerated by the reduction of the 2,3-epoxide catalysed by vitamin K 2,3-epoxide reductase (Olson 1984).

WATER-SOLUBLE VITAMINS

The B-vitamins and vitamin C are soluble in water and therefore are not easily stored in the animal body. The water-soluble B-vitamins are not an homogeneous family nor series of similar compounds. The

Table 8.10 Biochemical functions of the water-soluble vitamins

Common name	Metabolically active form: as coenzymes	Main reaction type
Vitamin B_1, thiamin	Thiamin pyrophosphate	Transfer of aldehyde groups
Vitamin B_2, riboflavin	Flavin mononucleotide and adenine dinucleotides	Transfer of electrons
Niacin, nicotinate	Nicotinamide adenine dinucleotide (NAD) and NADP	Transfer of electrons
Vitamin B_6 (pyridoxine, pyridoxal and pyridoxamine)	Pyridoxal-5-phosphate	Transfer of $-NH_2$ groups
Pantothenate	Part of coenzyme A	Transfer of acetyl groups
Biotin	Biotin–protein compound	Transfer of CO_2
Folate	Tetrahydrofolates	Transfer of $-CH_3$, $-CHO$, $-CH_2-$, $-CH=$ and $-CHNH-$ groups
Vitamin B_{12}	The 5'-deoxyadenosyl derivative	Methylation and isomerisation
Vitamin C,	Not known, but reduces Fe^{3+} to Fe^{2+} for prolylhydroxylase	Transfer of $-OH$ groups

chemical structures of each constituent vitamin of the vitamin B complex are quite different. Also their metabolic functions are diverse (Table 8.10). Generally the B-vitamin derivatives act as coenzymes in living tissues and post-harvest foods. There are a large number of enzymes with which certain coenzymes are associated, and therefore the biochemical functions are cited only in broad terms. Nevertheless a clear distinction is made in Table 8.10 between the vitamins originally discovered as dietary constituents and their metabolically active coenzyme forms. All the biochemical reactions requiring the B-vitamin-related coenzymes are very central to the metabolism of simple important organic compounds.

For dietary sources of the B-vitamins, insufficient attention has been given to the potential contribution available from the coenzyme and protein-bound forms which are present in varying amounts in all foods. During digestion in mammals, enzymes are available for the hydrolysis of the coenzymes. It is thought that the coenzyme NAD (App. I) is hydrolysed rapidly by intestinal enzymes to nicotinamide. Additionally, in secreted foods such as milk and eggs the vitamins are bound

Table 8.11 Loss of vitamins in the refining of whole wheat to white flour

Nutrient	Loss (%)
Thiamin	77
Riboflavin	80
Niacin	81
Vitamin B$_6$	72
Pantothenate	50
Folacin	67

(Bauernfiend 1977).

to specific binding proteins. For example, eggs are known to contain riboflavin- and biotin-binding proteins. Therefore the B-vitamin content of secreted foods like milk and eggs may be partly controlled through protein biosynthesis.

During food processing some of the B-vitamins as well as vitamin C are easily lost due to their solubility in water. Additionally thiamin, folates and ascorbate are thermolabile. The milling of cereals also results in very considerable losses (Table 8.11) of B-vitamins which are predominantly found in the seed coat.

The ultimate value of a B-vitamin must be determined by first, its absorption from the intestinal lumen, secondly, the circulation to target tissues and thirdly, the subsequent conversion of the vitamin to a metabolically active compound. Because vitamins form such a diverse group of chemically unrelated compounds, it is not surprising that the biochemical mechanisms of transport for each vitamin differ considerably. For the assimilation of water-soluble B-vitamins and vitamin C, specific carrier systems linked to an energy requiring Na$^+$ transport system seem to be operative, as demonstrated in experiments with inverted intestinal sacs. Although, at higher concentrations simple diffusion across the intestinal mucosal tissue also occurs. This indicates that at least a proportion of the high doses of water-soluble vitamins occasionally taken in pill form may be assimilated, although due to their high solubility in water they may also be rapidly excreted and thus might exert only transient effects on metabolism.

Thiamin pyrophosphate (TPP)

During heat processing and cooking thiamin is lost, partly due to its lability to heat and also its solubility in cooking water. Sterilisation of milk may result in a 25 to 40 per cent loss. Thiamin is also chemically

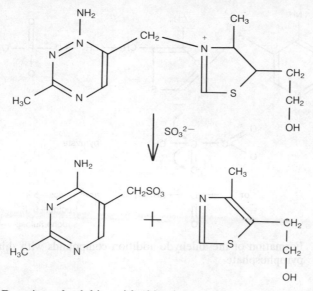

Fig. 8.9   Reaction of sulphite with thiamine

cleaved (Fig. 8.9) by sulphite anion to form a biologically inactive pyridinium sulphonate (Wedzicha 1984). Thiamin can also be lost through the action of enzymes.

Thiaminases are present in raw fish and catalyse the cleavage of the C–N bond to release the thiazole and pyrimidium moieties. The vitamin has been found in a wide range of foods including cereals, meat, milk and eggs. The use of high performance liquid chromatography for the separation of thiamin from other food constituents coupled to a specific fluorescent spectroscopic analysis has confirmed the order of magnitude of the values for thiamin in a selected number of foods (Table 8.12). The coenzyme form (TPP) is formed through the action of thiamin pyrophosphokinase (EC 2.7.6.2).

For α-keto acid dehydrogenases the coenzyme form acts as carrier of two carbon units by addition reactions with carbonyl groups present

Table 8.12   The vitamin B_1 content of
selected foods

Commodity	Thiamin (μg/100 g)
Bovine muscle	84
Liquid whole milk	32
Raw peas	305
Rolled oats	490

(Skurray 1981).

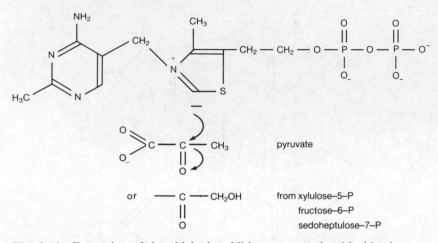

Fig. 8.10 Formation of the aldehyde addition compounds with thiamine pyrophosphate

in either α-ketoacids or ketoses. The acetylenic hydrogen atom between the nitrogen and sulphur atoms of TPP (Fig. 8.10) is acidic, and thus the carbanion forms an addition product with readily enolising carbonyl groups. Decarboxylation of the bound α-keto acid occurs to liberate carbon dioxide and the simultaneous formation of an α-hydroxyethylidene–TPP complex (active acetaldehyde) for pyruvate as substrate. Pyruvate dehydrogenase (EC 1.2.4.1) and α-ketoglutatate dehydrogenase (EC 1.2.4.2) transfer TPP-bound acyl groups to coenzyme A via a lipoyl intermediate (Fig. 8.11). These reactions are oxidative decarboxylations and are catalysed by a multienzymatic complex containing a decarboxylase, an acyl transferase and a dehydrogenase. They play a key role in the citric acid cycle for the formation of coenzyme A from pyruvate and the decarboxylation of α-ketogluarate to form succinyl coenzyme A.

pyruvate

$CH_3 - CO - CO_2H + NAD^+ + CoASH \rightleftharpoons CH_3COSCoA + NADH + H^+ + CO_2$

dehydrogenase

A flavin-linked enzyme couples the reaction to the reduction of NAD^+ (Fig. 8.11). For the transketolase catalysed reaction transfer of a two-carbon unit (as glycolaldehyde ($O=C–CH_2OH$)) from the TPP-complex (Fig. 8.10) to aldoses takes place. The biochemical symptoms of thiamin deficiency are accumulation of pyruvate, and an insufficiency of transketolase activity. Because of the key role of thiamin in oxidative metabolism the value for the recommended daily allowance (RDA) of 0.5 mg per 1000 kcal of food intake is coupled to a predicted energy intake.

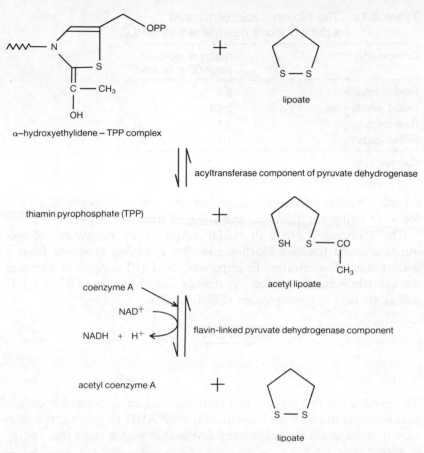

Fig. 8.11   Transfer of a TPP-bound acetyl group to form acetyl coenzyme A

Nicotinamide adenine dinucleotide

Nicotinic acid and nicotinamide, collectively known as niacin, are the precursors of the commonly occurring coenzymes, NAD and NADP (App. I). In cereals, niacin is present mainly in a bound form which is unavailable to man, although it is released on heating or treatment at alkaline pH values – as for the preparation of Mexican tortillas. Recently, high performance liquid chromatography has been used to estimate the vitamer, nicotinic acid (pyridine-3-carboxylic acid), in a small number of selected foods. Optical measurements for the estimation of nicotinic acid can be carried out at 250 nm after the chromatographic separation of nicotinate from other food constituents. The results (Table 8.13) obtained for nicotinate have confirmed the order of magnitude of the values obtained by chemical analysis. Unlike

Table 8.13 The nicotinic acid content of
selected foods determined by HPLC

Commodity	Nicotinic acid (mg/100 g of food)
Bovine muscle	5.1
Liquid whole milk	0.13
Raw peas	3.1
Rolled oats	1.1

(Skurray 1981).

thiamin, where microgram quantities are present, nicotinic acid is found in milligram quantities per 100 g of food.

The coenzymes, NAD or NADP (App. I) are derivatives of nicotinamide and function biochemically by accepting electrons from a wide range of substrates. Examples of NAD(P)-dependent enzymes are dehydrogenases typified by alcohol dehydrogenase (EC 1.1.1.1) and lactic acid dehydrogenases (EC 1.1.1.28).

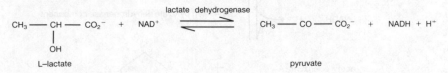

$$CH_3 \text{---} CH \text{---} CO_2^- + NAD^+ \overset{\text{lactate dehydrogenase}}{\underset{}{\rightleftharpoons}} CH_3 \text{---} CO \text{---} CO_2^- + NADH + H^+$$

L–lactate (with OH on the CH) / pyruvate

The pyridinium ring accepts two electrons and an associated hydrogen ion. For overall transfer of electrons from NADH to oxygen, the electron transfer chain is energetically favourable with a large free energy change.

$$H^+ + NADH + \tfrac{1}{2}O_2 = NAD^+ + H_2O \quad \triangle G^{o'} = -52.6 \text{ Kcal/mole}$$

A further, but less well known function of the coenzyme is a non-redox reaction in which the adenine diphosphoribose moiety of NAD (App. II) is transferred to protein-acceptor molecules. The cleavage of the β-N-glycosidic linkage liberates nicotinamide.

$$\text{Protein} + NAD^+ \overset{\text{transglycosidase}}{\underset{}{\rightleftharpoons}} \text{nicotinamide} + \text{ADPribose} - \text{protein}$$
acceptor / complex

Thus the nicotinate status may also affect – through such non-redox reactions – the extent of ribosylation of proteins that are partly responsible for regulation of DNA replication and cell differentiation.

Little attention has been given to the different forms in which nicotinate occurs in foods, although it is obvious that foods of both plants and animals must contain a large number of enzymes which are able to catalyse the interconversion and degradation of nicotinate-related vitamers. For example, a number of mammalian enzymes, like

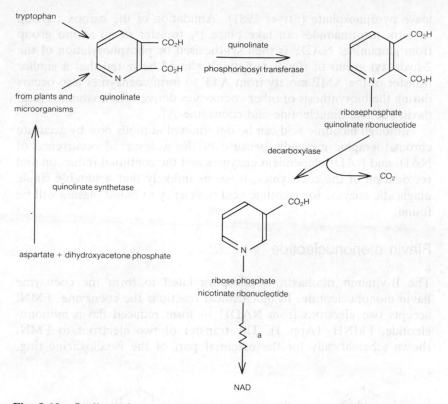

Fig. 8.12 Outline scheme for the biosynthesis of NAD from quinolinate (Stryer 1981)

NMN nucleosidase (EC 3.2.2.14), are known to degrade derivatives of nicotinate. It is generally thought that the vitamin is absorbed as nicotinamide, which is then transported to the liver where it is converted to NAD.

An alternative route for the biosynthesis in animals of nicotinate ribonucleotide arises from the metabolism of tryptophan (Fig. 8.12). However, owing to the large number of reactions required for the biosynthesis of nicotinic acid from tryptophan, and therefore an overall low conversion efficiency, such derived nicotinic acid is quoted to only one-sixtieth of the tryptophan content of a food. Nevertheless, to create a deficiency state, both niacin and tryptophan must be in short supply. Because of the widespread occurrence of the vitamin and coenzyme forms, deficiencies are rare, but they may arise indirectly from gastrointestinal disorders.

Unlike animals, plants and microorganisms are able to synthesise quinolinate more directly (Fig. 8.12) from aspartate and dihydroxyacetone phosphate where NAD is synthesised by a series of reactions terminating in the transfer of an AMP moiety from ATP (App. II) to leave pyrophosphate (Stryer 1981). Amidation of the carboxyl group to form nicotinamide can take place by transfer of an amino group from glutamine: NADP is then synthesised by phosphorylation of the 2-hydroxyl group of ribose moiety. It should be noted that a similar transfer of the AMP moiety from ATP to form coenzymes also occurs during the biosynthesis of other coenzymes derived from vitamins (e.g. flavin adenine dinucleotide and coenzyme A).

Although nicotinic acid can be determined in foods now by accurate chromatographic methods, because of the widespread occurrence of NAD- and NADP-dependent enzymes and the continual reduction and reoxidation of the coenzymes, it seems unlikely that a suitable single diagnostic enzyme for nicotinic acid deficiency in blood plasma will be found.

Flavin mononucleotide

The B-vitamin riboflavin is phosphorylated to form the coenzyme flavin mononucleotide. In biochemical reactions the coenzyme, FMN, accepts two electrons from NADH to form reduced flavin mononucleotide, $FMNH_2$ (App. I). The transfer of two electrons to FMN, shown schematically for the essential part of the isoalloxazine ring,

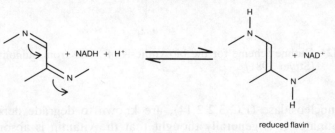

reduced flavin

is catalysed by NADH dehydrogenase (EC 1.6.99.3), which is one part of the electron transfer system by which electrons are transferred from NADH to oxygen.

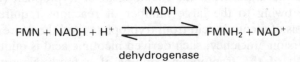

$$FMN + NADH + H^+ \rightleftharpoons FMNH_2 + NAD^+$$

The reduced flavin mononucleotide ($FMNH_2$) is oxidised, as two electrons are transferred to iron–sulphur proteins that form part of the oxidative electron transport chain.

$$FMNH_2 + 2(Fe^{3+}\text{–}S\text{–protein}) \rightarrow FMN + 2(Fe^{2+}\text{–}S\text{–protein}) + 2H^+$$

FMN is also a coenzyme for L-amino acid oxidases, where electrons are transferred directly from the substrate, without the involvement of NAD.

Flavin adenine dinucleotide

This is the second coenzyme derived from riboflavin. The coenzyme, FAD, acts as an electron acceptor for succinic dehydrogenase, xanthine oxidase, D-amino acid oxidases, acyl CoA dehydrogenase and mitochondrial FAD-linked glycerol dehydrogenases. As with FMN, the isoalloxazine ring of FAD is reduced by addition of one or two electrons. Glutathione reductase is an important FAD-dependent enzyme and is responsible for the formation of reduced glutathione. A deficiency of riboflavin may be detected by insufficiency of glutathione reductase (EC 1.6.4.2) activity.

$$\underset{\substack{|\\ \gamma\text{Glu–Cys–Glu}}}{FADH_2 + \gamma\text{Glu–Cys–Gly}} \overset{\text{glutathione}}{\underset{\text{reductase}}{\rightleftharpoons}} 2(\gamma\text{Glu–Cys–Gly}) + \underset{\substack{|\\ SH}}{\Gamma AD}$$

Riboflavin and vitamin B_6, as well as vitamin E, are partly destroyed by exposure to light. Therefore milk products and oils and fats that contain significant amounts of dietary riboflavin need protection from intensive illumination frequently found in retail display cabinets. The analysis of foods is complicated by the presence of protein-bound flavins to a number of enzymes, where both proteolysis or acid hydrolysis may be required to liberate FMN and FAD. Analyses (Skurray 1981), by high performance liquid chromatography to separate interfering compounds (Table 8.14), has indicated that the content of riboflavin in foods may have been previously overestimated. The previously used fluorescence methods of analysis which were carried out on unfractionated extracts are susceptible to interference by unknown substances. In particular, the errors may have been very appreciable for foods which contain the smaller quantities of riboflavin, such as bread and fish.

Table 8.14 The riboflavin content of selected foods determined by HPLC

Commodity	Riboflavin (mg/100 g of food)
Bovine muscle	0.15
Liquid whole milk	0.15
Raw peas	0.23
White bread	0.09
Rolled oats	0.14

(Skurray 1981).

Pyridoxal-5-phosphate

The six B_6-vitamers are related pyridinium compounds that are simply interconverted by oxidative and phosphorylation reactions (Fig. 8.13). Vitamin B_6 is the generic term for all 3-hydroxy-2-methylpyridine derivatives that exhibit the biological activity of pyridoxine. The coenzyme form of vitamin B_6 is pyridoxal phosphate, which contains the important free aldehyde group that reacts to form a Schiff base with the certain amino groups of associated enzymes. Consequently, it is reasonable to expect losses of vitamin B_6 in stored and processed foods as a result of similar condensation reactions with free amines, amino acids and other proteins. Pyridoxyllysine residues present in processed foods have a low vitamin B_6 activity. Dephosphorylation due to the action of phosphatases might also explain the loss of chemically determined vitamin B_6 during the storage and processing of foods. However, it has been established that pyridoxamine and pyridoxal can be absorbed in the unphosphorylated form through intestinal perfusion experiments. Also vitamin B_6 is believed to be synthesised by microorganisms in the human gastrointestinal tract. As the intestinal and liver cells are able rapidly to convert pyridoxine to pyridoxal-5'-phosphate, then the precise chemical form of the vitamer in the dietary source is less important. Pyridoxal kinase (EC 2.7.1.35) catalyses the phosphorylation of pyridoxine, pyridoxal and pyridoxamine and seems to be present in all mammalian tissues. The active metabolites are excreted as pyridoxic acid after hydrolysis by phosphatases and oxidation of the aldehyde group by aldehyde dehydrogenase (EC 1.2.1.3).

Unbound, or liberated B_6-vitamers, can now be individually determined after separation using high performance liquid chromatography. Values determined recently by these methods for the amounts of the various B_6-vitamers in some foods are given in Table 8.15. Animal muscles which contain up to 5 per cent of the total soluble protein as pyridoxal-dependent phosphorylase also act as a store for vitamin B_6. However, for ready-to-eat cereals only pyridoxine is present at any significant level (Vanderslice et al. 1981). The biological assay for all

Table 8.15   Amounts of B_6-vitamers[†] of selected foods[‡]

Commodity	PMP	PM	PNP	PN (μg/g)	PLP	PL	Total
Pork	3.9	—	0.09	0.17	2.1	—	6.3
Non-fat dried milk	1.3	0.8	—	0.21	1.4	2.2	6.0
Cereal	—	—	—	23	—	—	23

† PMP : pyridoxamine phosphate; PM : pyridoxamine; PNP : pyridoxine phosphate; PN : pyridoxine; PLP : pyridoxal phosphate; PL : pyridoxal.

(‡ Vanderslice et al. 1981).

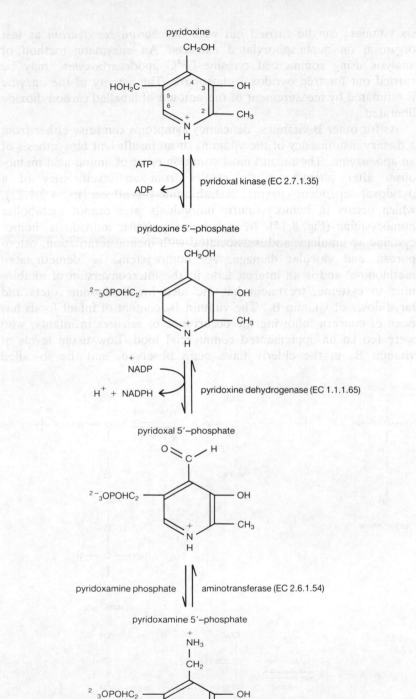

Fig. 8.13 The interconversion of B$_6$-vitamers

six vitamers can be carried out with *Saccharomyces ovarum* as test organism on dephosphorylated extracts. An enzymatic method of analysis using commercial tyrosine-1-^{14}C apodecarboxylase may be carried out for free pyridoxal phosphate. The activity of the enzyme is estimated by measurement of the amount of labelled carbon dioxide liberated.

As for other B-vitamins, deficiency symptoms can arise either from a dietary insufficiency of the vitamin, or an insufficient biosynthesis of an apoenzyme. The second most common error of amino acid metabolism after phenylketonuria results from an insufficiency of a pyridoxal-dependent enzyme, cystathionine β-synthase (EC 4.2.1.22), which occurs in homocystinuric individuals who cannot metabolise homocysteine (Fig. 8.14). In such homocystinuric individuals, homocysteine accumulates and is associated with mental retardation, osteoporosis and vascular damage. As homocysteine is 'demethylated methionine' and is an intermediate in the interconversion of methionine to cysteine, treatment has included low-methionine diets and large doses of vitamin B_6. The vitamin B_6 content of infant foods has been of concern following the occurrence of seizures in infants, who were fed an unsupplemented commercial food. Low tissue levels of vitamin B_6 in the elderly have been observed, and the so-called

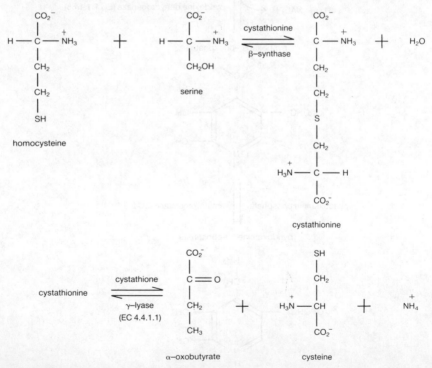

Fig. 8.14 The biosynthesis of cysteine

Chinese restaurant syndrome, due to excessive intake of glutamate can be alleviated by treatment with vitamin B_6. Because of the central role of vitamin B_6 for amino acid synthesis, the effects of deficiencies are widespread and include metabolic disturbances. Other groups at risk may include alcoholics and those taking oral contraceptives. For alcoholics, acetaldehyde, formed by oxidation of ethanol, may compete with pyridoxal for the binding sites of pyridoxal-dependent enzymes.

The vitamin B_6 status in humans may be assessed by measurement of either blood plasma pyridoxal-5'-phosphate, or the activity of some pyridoxal-5'-phosphate-dependent enzymes. These include:

glutamate : pyruvate aminotransferase (EC 2.6.1.2)
aspartate aminotransferase   (EC 2.6.1.1)
diamine oxidase   (EC 1.4.3.6)

For all pyridoxal-dependent enzymes there is a common mechanism for the formation of the enzyme–substrate complex. The coenzyme is tightly bound to the apoprotein in decarboxylases, aldolases, 1-amino-cyclopropane-1-carboxylic acid synthase in plants and mainly glycogen phosphorylase in animals. For most pyridoxal-dependent enzymes, with the exception of phosphorylase, during catalysis the methanal group of the coenzyme first forms a Schiff base with the α-amino group of substrates (Fig. 8.15). The pyridine ring nitrogen atom then attracts electrons which results in the formation of a ketimine and expulsion of a substituent group from the α-carbon atom of the amino acid. For transaminases, H^+ is released from the α-carbon atom of the substrate.

a–amino acid + enzyme → a–keto acid + enzyme-pyridoxamine

The covalently linked amino group is then transferred from pyridox-amine to the α-keto acid substrate to produce a new α-amino acid. For pyridoxal-dependent decarboxylases, the carboxyl group instead of

e.g. histidine → histamine + CO_2

H^+, is expelled from the α-carbon atom of the substrate. For the pyridoxal-dependent 1-aminocyclopropane-1-carboxylic acid synthase found in plants, the R-substituent group containing the electron-deficient sulphur atom of methionine, instead of H^+, is expelled to form an ethene precursor (Ch. 9).

Coenzyme A

Pantothenic acid forms the central part of the coenzyme A (CoA) molecule (Fig. 8.16), which is required for the metabolic transfer of two carbon atoms as acetyl groups. Although animals cannot syn-thesise the pantothenate moiety itself, the biosynthesis of coenzyme A,

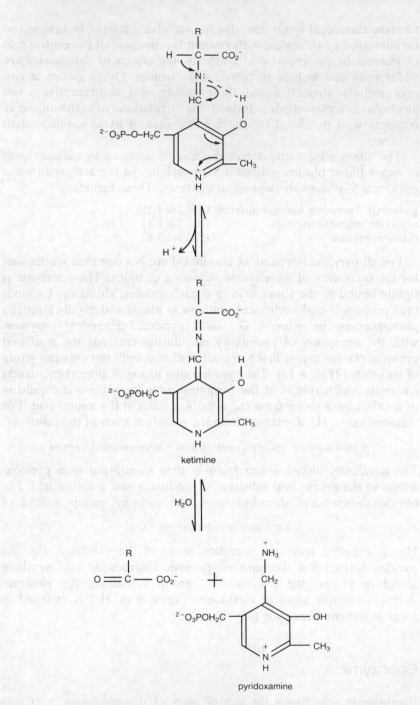

ketimine

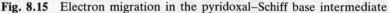

pyridoxamine

Fig. 8.15 Electron migration in the pyridoxal–Schiff base intermediate

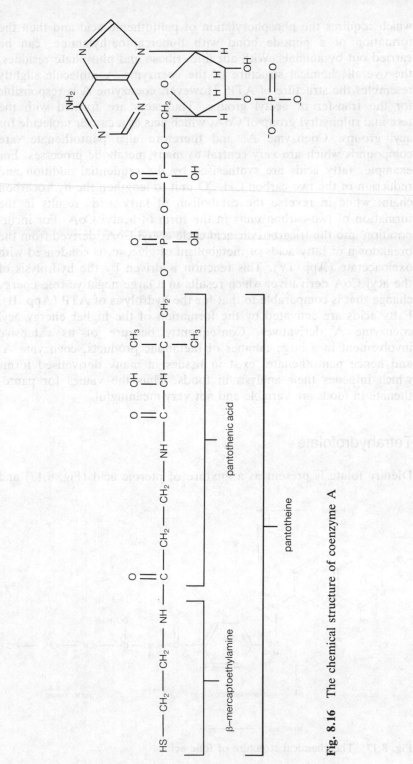

Fig. 8.16 The chemical structure of coenzyme A

which requires the phosphorylation of pantothenic acid and then the formation of a peptide bond with β-mercaptoethylamine, can be carried out by animals. With adenine, ribose and phosphate residues, the overall chemical structure of the coenzyme A molecule slightly resembles the structure of ATP. However, coenzyme A is responsible for the transfer of acetyl groups. Thioesters are formed with the terminal sulphydryl group of CoA, which acts as a carrier molecule for acyl groups. Coenzyme A, and therefore also pantothenate, are compounds which are very central to many metabolic processes. For example, fatty acids are synthesised by the sequential addition and reduction of the two-carbon CH_3CO unit to lengthen the hydrocarbon chain, while in reverse the catabolism of fatty acids results in the formation of two-carbon units in the form of acetyl CoA. For incorporation into the tricarboxylic acid cycle acetyl CoA, derived from the breakdown of fatty acids or metabolism of glucose, is condensed with oxaloacetate (App. IV). This reaction is driven by the hydrolysis of the acyl CoA derivative, which results in a large negative free energy change that is comparable to that for the hydrolysis of ATP (App. II). Fatty acids are activated by the formation of the higher energy acyl coenzyme A derivatives. Consequently because of its extensive involvement in a large number of metabolic products, coenzyme A, and hence pantothenate, exist in tissues in many derivatised forms which impedes their analysis in foods. Thus the values for pantothenate in foods are variable and not very meaningful.

Tetrahydrofolate

Dietary folate is present as a mixture of pteroic acid (Fig. 8.17) and

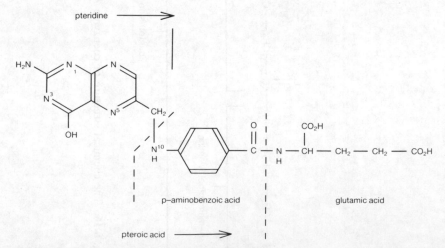

Fig. 8.17 The chemical structure of folic acid

derived polyglutamates, both of which can be destroyed during heat processing and the cooking of food. Some microorganisms can synthesise the vitamin from the p-aminobenzoic acid constituent, whereas others like *Lactobacillus spp.* require the complete vitamin for growth. Mammals are unable to synthesise the pteridine nucleus and therefore require dietary pteroylglutamates. The microbiological assays with *Lactobacillus casei*, which are still widely used, may underestimate the folate content of foods by failing to respond to various derivatives and in particular 5'N-methylfolate (Phillips *et al.* 1982). *Lactobacillus casei* only responds to free folate, and therefore food extracts require a preliminary treatment with conjugases to hydrolyse the polyglutamate moieties. Bound folate, which is present in microgram quantities in foods, is also released by autoclaving. Some values recently obtained using this technique are given in Table 8.16.

Table 8.16 The folate content of some green vegetables determined with *L. casei* after autoclaving

Vegetable	Folate (μg/100 g)
Lettuce	68
Cabbage	59
French beans	74
Brussels sprouts	174

(Nik-Dand and Bender 1983).

The coenzyme tetrahydrofolate derived from folates is simply formed by reduction. The reaction is catalysed by folic acid reductase and requires NADPH. Therefore, in common with other biosynthetic reactions, the formation of tetrahydrofolate may be controlled by the cellular content of NADPH. The coenzyme molecule accepts carbon units as either methyl CH_3-, methylene $-CH_2-$ or formyl $-CH=O$ groups, but not as carbon dioxide or hydrogen carbonate anion. The main pathway for the formation of one-carbon unit derivatives of tetrahydrofolate is from serine catalysed by serine hydroxymethylase (EC 2.1.2.1) (Fig. 8.18). The formyl and related transferases are classified under EC 2.1.2 by the Committee for Enzyme Nomenclature. The one-carbon methylene group $-CH_2-$ is substituted for each hydrogen atom on the N^5 and N^{10} nitrogen atoms of tetrahydrofolate. The substituted methylene group can be oxidised enzymatically to methenyl by transfer of electrons to NADP, or reduced enzymatically to an N^5-methyl derivative by NADH. As with other vitamins, the separate quantification of folates, which can be achieved now by improved chromatographic methods, should afford a better under-

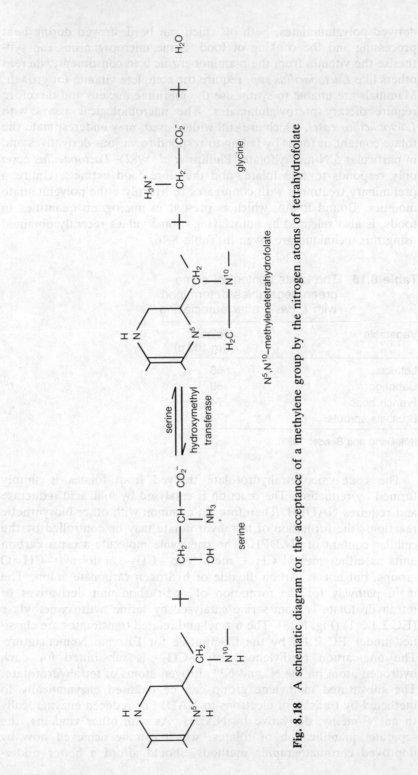

Fig. 8.18 A schematic diagram for the acceptance of a methylene group by the nitrogen atoms of tetrahydrofolate

Table 8.17 Folate coenzymes in selected foods determined by
high performance liquid chromatography[†]

Commodity	H₄–fol[‡]	5-CH₃–H₄fol	5-HCO–H₄fol (μg/100 g)	Folate	Total
Cabbage	31	5.1	—	—	36.1
Bovine liver	2132	160.5	90	33.5	2416
Orange juice	—	16.9	—	—	16.9

([†] Calculated from Gregory *et al*. 1983).

[‡] H₄–fol is the abbreviation for tetrahydrofolate.

standing of their distribution in all foods and eventually the nutritional
importance of each vitamer. Through the use of high performance
chromatography followed by fluorimetric detection, the amounts of
different coenzyme forms of tetrahydrofolate have been estimated for
some foods (Table 8.17). From these analyses, it seems that bovine
liver contains mainly tetrahydrofolate, whereas milk contains only the
5-methyl derivative. However, as folates occur as polyglutamates the
biological value of such foods is still difficult to determine because the
derivatives might not always be hydrolysed by intestinal pteroylpoly-
glutamyl hydrolases. Also feeding experiments carried out for a full
nutritional evaluation may be complicated by the intestinal microbial
biosynthesis of folates. After assimilation, folate is bound to enzymes
which are generally dehydrogenases responsible for demethylation
reactions. Folate-binding proteins can be detected and isolated through
the use of radioactive folates. Such proteins have been found in bovine
milk (Iwai *et al*. 1983), where they may affect the bioavailability of the
vitamin. For rat liver mitochondria the pentaglutamyl derivative of
folate was the most strongly protein-bound form of the vitamin.

The coenzyme tetrahydrofolate, as a carrier of one-carbon units, is
required for the biosynthesis of purines and thymine. The deficiencies
of folate primarily halt DNA synthesis and anemia may result. Also
uracil may be misincorporated into DNA while methionine may
accumulate in the liver.

Biotin

Biotin is a relatively simple cyclic molecule containing nitrogen and
sulphur. Biotin deficiency is rare as the vitamin is both ubiquitous in
the diet and synthesised by intestinal microorganisms. However, avidin
of egg white binds biotin so strongly that it can become unavailable
for absorption from diets containing raw egg white. Fortunately, heat-
treatment of egg white at 80 °C for 5 min. will denature avidin and
destroy its biotin-binding property. Deficiencies can also arise from

short bowel disposition due to failure to absorb the vitamin. Deficiency symptoms are dermatitis, alopecia, nervous irritability and anorexia with a marked fall in food intake. The deficiencies are similar to those induced by lack of dietary zinc or essential fatty acids.

Owing to the high affinity and tight binding to biotin, egg white avidin – or strepavidin from *Streptomyces spp.* – is now used as a test probe for the presence of biotin-dependent enzymes. Further, in immunological analyses antigens can be detected using a biotin-labelled antibody, which is then itself specifically detected with a synthetic avidin-coupled enzyme such as avidin–peroxidase. In the electron microscope, components labelled with biotin can be visualised with a ferritin–avidin complex.

As biotin is required as a covalently bound cofactor for the catalysis of important biosynthetic reactions, genetic deficiencies can also arise from defects in the biotin-dependent enzymes. Biotin-dependent enzymes catalyse the carboxylation reactions (Table 8.18). Pyruvate carboxylase (EC 6.4.1.1) participates in the regulated pathway for gluconeogenesis where phosphoenolpyruvate is the starting material for the biosynthesis of glucose.

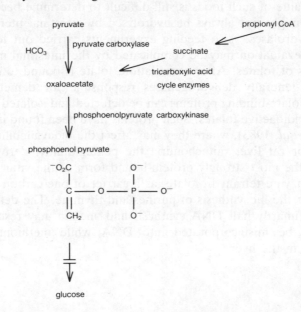

Also the first committed step in the biosynthesis of fatty acids is the biotin-dependent carboxylation of acetyl CoA to form malonyl CoA catalysed by acetyl CoA carboxylase (EC 6.4.1.2).

$$\underset{\text{acetyl CoA}}{CH_3COSCoA} + HCO_3^- + ATP \underset{\text{carboxylase}}{\overset{\text{acetyl CoA}}{\rightleftharpoons}} \underset{\text{malonyl CoA}}{{}^-O_2CCH_2COSCoA} + ADP + phosphate$$

Table 8.18 Biotin-dependent enzymes (EC 6.4 forming carbon–carbon bonds)

Enzyme	Substrate	Product
Acetyl CoA carboxylase	Acetyl CoA	Malonyl CoA
Pyruvate carboxylase	Pyruvate	Oxaloacetate
Propionyl CoA carboxylase	Propionyl CoA	Methylmalonyl CoA
Methylcrotonyl CoA carboxylase	Methylcrotonyl CoA	Methylglutaconyl CoA
Geranoyl CoA carboxylase	Geranoyl CoA	3-Isohexenylglutaconyl CoA
Oxaloacetate decarboxylase	Oxaloacetate	Pyruvate and carbon dioxide
Transcarboxylases	Carboxylic acids	Carboxylic acids

Biotin provides the means for introducing one-carbon units at the highest oxidation state (CO_2) into organic acids. The HCO_3 anion is used as the substrate by biotin-dependent enzymes, whereas tetra-hydrofolate is responsible for the transfer of reduced carbon atoms. The carboxylation of propionate to form methylmalonyl CoA is also catalysed by a biotin-dependent enzyme, propionyl CoA carboxylase (EC 6.4.1.3). Methylmalonyl CoA is then independently isomerised to succinyl CoA which is subsequently metabolised through the tricar-boxylic acid cycle.

Most biotin-dependent enzymes, like pyruvate carboxylase, possess three protein components: a biotin-dependent carboxylase, a biotinyl carrier protein and the carboxyl transferase. Halocarboxylase synthe-tase is the enzyme responsible for catalysing the linking of biotin to the ε-amino group of specific lysine residues in the biotinyl carrier proteins. In rat liver the allosteric activation of the biotin-dependent carboxylases is by a cyclic AMP-protein kinase and by citrate. First a conformational change in the carboxylase enzyme is induced by citrate and then the active enzyme is formed by dimerisation. The enzyme activity of the dimerised pyruvate carboxylase is also controlled by product inhibition which results from an accumulation of the enzyme-bound 1'N-carboxy-biotinyl group through the reversed catalysis of reaction (2) below. The biotin-dependent carboxylation reactions take place in two steps where the covalently attached biotin molecule serves as a carrier for a $^-O–C=O$ group (Fig. 8.19). The two partial reactions for the catalytic action of pyruvate carboxylase are:

$$\text{(1) Enzyme–biotin + ATP + HCO}_3^- \underset{\text{carboxylase}}{\overset{\text{pyruvate}}{\rightleftharpoons}} \text{Enzyme–biotin–CO}_2^- + \text{ADP + phosphate}$$

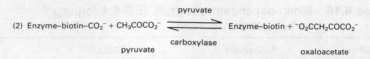

(2) Enzyme–biotin–CO$_2^-$ + CH$_3$COCO$_2^-$ $\rightleftharpoons$ Enzyme–biotin + $^-$O$_2$CCH$_2$COCO$_2^-$

pyruvate

carboxylase

pyruvate   oxaloacetate

Reaction (1) is dependent on the presence of Mg^{2+} and the enzyme is allosterically activated by acetyl CoA; the biotinyl group is carboxylated. Stabilisation of the biotinyl–carboxyl group by methylation with diazomethane has demonstrated the involvement of the ureido-1'-N atom. The 1'-N-carboxybiotin derivative is also an active carboxyl group donor. In reaction (2) the carboxyl group is transferred from the 1'-N-carboxybiotinyl to pyruvate to form oxaloacetate.

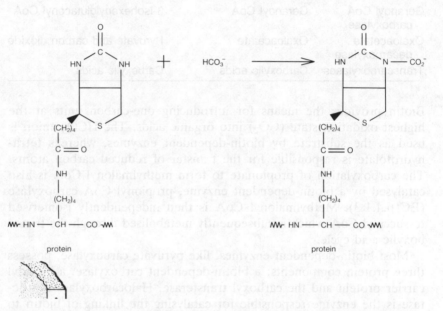

Fig. 8.19 The formation of an enzyme–biotin activated carboxyl group. Biotin is covalently linked to the enzyme through the ε-amino group of lysine residue

Owing to the role of biotin-dependent carboxylases for the metabolism of organic acids, deficiencies of the biotin-dependent enzymes result in the accumulation of toxic amounts of organic acids. The biochemical features of biotin deficiency can include lactic acidosis, increased excretion of 3-methylcrotonylglycine, 3-hydroxyisovaleric and 3-hydroxypropionic acids and methyl citrate. Both propionyl CoA carboxylase (Table 8.18) and methylcrotonyl CoA carboxylase are required for the metabolism of acids formed during the catabolism of amino acids. A deficiency of propionyl CoA carboxylase results in propionic acidosis, while a deficiency of methylcrotonyl CoA carboxylase results in β-methylcrotonylglycinuria due to the formation of a glycine conjugate of the organic acid. Biotin-deficient diseases are also coupled to immunodeficiency, which is possibly due to an insufficient synthesis of DNA: biotin is known to increase the cellular content of cyclic guanylate, as well as the activity of glucokinase in cultured rat hepatocytes.

Microbial biotin-dependent enzymes which catalyse the decarboxylation of oxaloacetate and methylmalonyl CoA to form pyruvate and propionyl CoA, respectively, are also known. Such catalysed reactions are important in some fermented foods.

Vitamin B$_{12}$

Vitamin B$_{12}$ occurs only in animal products, particularly meat, and is synthesised only by specific microorganisms. In view of the very small amounts of vitamin B$_{12}$ required by humans, dietary deficiencies of vitamin B$_{12}$ which result in pernicious anaemia are rare. However, a deficiency can arise from a vegetarian diet, but more commonly a deficiency results from defective assimilation of the vitamin. The latter can only be overcome by direct intramuscular injections of vitamin B$_{12}$. The vitamin B$_{12}$ content of some selected foods is given in Table 8.19. The data has been obtained using a competitive radioactive binding method for analysis (Osterdahl et al. 1986). The most important sources are animal liver, although significant amounts can be obtained from marine foods. No recommendations for daily allowances of vitamin B$_{12}$ have been made in the United Kingdom, but FAO/WHO (1974) and the United States have recommended 2 and 3 μg of dietary vitamin B$_{12}$, respectively, per day (NRC/NAS 1980). In foods, vitamin B$_{12}$ exists in the form of two types of coenzyme usually bound to both enzymes and vitamin B$_{12}$-binding proteins. A number of vitamin B$_{12}$-binding proteins have been found in human serum and saliva. The two coenzyme forms are the methyl derivative, found in the cytosol, and

Table 8.19 The vitamin B$_{12}$ content of some foods

Commodity	Vitamin B$_{12}$ (μg/100 g)[†]
Milk	0.4
Lamb's liver	104
Herring	10
Oyster	18
Crab	10
Egg yolk	3.8

([†] Janne 1982).

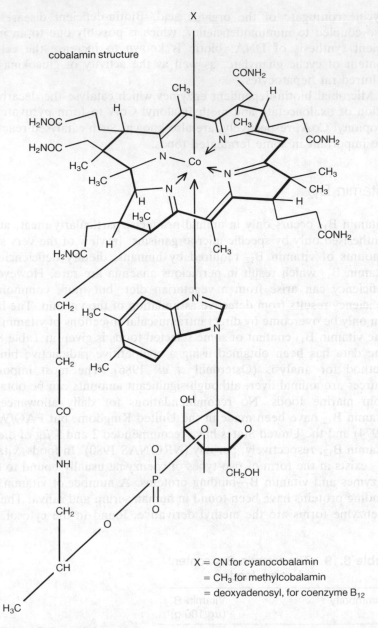

X = CN for cyanocobalamin
  = CH₃ for methylcobalamin
  = deoxyadenosyl, for coenzyme B₁₂

Fig. 8.20 Cobalamin structure

the 5′-deoxyadenosyl derivative, found in mitochondria. Vitamin B_{12} is an organocobalt compound containing a corrin ring (Fig. 8.20) containing partially saturated pyrolle rings joined directly and by methene bridges. The planar tetrapyrolle rings are substituted with acetamide and propionamide residues. The cobalt atom is centrally situated and linked by four coordinate bonds to the four pyrolle nitrogens and a fifth bond to the nitrogen atom of the benzimidazoyl ring. This large ring structure composed of 5,6-dimethylbenzimidazoyl, a substituted propionamide and ribofuranosyl-3-phosphate lies below the plane of the corrin ring (Fig. 8.20). The sixth axial ligand in the coenzyme is either the methyl, or the 5'-deoxyadenosine group, whereas commercial preparations, generally known as cyanocobalmin, contain a cyanide group in the sixth coordinate position.

Owing both to the occurrence of different chemical forms of vitamin B_{12} and the existence of various B_{12}-binding proteins, the vitamin B_{12} content of foods has been estimated frequently by microbiological assay with B_{12} requiring *Lactobacillus leichmannii*, or *Euglena gracilis*. Alternatively, high performance liquid chromatography can now be used to separate mixtures of cobalamins for radioisotopic competitive assays. For such assays a special intrinsic factor, which has a much higher specificity for vitamin B_{12} than the other binding proteins is used.

Assimilation of vitamin B_{12} in mammals requires first, the release of the bound vitamin from food proteins, secondly, the attachment of the released vitamin B_{12} to a mammalian binding protein, thirdly, transfer of the vitamin to a specific intrinsic factor, and finally absorption of vitamin B_{12} in the second half of the small intestine. The first stage requires the release in the stomach of vitamin B_{12} from food by the catalytic action of acid and pepsin. The released vitamin is then bound to special mammalian R-proteins which have been secreted in the saliva and gastric juices. The later transfer of the vitamin to the special intrinsic factor is mediated by proteolysis of the R-proteins catalysed by secreted mammalian pancreatic proteinases. The special intrinsic factor is a glycoprotein with a high affinity mainly for vitamin B_{12} ($K_a = 10^{-10}M^{-1}$). Degraded products of vitamin B_{12} formed by either deamidation of the acetamide and propionamide side chains or hydrolysis of the 5'-deoxyadenosinyl residue, are less firmly bound by the intrinsic factor but still strongly held by R-proteins (Seetharam and Alpers 1982). Absorption for only the vitamin B_{12}-intrinsic factor complex (Fig. 8.21) is believed to take place in the ileum which contains the specific calcium-receptor sites. Therefore an insufficiency of intrinsic factor can also result in vitamin B_{12} deficiency. However, also an excess of intrinsic factor can impede vitamin B_{12} uptake by presumably blocking the receptor sites. After absorption in the intestine, vitamin B_{12} is transported to the tissues by specific binding proteins called transcobalamines. The first step in the metabolism of vitamin B_{12} requires the reduction from Co^{3+} to Co^+ by NADH, from which the coenzyme forms of methyl- and deoxyadenosylcobalamin are synthesised.

Owing to the devastating effects of vitamin B_{12} deficiency in causing anaemia and neurological problems, it is surprising that only two

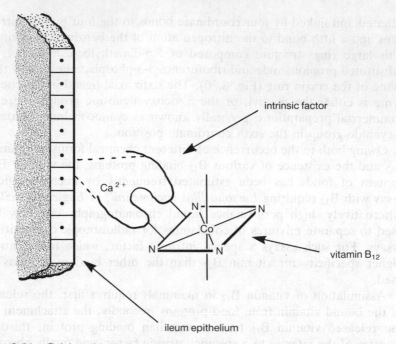

intrinsic factor

Ca^{2+}

vitamin B$_{12}$

ileum epithelium

Fig. 8.21 Calcium binding of intrinsic factor–vitamin B$_{12}$ complex

mammalian enzymes require vitamin B$_{12}$ derivatives: methylmalonyl
CoA mutase (EC 5.4.99.2) catalyses the intramolecular rearrangement
of methylmalonyl CoA to succinyl CoA for which the 5′-deoxy-
adenosyl derivative of vitamin B$_{12}$ is required.

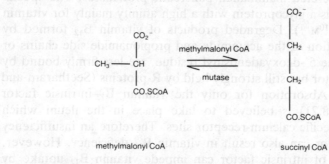

Homocysteine methyltransferase (EC 2.1.1.10) catalyses the
demethylation of N^5-methyltetrahydrofolate. Homocysteine acts as the
methyl group acceptor to form methionine. The formation of succinyl
CoA from the three-carbon carboxylic acid affords a link between the
catabolism of odd-numbered fatty acids, some branched chain amino
acids and the tricarboxylic acid cycle. In deficiency states methylmalonate is excreted in the urine of mammals.

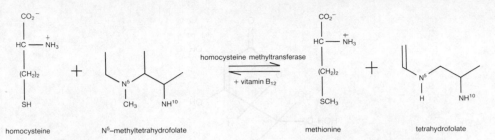

In view of the fact that folate deficiency also causes anaemia, it seems that vitamin B_{12} anaemia may be due to the lack of ummethylated folate. In vitamin B_{12} deficiency tetrahydrofolate is trapped as N^5-methyltetrahydrofolate, because the formation of the latter compound by reduction of methylene tetrahydrafolate is thermodynamically irreversible. The associated, but separate, neurological symptoms of vitamin B_{12} deficiency may arise from the separate accumulation of methylmalonate caused by the low enzymatic activity of methylmalonyl CoA mutase. However, in lactobacilli, 5′-deoxyadenosylcobalamin is also required for the reduction of ribonucleotides to deoxyribonucleotides by ribonucleotide reductase (Seetharam and Alpers 1982). As it is claimed that the RNA/DNA ratio is increased in megaloblastic anaemia, the significance of this observation also requires further investigation.

Vitamin C

Ascorbic acid is a polyol. It exists in solution as an unsaturated lactone (Fig. 8.22). The hydroxyl group attached to an ethylenic carbon atom is acidic with a pK value of 4.1; the alkene and carbonyl groups are conjugated. The immediate oxidation product dehydroascorbic acid (Fig. 8.23) is still biologically active and is believed to exist in solution as a bicyclic hydrated lactone. During enzymic browning of fruits and vegetables the quinone products rapidly oxidise ascorbate to dehydroascorbate, which may be converted to the ketogulonate by delactonisation. Also the copper-dependent enzyme ascorbate oxidase (EC

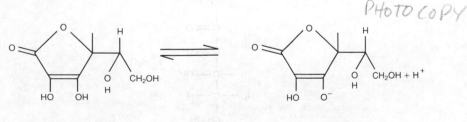

L-ascorbic acid   L-ascorbate anion

Fig. 8.22 The acidic property of vitamin C

PHOTOCOPY

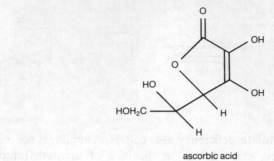

ascorbic acid

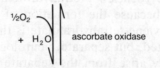

ascorbate oxidase

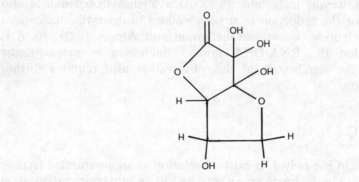

bicyclic hydrated dehydroascorbic acid

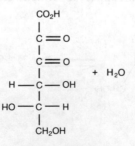

2.3-diketogulonic acid

Fig. 8.23 Oxidation of ascorbic acid

1.10.3.3) may catalyse the formation of dehydroascorbate. For non-enzymic browning first oxidation of ascorbate to dehydroascorbate may be catalysed by transition metals. Hydrolysis of the γ-lactone to form 2,3-ketogulonate, which is biologically inactive, is often followed by a series of rapid chemical reactions to produce tainting volatile and coloured compounds (Wedzicha 1984).

Fruits and vegetables, which provide 23 mg and 28.5 mg per day, respectively, are the chief sources of vitamin C in the United Kingdom dietary intake (MAFF 1984). Unfortunately, vitamin C dissolves in cooking water and is easily decomposed by heat. The chemical method of analysis using the oxidising agent 2,6-dichlorophenolindophenol for estimating the vitamin C content of food only measures the ascorbic acid content. However, dehydroascorbic acid can be determined separately using the fluorimetric assay with o-phenylenediamine, which depends on a condensation reaction with the α,α-dicarbonyl group present in dehydroascorbate and 2,3-diketogulonic acid. No single chemical method has yet been developed for the determination of total vitamin C. However, by high performance liquid chromatography it should be possible to determine both ascorbic and dehydroascorbic acids. Values for the amounts of both forms of vitamin C determined in some fruits are given in Table 8.20 to indicate the levels normally found in fresh and homogenised fruits. The data in Table 8.20 show that for banana, apple and guava purée after a short period, a rapid oxidation of ascorbate to dehydroascorbate occurs.

In the United Kingdom, potatoes represent a significant dietary source of vitamin C and therefore ascorbate is now added to dried potato powder in order to ensure the supply of vitamin from this staple food. Ascorbate is also used as a bread dough improver, where it is

Table 8.20 Changes in vitamin C content in fruit blends

Fruit blend	Ascorbate	Dehydroascorbate	Total vitamin C
	(mg/100 g of aqueous blend)		
Fresh orange juice	42	2	44
Fresh orange juice (30 min at 21 °C)	41	1	42
Fresh banana purée	8	4	12
Fresh banana purée (30 min at 21 °C)	1	9	10
Fresh apple purée	3	1	4
Fresh apple purée (30 min at 21 °C)	1	3	4
Fresh guava purée	108	0	102
Fresh guava purée (30 min at 21 °C)	60	45	105

(From Mokady et al. 1984).

thought to be oxidised to dehydroascorbate by wheat ascorbate oxidase. The generated dehydroascorbate may then oxidise glutathione and hence diminish its involvement in unwanted excessive disulphide interchange reactions in gluten proteins which reduce the elasticity of bread doughs (Ch. 5).

There is a nutritional requirement for ascorbate by primates, guinea-pigs, bats, many birds, trout, salmon, carp and probably many other fish and insect species. Radioautographic studies, in conjunction with tissue assay methods, have shown high levels of free ascorbate in the adrenal glands, brain and salivary glands. In healthy humans the pool size for ascorbate has been estimated to be between 2 and 3 g. The quantitative metabolism of ascorbate is estimated at approximately 40 mg per day and symptoms of scurvy appear when the pool size falls to a low value of 300 mg. The levels of ascorbate increase in tissues during regeneration of proteins, and in plants the quantities of ascorbate are highest in the growing tips and ripening fruits. These observations indicate that ascorbate concentration is in some way related to the regulation of growth.

An active coenzyme derivative of ascorbate has not been found, but it is now accepted that the most important role in animals for ascorbate is as a required constituent for enzymatic hydroxylation reactions during the biosynthesis of collagen. The reaction involves the hydroxylation of proline catalysed by prolylhydroxylases in procollagen and preelastin. In the presence of ascorbate, Fe^{3+} is reduced chemically to Fe^{2+} and in this way prolyl- and lysylhydroxylases are reactivated for the synthesis of hydroxyproline and hydroxylysine. In *Brassica spp.* ascorbate is an allosteric activator of glucosinolase. The reversible oxidation sequence of ascorbate–monodehydroascorbate–dehydroascorbate is considered to be central to the role of vitamin C as a redox compound and an antioxidant. Ascorbate, being a reducing agent, is able to maintain transition metal ions in a low oxidative state and is frequently used as an antioxidant in foods. Also the radical intermediate with one unpaired electron has a highly conjugated tricarbonyl system. It is generally accepted that ascorbate will act as a scavenger of free radicals in aqueous environments. Thus ascorbate is at the forefront for the protection of tissues and foods from free radical mediated oxidations.

RECOMMENDED DAILY ALLOWANCES

World wide, the recommended daily amounts (RDA) for vitamins and other nutrients vary between countries, and are under continual assessment and revision. Estimates of vitamin requirements are gained from knowledge of the minimum intakes of vitamins needed to prevent deficiencies, knowledge of the biochemical processes for assimilation and storage of vitamins, and the levels of vitamins required to saturate tissues. Generally, the recommendations made in different countries are merely judgements of the required needs of population groups over a period of time. Comparisons (Tables 8.21 and 8.22) of the RDAs by the United Kingdom, United States and FAO/WHO, illustrate how the values for the recommended amounts/allowances vary between countries. For example, the RDA values for vitamin A and vitamin C in the United States are higher than the values recommended both in the United Kingdom and by FAO/WHO. Also, RDA values are not now given in the United Kingdom (DHSS 1981) for vitamins B_{12}, B_6, pantothenate, folate, biotin and the fat-soluble vitamins E and K. Comparisons of the RDA values for different countries have been published by the International Union of Nutritional Sciences (IUNS 1983).

The RDA value should not be confused with the requirements of a specific individual who may continuously consume less than the recommended amounts of some nutrients, as the diet for such an individual may still be adequate. The recommended amounts are normally thought to exceed the estimated physiological requirements; the RDA values are considered large enough to reduce the risk 'that some people may not receive enough to meet their needs' to a minimum. Thus the RDA values are not precise targets for individuals, but mainly overall daily dietary goals for populations averaged over a period of weeks, months or seasons. Thus there is little concern in the United Kingdom that the dietary intake of some vitamins may fall below the RDA for a considerable number of people. Margins of safety which vary for the different vitamins also exist within the RDA value. The information on nutrient intake used to estimate RDA values is hindered by inadequate analytical techniques for measuring the nutrient content of such complex mixtures as whole foods. Further, sufficient information is not available on the bioavailability of the various vitamers of folate, B_6 and vitamins E and K. Consequently a single day's intake should not be compared with RDA values.

In the United States and the United Kingdom food consumption surveys (MAFF 1984, USDA 1982) and known analytical data for food composition provide the basis for estimating the dietary intake of vitamins. National Health and Nutrition Examination surveys (NHANES 1981) are also carried out in the United States. These surveys incorporate scientific measurements including clinical examinations and biochemical analyses. Among the latter group are measurements in blood serum of cholesterol, triglycerides, protein, iron and folate. NHANES-type surveys are valuable because they potentially allow a correlation between biochemical parameters and food consumption. Reports are also available of the nutrient intakes for special groups in the United States.

Table 8.21 Abbreviated recommended daily amounts of some vitamins for population groups in the United Kingdom[†]

Age range (years)	Thiamin (mg)	Riboflavin (mg)	Nicotinic acid equivalents (mg)[‡]
Boys			
under 1	0.3	0.4	5
5–6	0.7	0.9	10
Girls			
12–14	0.9	1.4	16
Men			
35–64	1.0	1.6	18
Women			
Pregnancy	1.0	1.6	18

([†] After DHSS 1981).

[‡] One nicotinic acid equivalent = 1 mg available nicotinic acid or 60 mg tryptophan.

[§] No dietary sources may be necessary for children and adults who are sufficiently exposed to sunlight, but during the winter children and adolescents should receive 10 μg (400 i.u.) daily by supplementation. Adults with inadequate exposure to sunlight, for example those who are housebound, may also need a supplement of 10 μg daily.

Table 8.22 Abbreviated recommended daily amounts of some vitamins for population groups in the United States of America (1980)[†]

Age (years)	Vitamin A (R. Eq.) (μg)	Vitamin D (μg)	Vitamin E (mg)	Vitamin K (μg)	Thiamin (mg)	Riboflavin (mg)
Males and females						
0–0.5	420	10	3	12	0.3	0.4
4–6	500	10	6	20–40	0.9	1.0
Males						
11–14	1000	10	8	50–100	1.4	1.6
23–50	1000	5	10	70–140	1.4	1.6
Females						
Pregnant	1000	10	10	70–140	1.5	1.6

([†] After NRC/NAS 1980).

R. Eq. = retinol equivalents; 1 μg of retinol = 6 μg of β-carotene = 12 μg of other biologically active carotenoids
N. Eq. = niacin equivalents; 1 mg of niacin = 60 mg of tryptophan.

Vitamin C	Vitamin A, retinol equivalents	Vitamin D (cholecalciferol)
(mg)	(μg)	(μg)[§]
20	450	7.5
20	300	[§]
25	725	[§]
30	750	[§]
60	750	10

Niacin (N. Eq.)	Vitamin B$_6$	Pantothenic acid	Biotin	Folacin	Vitamin B$_{12}$	Vitamin C
(mg)	(mg)	(mg)	(μg)	(μg)	(μg)	(mg)
6	0.3	2	35	30	0.5	35
11	1.3	3–4	85	200	2.5	45
18	1.8	4–7	100–200	400	3.0	60
18	2.2	4–7	100–200	400	3.0	60
16	2.6	4–7	100–200	800	4.0	80

Table 8.23 Daily dietary intake for staple food commodities in the United States

Food commodity	Use by proportion of population (%)
Beef	35
Poultry	18
Fish	9
Milk and milk drinks	69
Cheese	25
Potatoes	50
Other vegetables	17
Grains	16

(Swan 1983).

The surveys provide a useful guide for the actual dietary intake of nutrients for population groups and countries over a period of time and indicate dietary trends. However, a value for household intake needs to be corrected for waste, otherwise overconfident and misleading predictions may be obtained. Indeed food surveys have shown lower energy intakes compared to the amount of energy available in the total national food supplies. In the United States 3500 kcal per person per day is available, but only 2900 kcal is used. In the United Kingdom loss of available dietary energy as waste is estimated at approximately 25 per cent. The traditional foods, meat, dairy products and cereal-based foods in the United Kingdom continue to supply the staple foods of the diet. In the United States over 90 per cent of individuals consume meat, poultry or fish. Consumption of milk and milk drinks is also high and all the traditional food items are still being consumed in substantial amounts.

Table 8.24 Contributions to the dietary intake of some vitamins by staple foods in the United Kingdom in 1982[†]

Food type	Energy (kcal)	Thiamin (mg)
(1) Cereals	634 (29.2)	0.5 (42.7)
(2) Dairy Products	303 (14)	0.16 (13.4)
(3) Meat	354 (16.3)	0.18 (15.1)
Total of (1)(2)(3)	(59.5)	(71.2)
Total dietary intake for all foods	2172	1.16

([†] MAFF 1984).

The values in parentheses are percentages of the determined total dietary intake.

In the United Kingdom approximately 60 per cent of the dietary energy intake is provided by the staple foods (Table 8.24). For thiamin, riboflavin and nicotinic acid up to 70 per cent of the dietary intake is derived from cereals, dairy products and meat. However, the significant contributions for these vitamins made by cereals arises substantially from both the voluntary supplementation of breakfast cereals and the legal requirement in the United Kingdom for the fortification of white flour with thiamin and nicotinic acid. Bread alone provided approximately 22 per cent of the dietary intake of thiamin in the United Kingdom in 1982 (MAFF 1984). For vitamin C, approximately 22 per cent of the dietary intake in the United Kingdom is provided by potatoes, and therefore as a precautionary measure dried potato powder is now supplemented with ascorbic acid. For vitamin D, 13 per cent of the dietary intake is obtained from eggs. Margarine which is supplemented with vitamins A and D also makes a significant contribution to the dietary intake of these vitamins (Table 8.25). However, vitamin D is also provided by solar radiation and therefore the dietary need is small for most population groups. For nicotinic acid and tryptophan approximately 35 per cent of the dietary intake is provided from meat. Consequently, substantial changes in dietary habit which might include a lower energy intake, less fats and meat are likely to affect directly the vitamin status of the population: a decrease in intake of animal liver products would lower the dietary intakes of vitamin A, folate and vitamin B_{12}, although no values for the dietary intake of vitamin B_{12} and folate are available in the United Kingdom. Likewise, a change in the type of fat and vegetable oil consumed may influence the vitamin E status of the population: it has been claimed that olive oil and coconut oil contain smaller amounts of α-tocopherol than corn oil which also contains relatively high quantities of γ-tocopherol. On the other hand, appreciable quantities of

Riboflavin (mg)	Nicotinic acid (mg)	+	Tryptophan 60 (mg)
per person per day			
0.26 (14.9)	2.1→1	+	3.40 = (19.3)
0.69 (39.6)	0.3→1	+	3.72 = (14.1)
0.35 (19.8)	5.8→1	+	4.32 = (35.6)
(74.3)			(69)
1.74	13.6		14.8

Table 8.25 Contribution to the dietary intake of vitamins A, D and
C by some individual food items in the United Kingdom[†]

Food commodity	Retinol equivalent (vitamin A) (μg)	Vitamin D (μg)	Vitamin C (mg)
		per person per day	
(1) Whole egg	49 (3.5)	0.39 (13.0)	—
(2) Liver	450 (32.1)	0.02 (0.8)	0.3 (0.5)
(3) Milk	256 (18.2)	0.10 (3.3)	2.8 (5.9)
(4) Oranges	1 (0.1)	—	4.2 (7.4)
(5) Potatoes	—	—	12.7 (22.2)
Totals for (1) to (5)	(53.8)	(17.1)	(36.0)
Total dietary intake for all foods	1400	2.96	5.7

([†] MAFF 1984).
The values in parentheses are percentages of the total dietary intake.

vitamin E can be assimilated from the large quantities of milk
ingested, although the concentration of vitamin E in liquid milk is low.

KEY FACTS

1.   Vitamins, unlike hormones, are not synthesised by the human
body. Each vitamin exists in a number of chemically similar forms
(vitamers).
2.   More accurate analytical data for the amounts of vitamins in
foods is becoming available through the use of HPLC.
3.   Retinal is a metabolically active A-vitamer required for synthesis
of the visual pigment rhodopsin. Retinoic acids are now known to
control cell growth and cell division.
4.   β-Carotene, synthesised by plants and microorganisms, is a
terpene precursor of vitamin A. Liver and supplemented margarines
are good sources of vitamin A and carotenoids.
5.   For most of the human population the required amount of
vitamin D_3, cholecalciferol, is obtained by irradiation of the skin. Eggs
and margarine which are supplemented with vitamin D represent a
good dietary source.
6.   Vitamins D_3 and D_2 are secosteroids, which are hydroxylated
twice to produce compounds to regulate the biosynthesis of calcium-
binding proteins.
7.   E-Vitamers are fat-soluble antioxidants and protect cell

membranes against oxidation. Vegetables, oils and nuts are good sources of vitamin E.

8.   K-Vitamers are substituted 2-methylnaphthoquinones synthesised by plants and gut microorganisms. Cabbage and liver are important dietary sources of K-vitamers.

9.   Vitamin K is required for the γ-carboxylation of glutamate residues in bone proteins and blood clotting proteins.

10.   The B-vitamins are a very heterogeneous class of chemically unrelated water-soluble compounds.

11.   B-Vitamins are lost in the seed coat during the milling of cereals and in the cooking water during the cooking of foods. Thiamin and folates are thermolabile. Thiamin is degraded chemically by sulphur dioxide.

12.   B-Vitamins are readily converted by animals to the important coenzymes central to metabolism. TPP, NAD, FAD, coenzyme A, pyridoxa1-5-phosphate and tetrahydrofolate are all synthesised from different B-vitamins.

13.   Vitamin B_{12} occurs only in animal products and is synthesised by microorganisms. Assimilation of vitamin B_{12} requires specific binding proteins and an intrinsic factor. Absence of the intrinsic factor may also cause vitamin B_{12} deficiencies. Vitamin B_{12} is a cofactor for the enzyme-catalysed demethylation of N^5-methyltetrahydrofolate. Both folate and vitamin B_{12} deficiencies cause anaemia. Vitamin B_{12} is also a cofactor for methylmalonyl CoA mutase.

14.   Ascorbate and dehydroascorbate are biologically active forms of vitamin C which acts as an antioxidant in foods. Ascorbate is believed to act as a free radical scavenger.

15.   Food consumption surveys and analytical data for foods provide the basis for estimating the dietary intake of vitamins. In the United Kingdom 70 per cent of the estimated required dietary thiamin, riboflavin and nicotinic acid is provided by cereals, dairy products and meat.

REFERENCES

Bauernfiend, J. C. (1977) 'The tocopherol content of food and influencing factors', CRC Crit. Revs. Food Sci. Nutr., 8, 337–82.

Burton, G. W., Cheeseman, K. H., Doba, T., Ingold, K. U. and Slater, T. F. (1983) 'Vitamin E as an antioxidant in vitro and in vivo', in Biology and Vitamin E, Ciba Foundation 101. Pitman, London.

DHSS (1981) Department of Health and Social Security. 'Recommended daily amounts of food energy and nutrients for groups of people in the United Kingdom', Report on Health and Social Subjects no. 15, 2nd impr. HMSO, London.

FAO/WHO (1974) *Handbook of Human Nutritional Requirements*, FAO Nutritional Studies no. 28, Rome. WHO Monograph Series no. 61.

Gregory, J. F. III, Sartain, D. B. and Day, B. P. F. (1983) 'Fluorimetric determination of folacin in biological materials using high performance liquid chromatography', *J. Nutr.*, **114**, 341–53.

IUNS (1983) 'Recommended dietary intakes around the World', *Nutr. Abstr. and Rev.*, series A, **53A**, 939–1015.

Iwai, K., Tani, M. and Fushika, T. (1983) 'Electrophoretic and immunological properties of folate-binding protein isolated from bovine milk', *Agric. Biol. Chem.*, **47**, 1523–30.

Janne, K. (1982) 'Vitamin B_{12}', *Var. Foda*, **34** 280–6.

MAFF (1984) Ministry of Agriculture, Fisheries and Food. 'Household food consumption and expenditure 1982', Annual Report of the National Food Survey Committee. HMSO, London.

Mokady, S., Cogan, U. and Lieberman, L. (1984) 'Stability of vitamin C in fruits and fruit blends', *J. Sci. Food Agric.*, **35**, 452–56.

NHANES (1981) US Department of Health Education and Welfare. *Plan and Operation of the Second National Health and Nutrition Examination Survey*, 1976–80 (Hyathsville, A. D). DHEW Publ. no. (PHS) 81–1317.

Nik-Dand, N. I. and Bender, A. E. (1983) 'The content and stability of folic acid in foods', *Proc. Nutr. Soc.* **42**, 341–53.

NRC/NAS (1980) National Research Council Committee for Dietary Allowances. *Recommended Dietary Allowances*, 9th edn . . National Academy of Sciences Press, Washington DC.

Olson, R. E. (1982) 'Vitamin K', in *Hemostasis and Thrombosis* (ed. Coleman, R. W.). Annual Reviews, PaloAlto, California.

Olson, R. E. (1984) 'The function and metabolism of vitamin K', *Ann. Rev. Nutr.*, **4**, 281–337.

Osterdahl, B., Janne, K., Johansson, E., Johnsson, H. (1986) 'Determination of vitamin B_{12} in gruel by a radioisotope dilution assay', *Int. J. Vit. Nutr. Res.*, **56**, 95–9.

Paul, A. A. and Southgate, D. A. T. (1978) *McCance and Widdowson's The Composition of Foods*, 4th edn, of MRC Special Report no. 297. HMSO, London and Elsevier, Amsterdam.

Phillips, D. R., Wright, A. J. A. and Southgate, D. A. T. (1982) 'Values for folates in foods', *Lancet* 2, Sept. 11, 605.

Reynolds, S. L. (1985) 'The use of HPLC in the determination of fat soluble vitamins in a variety of milk-based food products', *Proc. Inst. Food Sci. and Technol. (UK)*, **18**, 43–50.

Seetharam, B. and Alpers, D. H. (1982) 'Absorption and transport of cobalamin (vitamin B_{12})', *Ann. Rev. Nutr.*, **2**, 343–69.

Sivell, L. M., Wenlock, R. W. and Jackson, P. A. (1982) 'Determination of vitamin D and retinoid activity in eggs by HPLC', *Human Nutr.: Appl. Nutr.* **36A** 430–7.

Sivell, L. M., Bull, N. L., Bush, D. H., Wiggins, R. A., Scuffam, D. and Jackson, P. A. (1984) 'Vitamin A activity in foods of animal origin' *J. Sci. Food Agric.*, **35** 931–9.

Skurray, G. R. (1981) 'A rapid method for selectively determining small amounts of niacin, riboflavin and thiamine in foods', *Food Chem.*, **7**, 77–80.

Speek, A. J., Schrijver, J. and Schreurs, W. H. P. (1985) 'Vitamin E composition of some seed oils as determined by high performance liquid chromatography with fluorometric detection', *J. Food Sci.*. **50**, 121–4.

Sporn, M. B., Roberts, A. B. and Goodman, D. S. (1984) *The Retinoids*, vols. 1 and 2. Academic Press, New York.

Stryer, L. (1981) *Biochemistry*, 2nd edn. W. H. Freeman and Co., San Francisco, California.

Swan, P. B. (1983) 'Food consumption by individuals in the United States: Two major surveys', *Ann. Rev. Nutr.*, **3**, 413–32.

Underwood, B. A. (1984) 'Vitamin A in animal and human nutrition', in *The Retinoids*, vol. 1 (eds. Sporn, M. B., Roberts, A. B. and Goodman, D. S.). Academic Press, New York.

USDA (1982) US Department of Agriculture. 'Food and nutrient intakes of individuals in 1 day in the United States, spring 1977. Nationwide Food Consumption Survey Reports 78, H-1 'Food consumption: households in the United States, spring 1977'. Washington DC.

Vanderslice, J. T., Maire, C. E. and Yakupkovic, J. E. (1981) 'Vitamin B_6 in ready-to-eat cereals: analysis by high performance liquid chromatography', *J. Food Sci..*, **46**, 943–6.

Wedzicha, B. L. (1984) *Chemistry of Sulphur Dioxide in Foods*. Elsevier Applied Science Publishers, London and New York.

ADDITIONAL READING

DeLuca, H. F. and Schnoes, H. K. (1983) 'Vitamin D: Recent advances', *Ann. Rev. Biochem.*, **52**, 411–35.

Englard, S. and Seifter, S. (1986) 'The biochemical functions of ascorbic acid', *Ann. Rev. Nutr.*, **6**, 365–406.

Goodwin, T. W. (1986) 'Metabolism, nutrition and function of carotenoids', *Ann. Rev. Nutr.*, **6**, 273–97.

Henderson, L. M. (1983) 'Niacin', *Ann. Rev. Nutr.*, **3**, 289–307.

Henry, H. L. and Norman, A. W. (1984) 'Vitamin D: metabolism and biological actions', *Ann. Rev. Nutr.*, **4**, 493–520.

Ink, S. L. and Henderson, L. M. (1984) 'Vitamin B_6 metabolism', *Ann. Rev. Nutr.*, **4**, 455–70.

IUNS (1983) 'Recommended dietary intakes around the World', *Nutr. Abstr. and Revs.*, series A, **53A**, 939–1015.

Korpela, J. (1984) 'Avidin: A high affinity biotin-binding protein as a tool and subject of biological research', *Med. Biol.*, **62**, 5–26.

Sporn, M. B., Roberts, A. B. and Goodman, D. S. (1984) *The Retinoids*, vols. 1 and 2. Academic Press, New York.

Wagner, C. (1982) 'Cellular folate binding proteins : function and significance', *Ann. Rev. Nutr.*, **2**, 229–48.

Part V

Enzymatic action in post-harvest and post-mortem foods

CHAPTER 9

Catabolic processes in food

INTRODUCTION

Many of the changes in flavour, colour and texture which occur in foods, and particularly in fresh foods, determine their immediate acceptability. Such changes are often caused by the action of enzymes naturally present in foods. In plant foods, some volatile aroma compounds are desirable. These are frequently produced by enzyme-catalysed reactions: in *Allium* and *Brassica* species the characteristic volatile sulphur compounds are rapidly formed when the cellular tissue is disrupted, whereas in other vegetables and fruits, short chain alcohols, aldehydes and esters may be formed by enzymatic degradation of amino acids and small quantities of unsaturated lipids. Bitterness in citrus products can arise from lactonisation of complex terpenes. Loss of colour in fruits may be due to the hydrolysis of anthocyanins and the oxidation of carotenoid pigments. Enzyme-catalysed reactions may also be responsible for the formation of undesirable taints: fish-like taints can be found occasionally in foods other than fish, such as eggs, and soap-like taints may result from the action of either microbial lipases or bovine lipoprotein lipases in milk-based products. In meat the most rapid and, therefore, the most significant enzyme-catalysed reactions, are those concerned with glycolysis. Also in animal foods and particularly in fish, enzyme-catalysed degradation of nucleotides results in the formation of desirable flavour compounds. In foods of both plant and animal origin, the enzyme-catalysed reactions cited above precede the more destructive hydrolytic reactions, like proteolysis and lipolysis.

The immediate effects of microbial spoilage are most evident in stored fish, where enzymes rapidly convert trimethylamine oxide into obnoxious trimethylamine. In fermented foods, microorganisms are responsible for the formation of desirable volatile compounds, which give rise to the more subtle characteristic flavours of such products like cheese and yoghurt. The cultured microorganisms used for the manufacture of fermented foods often include yeast and lactobacilli, many of which catalyse the formation of small volatile molecules such as methanol, ethanal, acetic acid and propionic acid and diacetyl. These simple organic molecules influence drastically the flavour and astringency of such foods.

Oxidative enzymes, such as peroxidases and polyphenol oxidases, are also present in foods of plant and animal origin. These constitutive enzymes, which catalyse the oxidation of small molecules, can be responsible for loss of colour and flavour in foods. Such oxidative reactions occur rapidly in fresh foods when the cellular tissue is disrupted, as for example during the manufacture of fruit juices or meat homogenates.

GLYCOGENESIS AND GLYCOLYSIS IN MEAT

Many sequential biochemical reactions that start with the activation of cellular ATPase are responsible for the physical changes, which take place when muscle is converted to meat. The stiff and inextensible state – rigor mortis – which arises from a depletion of ATP, is due to the contraction of the muscle myofibrils. The post-mortem changes occur because many of the native enzymes of the muscle retain much of their catalytic activity, for at least a short time after death. On the cessation of respiration in animals, glucose and oxygen are no longer supplied to resting muscle. At low blood glucose levels glycogen is mobilised, as the alternative metabolisable fuel. Glycogen is converted to glucose-1-phosphate and subsequently to pyruvate via the Embden–Meyerhoff–Parnas glycolytic pathway (App. III). During post-mortem glycolysis of meat, changes in the concentrations of the glycolytic intermediates, such as glucose-1-phosphate and glucose-6-phosphate can be followed by use of specific enzymatic assays for these substances in muscle extracts. Glucose-6- phosphate dehydrogenase is normally used as the detecting enzyme. Similarly, mixed enzyme prep-

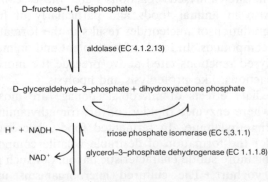

arations (Bergmeyer 1984) can be used to determine the concentrations of fructose-1,6-diphosphate, glyceraldehyde-3-phosphate and dihydroxyacetone phosphate in meat. In this case the detecting enzyme is glycerol-3-phosphate dehydrogenase (EC 1.1.1.8)

The rate of reaction is followed by the decrease at 340 nm due to oxidation of NADH. Other glycolytic intermediates, including glycerate-3-phosphate, glycerate-2-phosphate and phosenolpyruvate, can be estimated with phosphoglyceromutase (EC 2.7.5.3), enolase (EC 4.2.11), pyruvate kinase (EC 2.7.1.40) together with lactate dehydrogenase (EC 1.1.1.27) as the detecting enzyme.

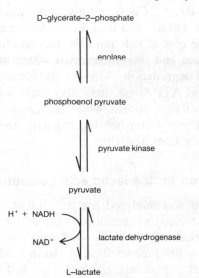

Again the rate of reaction is determined by measurements at 340 nm.

Post-mortem glycolysis, due to the cessation of respiration in the muscle tissue, is anaerobic and therefore NADH is no longer oxidised through the respiratory chain and accumulates as a result of the continued oxidation of D-glyceraldehyde-3-phosphate catalysed by glyceraldehyde phosphate dehydrogenase (EC 1.2.1.12). Although this reaction is thermodynamically unfavourable and results in the formation of 1,3-diphosphoglycerate as a higher energy phosphate compound – the reaction is driven by the energy released from the oxidation of the aldehyde group. Pyruvate, as the terminal product of

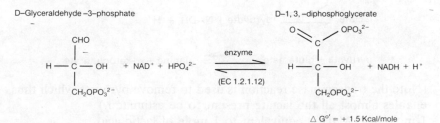

glycolysis, cannot enter the tricarboxylic acid cycle because the accumulating NADH inhibits the key enzyme, citrate synthase (EC 4.1.3.7). However, in the presence of accumulating amounts of pyruvate, NADH is reoxidised by lactic acid dehydrogenase in the coupled reduction of pyruvate to lactate: thus glycolysis proceeds through the recycling of NAD. Lactate continues to accumulate until the glycogen supply is exhausted, as small amounts of ATP (3 moles per hexose unit) are resynthesised during glycolysis. The low pH value of approximately 5.5 for meat results from the accumulation of lactate. The amounts of lactate formed are proportional to the reserves of muscular glycogen before death. Consequently, any depletion of muscular glycogen reserves before death due to, for example, unrestrained struggling as in the case of fish and incorrect handling of cattle, results in higher pH values and therefore meats which are more susceptible to microbiological degradation. Also the stress condition, which causes lower glycogen and ATP levels, may also cause a more rapid onset of both glycolysis and rigor mortis while the carcase is still 'hot'. Such meats possess a lower water-holding capacity and produce excessive exudate, commonly known as drip.

Sample calculation for the lactic acid content of meat

A sample of meat was analysed for its content of lactic acid. Meat (5 g) was homogenised in perchloric acid and made up to 50 cm^3. After cooling to remove perchloric acid, the supernatant was diluted twenty-five times to produce solution A. Buffer solution, NAD, glutamate and glutamate : pyruvate transaminase and 0.2 cm^3 of solution A (total volume 2.80 cm^3) were placed in a dry spectrophotometric cell (1 cm path length). The absorbance at 340 nm was 0.030 when read against distilled water. A solution (10 μl) of lactate dehydrogenase was added to the cell and 15 min. later the absorbance was 0.130. When the procedure was repeated using water in place of solution A the absorbance values recorded were 0.02 and 0.03, respectively. A calibration curve for concentration of lactic acid in the cuvette has shown that $\Delta A_{standard} = 5.63$ μmole^{-1}/cm^3.

Calculate the concentration of lactic acid per 100 g of meat.

$$\text{lactate} \underset{}{\overset{NAD^+}{\rightleftharpoons}} \text{pyruvate} + \text{NADH} + \text{H}^+$$

$$\text{pyruvate} + \text{glutamate} \rightleftharpoons \text{alanine} + \alpha-\text{ketoglutarate}$$

(Note the transaminase reaction is used to remove pyruvate which thus enables almost all the lactate present to be estimated.)

1 mole of NADH is equivalent to 1 mole of lactic acid

The change in absorbance (ΔA_{340}) for NADH produced
= (0.130 − 0.03) minus change for water blank (0.03 − 0.02) = 0.09
For $\Delta A_{standard}$ 5.63 = 1 μmole of lactate/cm^3

Therefore the concentration of lactate in the cuvette $= \dfrac{0.09}{5.63}$ μmole/cm^3

Therefore total lactate in the cuvette $= \dfrac{0.09}{5.63} \times 2.81 = 0.045$ μmole

Therefore total lactate in 50 cm^3 of perchlorate extract (5 g of meat)

$= \dfrac{0.045 \times 25 \times 50}{0.2}$

$= 281.2$ μmole

Therefore 100 g of meat contained $281.2 \times 20 \times 90 \times 10^{-6}$ g

= 0.51 g of lactic acid

It is now known for the live and immediate post-mortem muscle that
the mobilisation of glycogen (Cohen 1976) and the utilisation of ATP
are both initiated by increased concentrations of cytoplasmic Ca^{2+} ion.
In the resting live muscle the concentration of Ca^{2+} in the cytosol is
maintained at a very low level (10^{-7}M) by a complex Ca storage and
ATP-dependent pumping system in the sarcoplasmic reticulum. This
is a collection of vesicles which are wrapped around the muscle
myofibrils and discharge Ca^{2+} in response to nerve stimuli. In the live
resting muscle the concentrations of ATP and creatine phosphate (a
reserve supplementary store of high-energy phosphate) are approximately 5 mM and 20 mM, respectively, where the muscle remains in a
relaxed state due to the plasticising effect of ATP on the interaction
of actin with myosin.

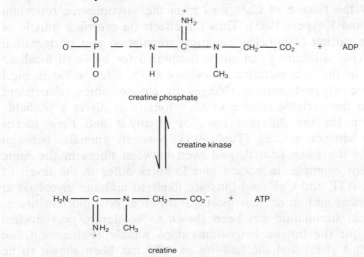

Measurements of cellular Ca^{2+}, using a dye-binding technique (Jeacocke 1982), have shown that when the concentration of Ca^{2+} in the cytosol rises to even $10^{-6}M$ mild contraction of muscle is stimulated as follows. For a short time after death the concentration of muscular ATP is maintained by further phosphorylation of ADP from creatine phosphate catalysed by creative kinase (EC 2.7.3.2). First, as the concentration of ATP is depleted to $10^{-4}M$, when ATP and creatine phosphate reserves are used up, stiffening of the muscle fibres occurs with the consequent onset of rigor mortis. Secondly, the conversion of glycogen to glucose-1-phosphate by phosphorylase-a (EC 2.4.1.1) is also activated indirectly by the small amounts of Ca^{2+} ($10^{-6}M$) present in the muscle cells: Ca^{2+} activates phosphorylase kinase (EC 2.7.1.38), which is the enzyme responsible for the ATP-dependent phosphorylation of inactive phosphorylase-b to form enzymatically active phosphorylase-a (App. V). This activated dimer, phosphorylase-a, possesses binding sites for pyridoxal phosphate, AMP and glycogen. AMP is an allosteric activator (App. VII), which therefore enhances the hydrolysis of glycogen by phosphorylase-a as the levels of ATP decrease and those of AMP increase. Although the hydrolysis is thermodynamically unfavourable and the equilibrium constant (0.27) is relatively close to unity at pH 6.8, the reaction proceeds towards completion due to the high reactant-to-product ratio (100 : 1) of cellular orthophosphate (Pi) to glucose-1-phosphate. The α-1,6-glycosidic bonds of the branch points of glycogen are hydrolysed after transfer of a terminal block of three glucose residues to leave a single α-1,6-linked glucose residue which is removed by amylo-α-1,6-glucosidase (EC 3.2.1.33). Both the transferase and glucosidase activity are associated with the same protein (Fig. 9.1).

Overall, the increased rates of glycolysis, caused by physical treatment of muscle, are attributed to the initial activation of phosphorylase kinase by the release of Ca^{2+} ions from the sarcoplasmic reticulum (Horgan and Kuypers 1985). Thus the effects on pre-rigor muscle of transverse cutting of muscles, electrical stimulation and refrigeration inducing cold shortening can all be accounted for by small localised increases in the concentration of cytosol Ca^{2+}. Such a biochemical explanation of post-mortem changes in muscle fibres, dependent largely on the variable release of Ca^{2+} ions, also offers a probable explanation for the different rates of glycolysis and rigor mortis observed between species (Table 9.1), between animals, between muscles of the same animal, and even between fibres in the same muscle. For example, individual muscle fibres differ in the levels of glycogen, ATP and Ca^{2+} and thus are likely to undergo glycolysis at different rates and enter rigor mortis at different post-mortem times.

Electrical stimulation has been shown to accelerate post-mortem glycolysis for the bovine longissimus dorsi muscle (Fabiansson and Reuterswärd 1985) and the half-life of ATP has been shown to be

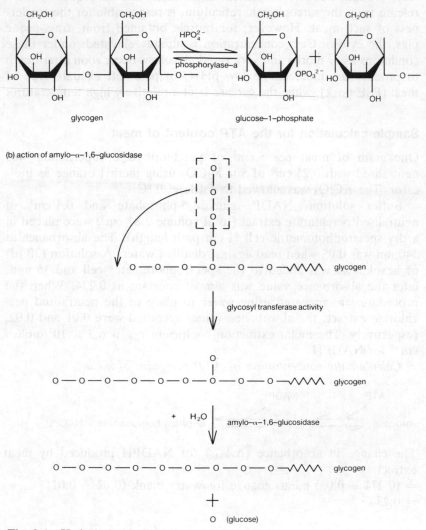

(a) action of phosphorylase–a

glycogen

glucose–1–phosphate

(b) action of amylo–α–1,6–glucosidase

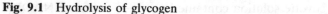

Fig. 9.1 Hydrolysis of glycogen

Table 9.1 Time scale for post-mortem rigor

Animal	Time period after death
Fish	30 min.–2 hours
Chicken	1–4 hours
Turkey	up to 24 hours
Lamb	4–24 hours
Pig	4–8 hours
Beef	24–48 hours

reduced from 10 to 5 hours. It is claimed that the increased catabolic rate, brought about by electrical stimulation and subsequently Ca^{2+} release from the sarcoplasmic reticulum, is responsible for the tenderness of such meat. However, for muscle obtained from stress-prone pigs, the cytosol Ca^{2+} concentration is already elevated: under these conditions rigor mortis and very rapid glycolysis occur soon after death to produce an unacceptable low pH (4.8) pale soft exudate type of meat (PSE pork), while the carcase is at a relatively high temperature.

Sample calculation for the ATP content of meat

One gram of meat per 5 cm^3 of perchloric acid supernatant was neutralised with 0.25 cm^3 of 5 M K_2CO_3 using methyl orange as indicator. The $KClO_4$ was allowed to settle at 0 °C.

Buffer solution, NADP, glucose-6-phosphate and 0.1 cm^3 of neutralised perchlorate extract (total volume 2.81 cm^3) were placed in a dry spectrophotometric cell (1 cm path length). The absorbance at 340 nm was 0.03 when read against distilled water. A solution (20 μl) of hexokinase was added to the spectrophotometer cell and 15 min. later the absorbance value was almost constant at 0.274. When the procedure was repeated using water in place of the neutralised perchlorate extract, the absorbance values recorded were 0.01 and 0.02, respectively. The molar extinction coefficient ε_{340} is 6.3×10^3 $mole^{-1}$ cm^{-1} for NADPH.

Calculate the concentration of ATP per gram of meat.

$$\text{glucose} \xrightarrow[]{ATP} \text{G-6-P} \xrightarrow[]{NADP^+} \text{6-phosphogluconate + NADPH + H}^+$$

The change in absorbance (ΔA_{340}) for NADPH produced by meat extract
= (0.274 − 0.03) minus change for water blank (0.02 − 0.01)
= 0.234

Therefore the cuvette solution contained $\dfrac{0.234}{6.3 \times 10^3}$ moles of NADPH per litre

Therefore 100 μL of the neutralised extract
contained $\dfrac{0.234}{6.3 \times 10^3} \times \dfrac{2.83}{1000}$ moles of ATP = 0.105 μmoles of ATP

(1 mole of ATP produces 1 mole of NADPH)

Therefore 1 g of meat contained $\dfrac{0.105 \times 5.25}{0.1} = 5.52$ *μmoles of ATP.*

Sample calculation for the ADP and AMP content of meat

One gram of meat homogenised in 5 cm³ of perchloric acid supernatant was neutralised with 0.25 cm³ of 5 M K_2CO_3 using methyl orange as indicator. The $KClO_4$ was allowed to settle at 0 °C.

Buffer solution, NADH, ATP, phosphoenol pyruvate, L-lactate dehydrogenase and 0.5 cm³ of neutralised perchlorate extract (total volume 2.80 cm³) were placed in a dry spectrophotometric cell (1 cm path length). The absorbance at 340 nm was 0.404 when read against distilled water. A solution (20 μL) of pyruvate kinase suspension was added to the spectrophotometric cell and after 8 min. the decreased absorbance value was almost constant at 0.240. When distilled water (0.5 cm³) was used instead of the neutralised perchlorate extract the change in absorbance was −0.04 units at 340 nm.

To find the amount of AMP in the spectrophotometric cell, myokinase suspension (20 μL) was added and decreases in absorbance of 0.106 and 0.02 were observed, respectively, for the neutralised extract and water blank at 340 nm. The molar coefficient ε_{340} is 6.3×10^3 mole^{-1} cm^{-1} for NADH.

Calculate (a) the concentration of ADP per gram of meat
(b) the concentration of AMP per gram of meat.

(a)

$$\text{ADP + phosphoenolpyruvate} \rightleftharpoons \text{ATP + pyruvate}$$

$$\text{H}^+ + \text{pyruvate + NADH} \rightleftharpoons \text{L-lactate + NAD}^+$$

Decrease in absorbance (ΔA_{340}) for loss of NADH by meat extract
= (0.404 − 0.240) minus 0.04 (for water blank)
= 0.124

Therefore the cuvette solution lost $\dfrac{0.124}{6.3 \times 10^3}$ moles of NADPH per litre

Therefore 0.5 cm³ of the neutralised extract contained

$\dfrac{0.124}{6.3 \times 10^3} \times \dfrac{2.82}{1000}$ moles of ADP = 0.055 μmole of ADP

(1 mole of ADP results in the oxidation of 1 mole of NADH)

Therefore 1 g of meat contained $\dfrac{0.055 \times 5.25}{0.5} = 0.58$ μmole of ADP.

(b)

$$AMP + ATP \rightleftharpoons 2ADP$$

$$ADP + \text{phosphoenolpyruvate} \rightleftharpoons ATP + \text{pyruvate}$$

$$H^+ + \text{pyruvate} + NADH \rightleftharpoons L\text{–lactate} + NAD^+$$

Therefore 1 mole of AMP is equivalent to 2 moles of NADH.
Decrease in absorbance (ΔA_{340}) for loss of NADH by meat extract
$= 0.106 - 0.02 = 0.086$
Therefore the cuvette solution lost

$\dfrac{0.086}{6.3 \times 10^3}$ moles of NADH per litre

Therefore 0.5 cm^3 of the neutralised extract contained

$$\frac{1}{2} \times \frac{0.086}{6.3 \times 10^3} \times \frac{2.84}{1000} \text{ moles of AMP} = 0.019 \ \mu\text{mole of AMP}$$

(2 moles of NADH are formed from 1 mole of AMP)

Therefore 1 g of meat contained $\dfrac{0.019 \times 5.25}{0.5} = 0.20 \ \mu\text{mole of}$
AMP.

NUCLEOTIDE-DEGRADING ENZYMES

The biochemistry of nucleotides, and particularly the aspect of the subject concerned with their biosynthesis, has been of only limited interest to food scientists. However, because of the widespread occurrence of ATP in animal muscle, significant amounts of nucleotide degradation products such as inosine-5′-phosphate (IMP) and hypoxanthine can arise as a result of post-mortem autolysis. IMP is claimed to enhance the flavour of animal foods, while the concentration of the further degradation product, hypoxanthine, which is tasteless, can be used as an indicator of substantial autolysis, particularly in fish. Generally, for fresh fish very little is present in the muscle, whereas after 14 days storage at 0 °C up to 6 μmole of hypoxanthine per gram of fish may accumulate. The two major purine bases in biological tissues, adenine and guanine, occur as nucleotides, where the purine base is covalently linked to ribose-5-phosphate. The nucleotides can be catabolised in three different ways: simple dephosphorylation, cleavage of the N-glycosidic bond or by oxidative deamination. The chief source of IMP in animal foods arises from the rapid temperature-dependent oxidative deamination of adenosine 5′-phosphate (AMP)

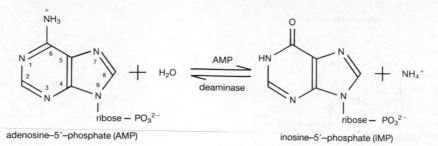

Fig. 9.2 Deamination of adenosine-5'-phosphate (AMP)

catalysed by AMP deaminase (EC 3.5.4.4). AMP is formed from the hydrolysis of the intracellular ATP reserve, where the normal concentration is approximately 5 mM. Also during anaerobic glycolysis 3 moles of ATP are formed per hexose unit and therefore a concentration of up to 100 mM of IMP can accumulate as a result of postmortem glycolysis and the subsequent oxidative deamination of AMP. Other sources of AMP are DNA and RNA, which are hydrolysed by ribonucleases.

The phosphate sugar bonds of the nucleotides can be cleaved by ribonucleases (DNAase and RNAase) which exhibit a specific action towards the phosphate ester bonds of the hydroxyl group of either the C-3 atom or C-5 atom of ribose and 2-deoxyribose. The nucleases are strictly phosphodiesterases and hydrolase only one of the ester bonds. The hydrolysis of the C-3 phosphate ester results in the formation of 5'-nucleotides, such as adenosine-5'-phosphate (AMP). There are exo- and endonucleases for hydrolysis of the terminal and central nucleotide residues, some of which are specific for the different purine and pyrimidine bases. The phosphate residue of a liberated nucleotide can be removed by the hydrolytic action of 5'-nucleotidases (EC 3.1.3.5) to form nucleosides, which consist of a purine or pyrimidine base linked to ribose or deoxyribose (Fig. 9.3). Thus, IMP may not accumulate in animal meats, due to either the use of the above reaction for the degradation of the precursor (AMP) to form adenosine, or the hydrolysis of the phosphate ester bond in IMP itself by 5'-nucleotidases. Subsequently, inosine formed from either adenosine or IMP is converted to hypoxanthine by cleavage of the glycosidic bond catalysed by inosine ribohydrolase (EC 3.2.2.2). Thus the desirable flavour compound (IMP) of meat is easily lost through the action of a number of endogenous enzymes.

For fish the level of hypoxanthine is often used as an index of quality. Enzymatic analysis for hypoxanthine is easily carried out using xanthine oxidase (EC 1.1.3.22) which catalyses the oxidation of both xanthine and hypoxanthine to uric acid (Fig. 9.4). Catalase is added to the assay solutions in order to remove hydrogen peroxide formed

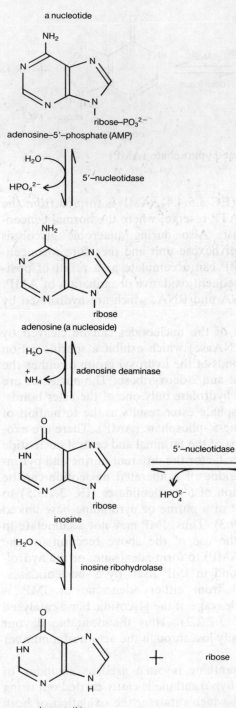

a nucleotide

adenosine–5'–phosphate (AMP)

H_2O ⟶
HPO_4^{2-} ←   5'–nucleotidase

adenosine (a nucleoside)

H_2O +
NH_4 ←   adenosine deaminase

inosine

5'–nucleotidase ⟶
HPO_4^{2-} H_2O inosine–5'–phosphate (IMP)

H_2O ⟶
inosine ribohydrolase

hypoxanthine   +   ribose

Fig. 9.3 Degradation of purine nucleotides

The main catabolic routes are characterised by

(1) deamination

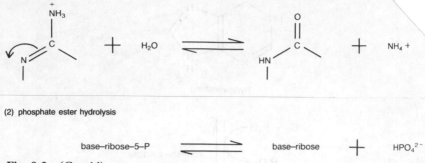

(2) phosphate ester hydrolysis

$$base–ribose–5–P \rightleftharpoons base–ribose + HPO_4^{2-}$$

Fig. 9.3 (Cont'd)

and the initial rate of reaction can be measured at 290 nm. Early heat-treatment of fish homogenates before analysis is desirable in order to denature the nucleotide-degrading enzymes. Further, to improve the sensitivity of the reaction and eliminate non-specific absorption at 290 nm, deproteinised extracts should be used. Alternatively, 2,6-dichlorophenolindophenol can be used, instead of oxygen, as electron acceptor with measurements for the rate of oxidation made at 618 nm.

ORIGIN OF AMINES

Trimethylamine and dimethylamine

The fishy odour of spoiled fish is correlated with the formation of amines. Therefore amines, ammonia and in particular trimethylamine (TMA) have also been used as an index of fish spoilage. TMA arises from the reduction of the non-volatile trimethylamine oxide (TMAO), which is present in the blood and muscle (approximately 10 mg/100 g of tissue) of many salt-water fish. TMA may be produced by the catalytic action of endogenous enzymes in some fish. However, owing to the rapid growth of psychrotropic microorganisms which are always naturally associated in substantial numbers with cold-water fish, the spoilage of fish held in ice is mainly bacteriological. Specific microbial enzymes are frequently present which can reduce TMAO to TMA. Either lactate, the reduced cofactor FADH, or cytochromes may act as electron donors for trimethylamine N-oxide reductase (EC 1.6.6.9).

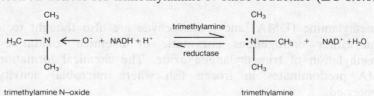

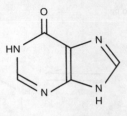

hypoxanthine

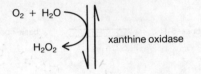

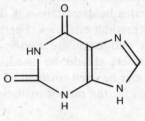

xanthine

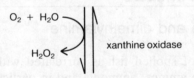

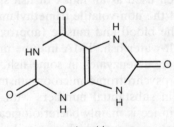

uric acid

Fig. 9.4 Oxidation of hypoxanthine by xanthine oxidase

Dimethylamine (DMA) and formaldehyde are also thought to arise from either endogenous enzymatic or chemical oxidative N-demethylation of trimethylamine oxide. The chemical formation of DMA predominates in frozen fish where microbial activity is suppressed.

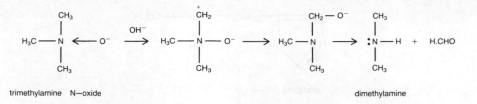

trimethylamine   N—oxide   dimethylamine

Total volatile nitrogen bases which include ammonia, dimethylamine and trimethylamine can be measured routinely and therefore these substances are frequently used as determinants of fish quality. Trimethylamine can be estimated separately by means of a simple and inexpensive enzymatic method using trimethylamine dehydrogenase (EC 1.5.99.7) and 2,6-dichlorophenolindophenol as electron acceptor can be used (Large and McDougall 1975). Alternatively, both TMA and DMA can be detected with a gas sensor by measurement of a decreased resistance in the presence of volatile amines (Storey *et al.* 1984).

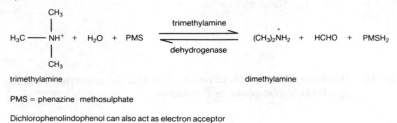

trimethylamine   dimethylamine

PMS = phenazine methosulphate

Dichlorophenolindophenol can also act as electron acceptor

Action of amino acid decarboxylases

Amines in fermented foods and ingredients can arise from the action of microbial amino acid decarboxylases.

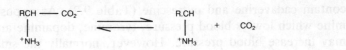

Amines derived from most of the amino acids are found in a wide variety of foods, but those present in cheese, chocolate and particularly contaminated Scombroid fish, have been implicated as hazardous to health. The major cause of Scombroid food poisoning is histamine (Fig. 9.5) which is a very potent capillary dilator in man, although normally 1000 mg are required to produce a response. Histamine is formed by the microbial decarboxylation of histidine, which is present in relatively large amounts in the muscles of tuna and mackerel. Although several types of microorganisms can synthesise histidine decarboxylase (EC 4.1.1.22), only a limited number of such bacteria have been isolated from fish: *Proteus morganii* is considered to possess the greatest capacity to decarboxylate histidine to produce histamine.

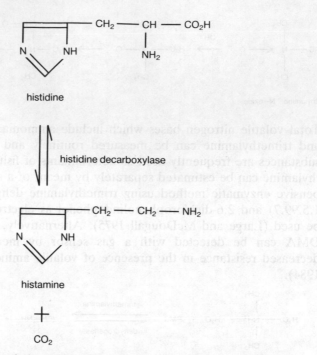

histidine

histidine decarboxylase

histamine

+

CO_2

Fig. 9.5 Decarboxylation of histidine. Amino acid decarboxylases require pyridoxal 5'-phosphate as a cofactor

For stored fish a simple test using pyridoxal-5'-phosphate has been claimed to be useful for the detection of diamines. This simple chemical test is much quicker but less specific than chromatographic methods (Jacober and Rand 1984).

Other foods like cocoa and chocolate may contain up to 10 ppm of phenylethylamine, while cheese contains tyramine and meats may contain cadaverine and putrescine (Table 9.2). As opposed to histamine which lowers blood pressure, tyramine, dopamine and serotonin may increase blood pressure. However, normally the small amounts of these amines are removed from the blood by the action of mammalian amine oxidase (EC 1.4.3.4).

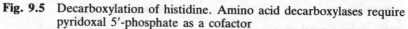

$$^-O_2C.CH_2CH_2CH_2NH_2 + O_2 \rightleftharpoons O_2^-C\,CH_2CH_2CHO + NH_4^+ + H_2O_2$$

γ–aminobutyrate

monoamine oxidase

succinyl semialdehyde

Nevertheless, some antidepressant drugs also inhibit monoamine oxidase and so prevent deamination. Under these conditions even small quantities of ingested tyramine may cause an increase in blood pressure.

In fermented products like yoghurt and cheese, keto acids, aldehydes and thiols can be formed directly by enzymatic deamination of

Table 9.2. Some commonly occurring amines in foods

Source amino acid	Decarboxylated product†
Histidine	Histamine
Tyrosine	Tyramine
Tryptohan	Tryptamine
Phenylalanine	Phenylethylamine
Dihydroxyphenylalanine (DOPA)	Dopamine
Glutamic acid	γ-Aminobutyric acid
Lysine	Cadaverine
Ornithine	Putrescine
Arginine	Agmatine
Serotonin	5-Hydroxytryptophan

† The carboxyl group is removed from the α-carbon atom by a specific decarboxylase for each amino acid.

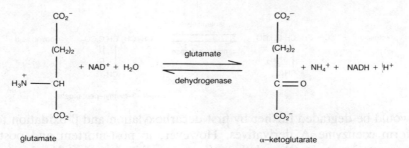

amino acids. While small amounts of thiol compounds, including hydrogen sulphide, may be advantageous in the more common Cheddar cheeses, ammonia is believed to contribute to the aroma of some cheeses such as Camembert. Ammonia easily arises from the oxidative deamination of amino acids as exemplified by the action of glutamate dehydrogenase (EC 1.4.1.2). The keto acid can recycle as an acceptor of amino groups donated from other amino acids through the catalytic action of pyridoxal-dependent transaminases: thus glutamate is the prime source of ammonia. In mammals, the glutamate–α-ketoglutarate reaction plays a central role for the synthesis and degradation of amino acids mediated by transaminases.

$$\text{a–ketoglutarate + a–amino acid} \underset{\text{transaminase}}{\overset{}{\rightleftharpoons}} \text{a–ketoacid + glutamate}$$

Glutamate can also be formed by degradation of arginine, proline and histidine (Stryer 1981).

Pyruvate and oxaloacetate are also formed by deamination of alanine and aspartate, respectively, catalysed by transaminases. While serine and threonine can be oxidatively deaminated directly by serine dehydratase (EC 4.2.1.13) and threonine dehydratase (EC 4.2.1.16).

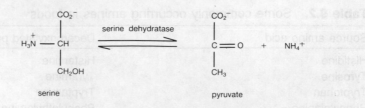

Sulphur compounds, including hydrogen sulphide and sulphite, can arise from oxidative deamination of cysteine to form pyruvate. Volatile six-carbon compounds arise from deamination of leucine and iso-leucine. These products, during controlled metabolism in living tissues,

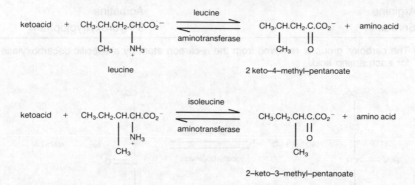

would be degraded further by first decarboxylation and β-oxidation to form coenzyme A derivatives. However, in post-mortem and post-harvest tissues decarboxylation of α-keto acids either catalysed enzymatically, or occurring under acidic conditions, may produce aldehydes which are important volatile aroma compounds in a large number of foods including cheese and fruits.

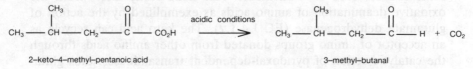

Amines formed by the catalytic action of decarboxylases can also be oxidatively deaminated by monoamine oxidases, which may account for the presence of aldehydes and alcohols, particularly present in some varieties of surface-ripened cheeses. 3-Methyl-1-butanol, phenyl-ethanol and phenol are expected to arise from leucine, phenylalanine and tyrosine, respectively, through the action of enzymes present in contaminating yeasts and bacteria such as *Geotrichum* and *Brevibac-terium spp*. Reduction of the aldehydes to alcohols catalysed by

$$RCHO + NADH + H^+ \rightleftharpoons RCH_2OH + NAD^+$$

dehydrogenases, and subsequent esterification also influences the aroma of fruits (Table 9.3).

Table 9.3 Fruit-like aroma of esters

Ester	Fruit
Ethylbutyrate	Orange
Ethyl-2-methyl butanoate	Melon
Isopentylacetate	Apple
Methyl-β-methiopropionate	Pineapple
Methyldecadienoate	Pear

Esterification of the alcohols may occur with acyl CoA derivatives of fatty acids acting as acyl donator. Such a reaction would be energetically favourable due to the energy released on hydrolysis of the coenzyme A derivatives. It is possible that the enzymes normally involved in the β-oxidation of fatty acids, namely acyl coenzyme A transferase and the β-ketothiolase (see App. V) adsorb alcohols at their hydrophobic sites. The adsorbed alcohols may compete with a molecule of water normally required for the hydrolysis of the coenzyme A derivatives and thus instead accept the fatty acid acyl groups to form volatile esters. However, no definite scheme for ester formation in fruits has been elucidated, but the branched chain alkyl groups found in esters are likely to be formed from the alcohols derived from α-amino acids that can provide the carbon skeletons as outlined above.

HYDROPEROXIDE DEGRADATION IN PLANTS

The hydroperoxides present in plant tissues derived from the polyunsaturated fatty acids, linoleic or linolenic acids, may be either isomerised to isomeric ketols, cyclised, or degraded to produce C-6 and C-9 aldehydes. The hydroperoxides are formed through the catalytic action of lipoxygenases (see Ch. 10) on polyunsaturated fatty acids such as linoleic and linolenic acids.

Hydroperoxide isomerase (EC.5.3.99.1)

Hydroperoxide isomerase has been reported to be present in a number of plants, including barley, cauliflower, corn germ and cotton seedlings. Although the activity of lipoxygenases is low in dormant seeds, for many seeds rapid synthesis occurs shortly after germination, which supports the view that the enzymes involved with the oxidation, isomerisation and degradation of unsaturated fatty acids have a special metabolic function during germination. The overall properties and mode of action of many of the plant hydroperoxide isomerases are similar and detailed studies have been carried out on purified linoleate hydroperoxide isomerase obtained from eggplant fruit using affinity chromatography with soybean lipoxygenase antibody (Grossman *et al*. 1983). The linoleate hydroperoxide isomerase from eggplant fruit was active towards both the 9-hydroperoxyoctadeca-10,12-dienoic and the 13-hydroperoxyoctadeca-9,11-dienoic acids, whereas the enzyme from flax and cotton seedlings utilises the 13-hydroperoxy isomer preferentially. The main reaction products are the α-ketols with small amounts of γ-ketols. Specifically for the 13-hydroperoxy substrate, the 13-hydroxy-12-oxo-*cis*-9-octadecenoic acid (α-ketol) is formed (Fig. 9.6).

Small amounts of the γ-ketol may arise during the isomerisation from the intermediate ion or radical. The products can be specifically identified as trimethylsilyl derivatives by gas chromatography and mass spectrometry. The function of oxygenated acids in plants is unknown, although for cotton seedlings the formation of a cyclic oxidation

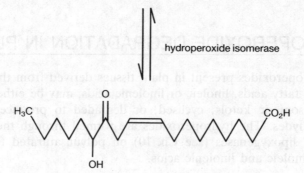

13–hydroperoxy–cis–9,trans–11–octadecadienoic acid

hydroperoxide isomerase

13–hydroxy–12–oxo–cis–9–octadecenoic acid (α–ketol)

or

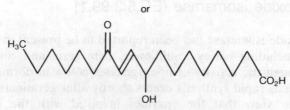

9–hydroxy–12–oxo–trans–10–octadecenoic acid (γ–ketol)

Fig. 9.6 Action of hydroperoxide isomerase on linoleate-13-hydroperoxide

product from linolenic-13-hydroperoxide has been claimed (Vick and Zimmerman 1981).

The eggplant hydroperoxide isomerase has a low K_m value (2.4 × 10^{-5}M) which indicates a high affinity of the enzyme for the substrates and hence their rapid removal from plant tissue. Separate studies with the sulphydryl inhibitors, iodoacetate and methylmercuric iodide, indicate the presence of an essential sulphydryl group in the eggplant hydroperoxide isomerase.

Hydroperoxide lyase

The characteristic grassy odours of leafy plants are believed to be mainly due to the formation of C-6 and C-9 alcohols and aldehydes derived from the unsaturated fatty acid hydroperoxides. Enzymes which cleave the hydroperoxides have been found in cucumbers, tomatoes, tea and kidney bean leaves, and have been investigated in cultured tobacco cells (Sekiya et al. 1984).

Degradation, catalysed by lyases, of the 13-hydroperoxides derived from the commonly occurring polyunsaturated fatty acids, such as linoleic acid, results in the formation of hexanal (Fig. 9.7) by cleavage of the carbon–carbon bond between the hydroperoxide group and the trans-double bond. Alternatively, the action of the 13-hydroperoxide lyases on the 13-hydroperoxides of the trienoic acid (linolenic acid) results in the formation of cis-3-hexenal. The hydroperoxide lyases can also catalyse the symmetrical cleavage of 9-hydroperoxides to form products containing nine carbon atoms. The carbon–carbon bond between the hydroperoxide trans-double bond (Fig. 9.7) is again cleaved by the hydroperoxide lyase.

Therefore the proportions of the C-6 and C-9 type products in vegetables or fruits is determined first, by the specificity of the lipoxygenase to produce various hydroperoxides and secondly, by the subsequent action of the lyase enzymes to form different volatile C-6 and C-9 aldehydes. Cowpea lipoxygenase has been reported only to catalyse the oxidation of linoleic acid and thus cis-3-hexenal cannot be produced in the cowpea. On the other hand the tomato fruit lyase enzyme is specific for only the 13-hydroperoxides and thus a mixture of hexanal and cis-3-hexenal may be produced. For cucumber, the lyase is claimed to catalyse equally the cleavage of the 9- or 13-hydroperoxides. However, the observable different aromas of various fruits is not simply due to the presence or absence of C-6 or C-9 aldehydes or corresponding alcohols, but also due to the modulating effect of these compounds on other key components, like isobutylthiazole found in the leaves and fruits of tomatoes.

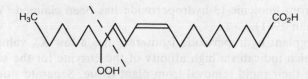

13–hydroperoxy–cis–9,trans–11–octadecadienoic acid

hydroperoxide lyase

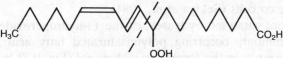

CH₃–(CH₂)₄–CHO $+$ OHC–CH₂–CH = CH–(CH₂)₇CO₂H

hexanal   12–oxo–cis–9–dodecenoic acid

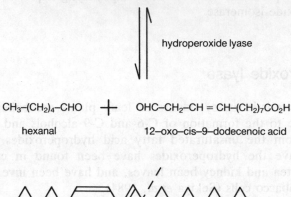

9–hydroperoxy–trans–10,13–cis–octadecadienoic acid

hydroperoxide lyase

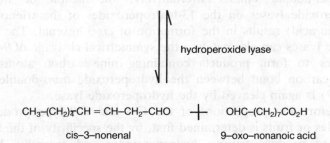

CH₃–(CH₂)₄CH = CH–CH₂–CHO $+$ OHC–(CH₂)₇CO₂H

cis–3–nonenal   9–oxo–nonanoic acid

Fig. 9.7 The action of hydroperoxide lyases on linoleate-9- or-13-
hydroperoxides

Degradation of chlorophyll

The green colour of vegetables is substantially retained during frozen
storage. However, blanching, canning and controlled atmosphere
storage of vegetables of fruits can cause or initiate the loss of chlorophyll colour.

The most significant way in which chlorophyll is degraded involves
the replacement of the magnesium atom by H⁺ to form unattractive
yellow-to-brown colours

$$\text{chlorophyll} \xrightarrow[\text{heat}]{H^+} \text{pheophytin} + Mg^{2+}$$

In chlorophyll Mg^{2+} interacts strongly with the nitrogen atoms of pyrolle ligands, where the coordination is primarily planar – with the magnesium ion centrally placed between four pyrolle residues and axially coordinated with water molecules. The porphyrin ring contains a phytol ester and a cyclopentanone ring is added to one pyrolle residue. Chlorophyll-a, contains a methyl substituent whereas chlorophyll-b, contains the formyl group (Fig. 9.8). Replacement of the magnesium atom by copper or zinc results in more stable green colours which may form during the storage of canned vegetables. The copper and zinc atoms would normally be released from the various metal-containing enzymes present.

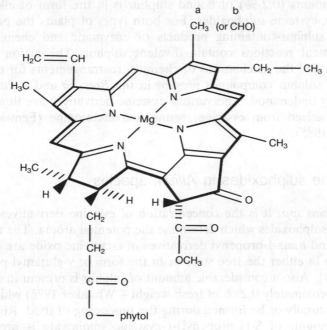

Fig. 9.8 Structure of chlorophyll

Removal of the phytol ester by the action of chlorophyllase (EC 3.1.1.14) does not cause loss of colour which is still retained in the chlorophyllide. However, the magnesium atom may again be lost in the presence of acid and heat from the chlorophyllide to form a colourless pheophoride (devoid of phytol and Mg^{2+}).

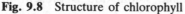

$$\text{chlorophyll} \underset{}{\overset{\text{chlorophyllase}}{\rightleftharpoons}} \text{chlorophyllide} + \text{phytol}$$

Lipoxygenses, and possibly the hydroperoxide-degrading enzymes, may also cause bleaching of chlorophyll. Although the mechanisms of such reactions are not understood, it is possible that such oxidative reactions may involve the cyclopentanone ring that contains an activated methylene group.

SULPHUR COMPOUNDS IN *ALLIUM* AND *BRASSICA* SPECIES

Volatile sulphur compounds which arise from the action of enzymes on precursor molecules, are responsible for the odour characteristics of *Allium* and *Brassica spp*. Non-volatile glucosinolate precursors are mainly found in *Brassica spp*. whereas in onions and garlic relatively large amounts (0.2 %) of bound sulphur is in the form of alkyl and alkenyl-L-cysteine sulphoxides. For both types of plants the principal volatile sulphur-containing products of enzymatic and chemical rearrangement reactions contain divalent sulphur. The action of the enzymes and the mechanisms of chemical rearrangements for the two types of sulphur compounds present in the *Brassica* and *Allium spp*. is mainly understood. The various cysteine derivatives are thought to be synthesised from cysteine, serine and methionine (Fenwick and Hanley 1985).

Cysteine sulphoxides in *Allium* species

For *Allium spp*. it is the concentration of cysteine derivatives in the form of sulphoxides which determine the potential aroma. The methyl, propyl and *trans*-1-propenyl derivatives of L-cysteine oxide are present in onion in either the free state or in the form of γ-glutamyl peptides (Fig. 9.9). Also a considerable amount of sulphur is present in cycloalliin (approximately 0.2 % of fresh weight – Whitaker 1976) which may occur naturally or be formed during the processing of food. Relatively large amounts of S-(1-propenyl)-L-cysteine sulphoxide is present in

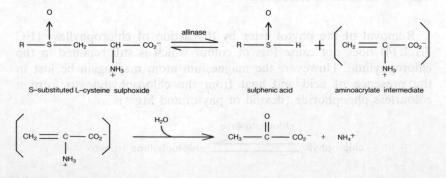

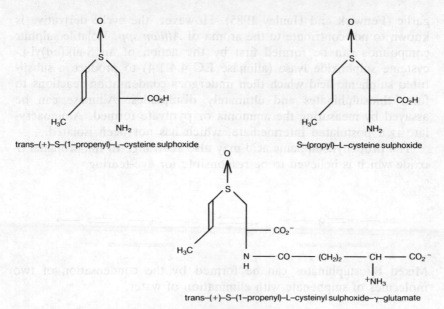

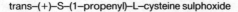

trans–(+)–S–(1–propenyl)–L–cysteinyl sulphoxide–γ–glutamate

Fig. 9.9 Some sulphoxides of *Allium* species

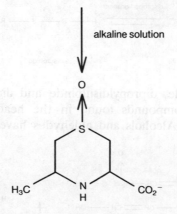

Fig. 9.10 The formation of cycloalliin (3-methyl-1,4-thiazane-5-carboxylic acid-S-oxide)

garlic (Fenwick and Hanley 1985). However, the cyclic derivative is known to not contribute to the aroma of *Allium spp*. Volatile sulphur compounds can be formed first by the action of an S-alk(en)yl-L-cysteine sulphoxide lyase (alliinase EC 4.4.1.4) to produce a substituted sulphenic acid which then undergoes condensation reactions to form thiosulphinates and ultimately disulphides. Alliinase can be assayed by measuring the ammonia or pyruvate formed. Aminoacrylate is a postulated intermediate, which has not been isolated.

The propenyl sulphenic acid may also rearrange to thiopropanal S-oxide which is believed to be responsible for eye-tearing.

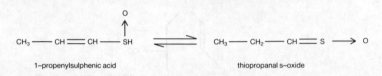

Mixed thiosulphinates can be formed by the condensation of two molecules of sulphenate with elimination of water.

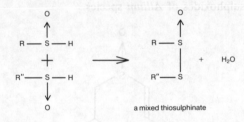

Disulphides can be formed by a disproportionation reaction of the unstable thiosulphinates.

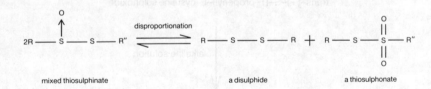

Dimethyldisulphide, dipropyldisulphide and diallyldisulphide are the major sulphur compounds found in the headspace vapours above chopped onions. Alcohols and aldehydes have also been found and

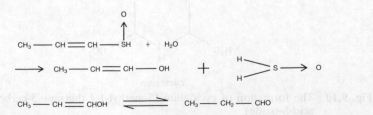

may be formed from the decomposition of *trans*(1-propenyl)sulphenic acid (Whitaker 1976). Thiosulphinates such as diallylthiosulphinate (allicin) in garlic and disulphides such as allylallyldisulphide are believed to be responsible for the aroma in garlic.

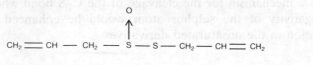

diallyl thiosulphinate (allicin)

While it is accepted that many of the sulphur products arising from the action of allinase contribute to the flavour of onion, garlic and other *Allium spp.*, the nature and amounts of individual compounds responsible for aromas characteristic of individual plants remains largely unknown. The reasons for this lack of knowledge are twofold: first, many of the compounds (thirty or more) have only been detected after thermal treatment by gas chromatography during which chemical re-arrangement and degradation reactions can occur; secondly, the specificity and affinity of various alliinases to many of the different sulphoxides present in the plants is unknown. Additionally, the sulphoxides often occur as γ-glutamylpeptides which are only cleaved by alliinases after removal of the γ-glutamyl residue by hydrolases. All these changes catalysed by enzymes can occur during the post-harvest storage of *Allium spp*.

Cold extraction techniques, followed by analysis using thin layer chromatography have now revealed S-1-propyl-L-cysteine sulphoxide (Table 9.4). to be the predominant free sulphoxide in white onion bulbs. Nevertheless, other sulphoxides trapped as γ-glutamyl peptides may be present in greater amounts which might be released slowly through the catalytic action of hydrolases which may change the aroma of stored products. Furthermore the amount of volatile product formed is dependent on the affinity (K_m) of alliinases for the various substrates, V_{max}, and the relative rates of the various chemical rearrangement reactions, which are likely to vary for different sulphoxides.

Alliinases and expected isoenzymes have not been thoroughly investigated, although it is known that alliinase is a pyridoxal-dependent

Table 9.4 Sulphoxides of white onion bulbs

Sulphoxide	Amount (mg/g fresh weight)
S-1-Propyl-L-cysteine sulphoxide	2.9
S-1-Methyl-L-cysteine sulphoxide	0.9
trans-S-1-Propenyl-L-cysteine sulphoxide	0.6

(After Lancaster and Kelly 1983).

enzyme. The enzyme is not active towards the γ-glutamyl peptides of L-cysteine, but more active towards substrates with unsaturated S-substituents. Schiff base formation between the amino group of cysteine and the aldehyde group of pyridoxal phosphate probably offers a mechanism for the cleavage of the C–S bond where the electronegativity of the sulphur atom would be enhanced by electron migration in the unsaturated derivatives.

Glucosinolates in *Brassica* species

Isothiocyanates, thiocyanates and nitriles contribute to the characteristic volatile aroma compounds present in members of the Cruciferae. However, for Brassica vegetables, like Brussels sprouts, cabbage, cauliflower, broccoli, swedes, turnips and condiments such as mustard, the desirable flavours are due mainly to the presence of volatile isothiocyanates. These compounds are the products most frequently formed by the hydrolytic action of thioglucoside glycohydrolase (glucosinolase or myrosinase EC 3.2.3.1) on naturally occurring glucosinolates after disruption of plant tissue. Although a large number of different glucosinolates are found in Cruciferae as a whole a much more limited number (from five to ten) occur in *Brassica spp.* However, unfortunately, four of the glucosinolates found in *Brassica* vegetables may give rise to small amounts of goitrogenic substances (Table 9.5). Also in dry flours and concentrates manufactured from *Brassica* seeds, such as rape, mustard and crambe flours, the isothiocyanate aroma is undesirable as such powders are required to possess a bland flavour.

Glucosinolase catalyses the hydrolysis of the β-thioglucoside bond to form firstly glucose and an unstable intermediate (thiohydroxamic O-sulphonate). The plant glucosinolases are allosterically activated by ascorbate, approximately (10^{-3} M), which decreases the K_m value of the enzyme. Thioglucosidase activity also occurs in a number of microorganisms. The unstable O-sulphonate intermediate normally undergoes a Lossen rearrangement to form isothiocyanates, hydrogen sulphate and glucose. Small amounts of thiocyanates, which for benzylthiocyanate has a garlic odour, are occasionally formed and may arise from either a geometric isomer of the original glucosinolates (Schwimmer 1981) or by isomerisation of the isothiocyanate. Under acidic conditions and enhanced by the presence of Fe^{2+}, nitriles are formed. These are found in fermented vegetable products like sauerkraut and coleslaw where the pH value is approximately 3.8. Epithiobutyl- and pentylnitriles have also been isolated from autolysing turnip. Indoylglucosinolates are believed to form unstable isothiocyanates which are rapidly degraded to release the thiocyanate anion. The indoylmethyl alcohol might react chemically with ascorbic acid, but

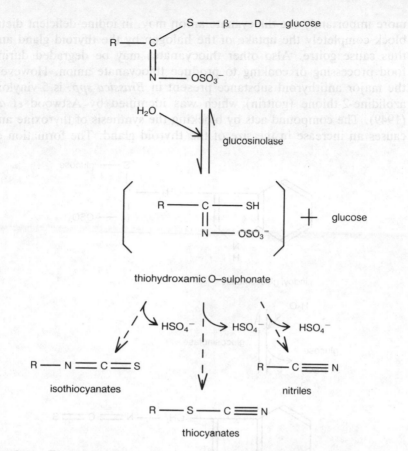

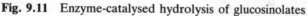

Fig. 9.11 Enzyme-catalysed hydrolysis of glucosinolates

Table 9.5 The average content of progoitrins and thiocyanate precursors in some *Brassica* species (mg/100 g fresh weight)[†]

| Brassica species | Glycosinolates | | |
| | Common names | | |
	Progoitrin[‡]	Gluconapoleiferin[§]	Glucobrassicins[¶]
Cabbage	3.8	—	32
Cauliflower	2.3	—	27.5
Brussels sprouts	47.8	—	73.4
Swede/turnip	37.1	4.2	14.4

([†] From Sones *et al.* 1984).

[‡] 2-Hydroxy-3-butenylglucosinolate.

[§] -2-Hydroxy-4-pentenylglucosinolate.

[¶] 3-Indoylmethyl- and 1-methoxyl-3-indoylmethylglucosinolates.

more importantly the thiocyanate anion may, in iodine-deficient diets, block completely the uptake of the halogen by the thyroid gland and thus cause goitre. Also other thiocyanates may be degraded during food processing or cooking to produce thiocyanate anion. However, the major antithyroid substance present in *Brassica spp.* is 5-vinylox-azolidine-2-thione (goitrin) which was identified by Astwood *et al.* (1949). The compound acts by blocking the synthesis of thyroxine and causes an increase in the size of the thyroid gland. The formation of

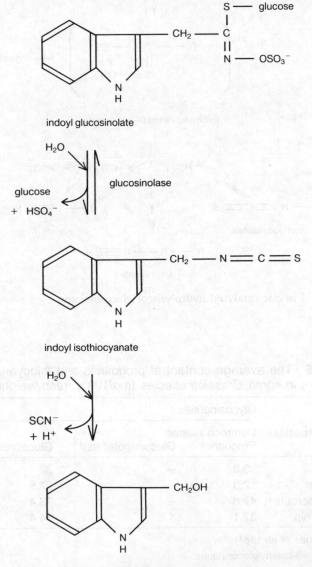

indoyl glucosinolate

indoyl isothiocyanate

3–indoylmethyl alcohol

Fig. 9.12 Formation of thiocyanate anion from indoyl glucosinolate

vinyloxazolidine-2-thione arises from the spontaneous cyclisation of the 2-hydroxyisothiocyanates liberated from β-hydroxyglucosinolates (Fig. 9.13). Although there are a large number of glucosinolate hydrolysis products, for 2-oxo-substituted compounds only 2-hydroxy-3-butenylglucosinolate and 2-hydroxy-4-pentenylglucosinolate, have been identified (Table 9.5). The toxicity of the hydrolysis products of

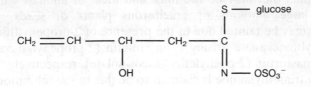

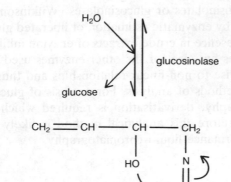

2–hydroxy–3–butenyl glucosinolate (progoitrin)

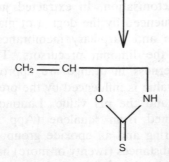

2–hydroxy–3–butenyl isothiocyanate

5–vinyloxazolidine–2–thione (goitrin)

Fig. 9.13 Formation of goitrin

glucosinolates, and in particular the goitrins, is not known, although the incidence of goitre is relatively low. The mean daily intake per person in the United Kingdom of total glucosinolates has been estimated to be approximately 29 mg for cooked *Brassica* species (Sones *et al*. 1984), although there are large variations due to the seasonal nature of the products. Alternative sources of goitrins and thiocyanates in the human diet may be the milk and meat of animals which have ingested large amounts of cruciferous plants or seeds. Milk in particular may be tainted due to the presence of 2-propenylthiocyanate and benzylthiocyanate arising from sinigrin (2-propenylglucosinolate) and gluconasturtiin (2-phenylethylglucosinolate), respectively. Tainting of eggs by trimethylamine is claimed to be due to the inhibition of liver trimethylamine oxidase by goitrin (5-vinyloxazolidine-2-thione) in a small number of genetically disposed laying hens.

Analysis for total glucosinolates or glucosinolases (Wilkinson *et al*. 1984) may be carried out by enzymatic estimation of liberated glucose. However, the possible presence in crude extracts of enzyme inhibitors, not only for glucosinolases but also for the other enzymes used in the glucose assay, may give rise to non-linear relationships and thus limit the usefulness of such methods of analysis. For analysis of glucosinolates by gas chromatography, derivatisation is required which gives variable results, and therefore this analytical method is likely to be superseded by high performance liquid chromatography.

FORMATION OF LIMINOIDS

In citrus fruit and leaf tissue the naturally occurring salt of limonoic acid (Fig. 9.14) is tasteless, but during the extraction of juice, lactonisation of limonoic acid, catalysed by liminoate D-ring lactonase (EC 3.1.1.36), can occur to form a very bitter compound, limonin. Cellular disruption caused by both bruising and freezing of citrus fruits also induces the enzyme-catalysed lactonisation. In extracted juices the amount of limonin present is influenced by the degree of maceration and incorporation of the albedo and carpillary membranes, which contain high concentrations of the limonin precursors. Threshold values for the detection of bitterness in orange are approximately 6 ppm of limonin, although this value is influenced by the presence of flavonoid glycosides, citric acid and the pH value. Limonoate is a triterpine (C-30) derivative formed from squalene (App. X), and contains a furan ring, a lactone ring and an epoxide group. A large number of other closely related substances (twenty or more) have been isolated from a range of citrus fruits. These include 7-liminol, deoxy-liminol and isolimonic acid and many other related compounds – some of which are precursors of limonoate or nomilin – which is also known

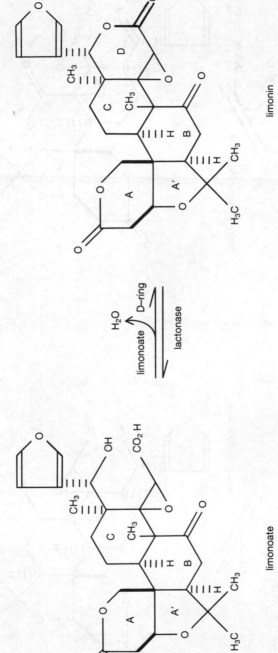

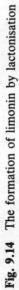

Fig. 9.14 The formation of limonin by lactonisation

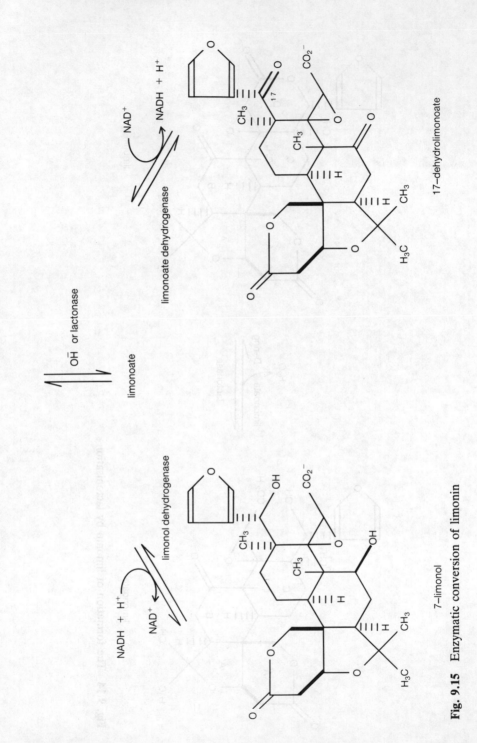

Fig. 9.15   Enzymatic conversion of limonin

to be bitter. The use of ^{14}C-labelled compounds, has indicated that limonoate is most likely synthesised in citrus leaves and translocated to the fruit and seeds. Possible precursors are those compounds which lack the lactonised A-ring, or the dihydrofuran A'-ring. The D-lactone-ring of limonin is hydrolysed under alkaline conditions, whereas protonation of the carboxyl group enhances lactonisation (Fig. 9.15).

Although limonin can be determined in extracts by HPLC, as microbial dehydrogenases specific for limonin are now known, rapid enzymatic analysis of larger numbers of samples should be possible. Furthermore, microorganisms may provide a source of purified enzymes for the removal of limonin precursors. Limonoate dehydrogenase (Fig. 9.15) catalyses the oxidation of the acid to 17-dehydrolimonoic acid which prevents the formation of limonin by lactonisation. Also, immobilised cells of *Corynebacterium fascians* have been used for debittering of citrus products; limonol dehydro-genase catalyses the reduction of limonin to 7-liminol; an acetyl lyase catalyses the deacetylation (Fig. 9.16) of another bitter compound, nomilin (Hasegawa *et al.* 1985). Nomilin, which is present in oranges and grapefruit, is effectively converted to a non-bitter compound by nomilin acetyllyase (Fig. 9.16) that is then hydrolysed by an A-ring lactone hydrolase to form obacunoate. The enzymes from *Corynebac-terium spp.* are claimed to be constitutive and therefore are potentially useful, as substantial quantities of the organism may be obtained by growth on low-cost substrates.

Many plants contain a substantial number of glycosides such as the flavanoids, betalaines and cyanogenic compounds; narginin, respon-sible for the bitterness in grapefruits, is also a glycoside of 4,5,7-tri-hydroxyflavanone. All these compounds, because of their predominant glycosidic nature, are described fully in Ch. 1. The enzymatic changes given there for the release of cyanide and the decolorisation of antho-cyanins, can all occur in post-harvest fruits and vegetables as a conse-quence of the disruption of the cellular tissues.

ETHENE BIOSYNTHESIS

While there are many post-harvest changes in harvested foods which reveal intriguing metabolic pathways, such as purine degradation and the formation of volatile C-6 compounds from polyunsaturated fatty acids, the catabolism of methionine to liberate ethene (ethylene) reveals a precisely controlled pathway and ingenious investigative science particularly by Liebermann, Yang and the late Leslie Mapson at the Low Temperature Research Station in Cambridge. Richard Gane from the same laboratory had discovered in 1934 that ethylene was produced by apples. Subsequently ethylene was shown to stimu-

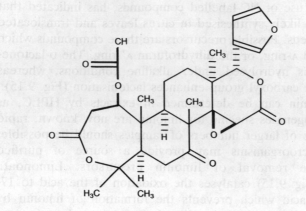

nomilin

nomilin acetyl lyase

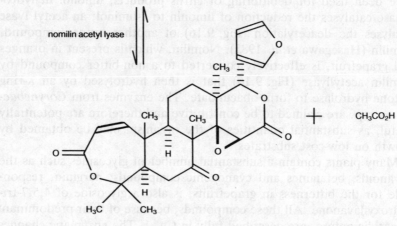

obacunone

$+ \quad CH_3CO_2H$

obacunone A–ring lactonase

$+ \quad H_2O$

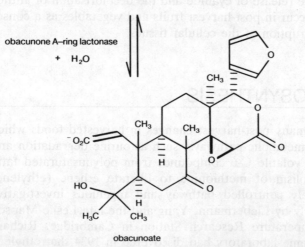

obacunoate

Fig. 9.16 Enzymatic conversion of nomilin (Herman *et al*. 1985)

late the ripening of fruit; the use of labelled ^{14}C identified the $-CH_2-CH_2$-group of methionine as the precursor of ethylene; biochemical intermediates were identified by the use of test substrates for ethylene biosynthesis; oxygen was shown to be required for the biochemical utilisation of the intermediate 1-aminocyclopropane-1-carboxylic acid; and more recently the sulphur atom of methionine has been shown to be recycled.

All plant tissues are able to generate ethene and climacteric fruits produce an ethene spurt of several hundred orders of magnitude at the onset of ripening. Small amounts of ethene are also able to trigger both the ripening process and the production of ethene itself; thus the molecular mechanism for ethene liberation is autocatalytic. 'Stress' caused by physical damage to plant tissues such as bruising, cutting, drought or chilling also induces ethene production. Moreover, indole acetic acid induces ethene production.

Methionine is activated by enzymatic conversion to S-adenosyl-methionine and subsequently to the active intermediate, 1-aminocyclo-propane-1-carboxylic acid, through the action of a synthase (EC 4.4.1.14) with a very high affinity (K_m, 13 μM) for the activated methionine. The synthase enzyme is a pyridoxal phosphate-dependent enzyme which catalyses first the formation of a typical pyridoxal Schiff base intermediate and subsequent liberation of the substituent electro-

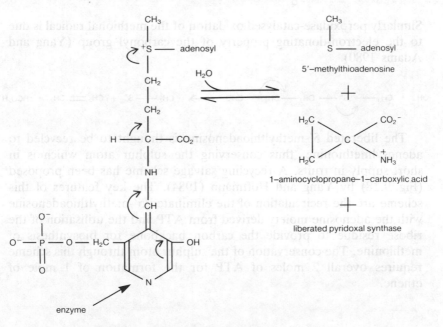

Fig. 9.17 Formation of 1-aminocyclopropane-1-carboxylic acid from S-adenosyl methionine synthase complex

philic group, as 5'-methylthioadenosine (Fig. 9.17). The formation of ethene from 1-aminocyclopropane-1-carboxylic acid requires oxygen and is believed to be catalysed by an ethene-forming enzyme. The mechanism is proposed to involve the oxygenation of the amino group and the subsequent liberation of ethene by the concerted action of the electron-deficient nitrogen atom and the electron-donating tertiary carbon atom (Yang and Adams 1980).

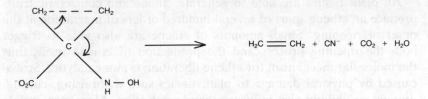

$$H_2C = CH_2 + CN^- + CO_2 + H_2O$$

A similar concerted electron migration reaction occurs during the chemical liberation of ethene from a number of compounds, which also contain electron-donating and electrophilic groups in the 1,2-substituent position, respectively. For example with chloroethyl-2-phosphate:

$$Cl-CH_2-CH_2-\overset{\displaystyle O}{\underset{\displaystyle O_-}{\overset{\displaystyle \|}{P}}}-O^- + H_2O \longrightarrow \tfrac{1}{2}Cl_2 + H_2C = CH_2 + H_2PO_4^-$$

Similarly peroxidase-catalysed oxidation of the methional radical is due to the electron-donating property of the carbonyl group (Yang and Adams 1980).

$$OH^- + CH_3-{}^+S^\bullet-CH_2-CH_2-CHO \longrightarrow CH_3-S^\bullet + CH_2 = CH_2 + HCO_2H$$

The liberated 5'-methylthioadenosine is thought to be recycled to adenosylmethionine, thus conserving the sulphur atom which is in short supply in fruits. A recycling salvage scheme has been proposed (Fig. 9.18) by Yang and Hoffmann (1984). The key features of this scheme are the recirculation of the eliminated 5'-methylthioadenosine with the adenosine moiety derived from ATP and the utilisation of the ribose residue to provide the carbon backbone for biosynthesis of methionine. The conservation of the sulphur atom through this scheme requires overall 2 moles of ATP for the formation of 1 mole of ethene.

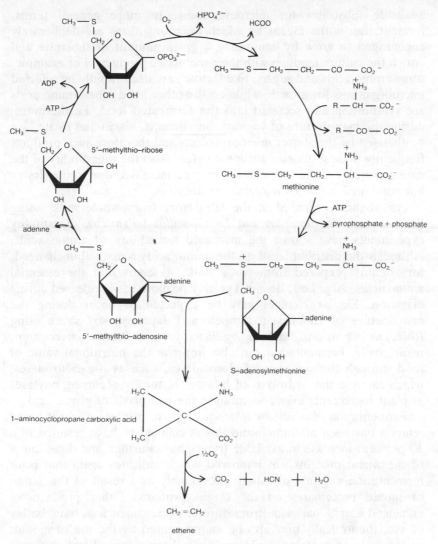

Fig. 9.18 Ethene biosynthesis and the methionine cycle (from Yang and Hoffman 1984, reproduced with permission from *The Annual Review of Plant Physiology*, **34** © 1984 by Annual Reviews Inc.)

ENZYME-CATALYSED REACTIONS IN FERMENTED FOODS

The nutritional value, texture and flavour of raw materials and foods is changed by fermentation. In yoghurt, cheese, tempeh, soy sauce and bread the growth of selected microorganisms first causes rapid changes in the free sugars and amino acids, as these substances are readily available substrates for microorganisms. In more general terms, fermentation is the means by which microorganisms are deliberately encouraged to grow by consuming a given amount of substrate and enrich the culture medium with their metabolic products. For example, some amino acids and sugars, like lactose, are used rapidly by selected microorganisms for growth, while on the other hand other amino acids are synthesised and secreted into the fermented food. Furthermore, during the manufacture of yoghurt the vitamins, niacin and folate, are synthesised by the starter microorganisms and therefore such products frequently possess added nutritional value. Also the digestibility of the native proteins of the raw material may be increased due to the slower but continued action of microbial proteinases.

For yoghurt prepared in the laboratory from whole milk, using *Streptococcus thermophilus* and *Lactobacillus bulgaricus*, digestibility experiments have shown the increased availability of amino acids. Although the distribution of all the amino acids remained unchanged, for yoghurt prepared from cow's milk, it seems that the essential amino acids, Arg, Leu, Ile and Tyr may be more easily released during digestion. Similar changes may be expected to occur during the manufacture of Indonesian tempeh and Japanese soy sauce using *Rhizopus oligosporus*, and *Aspergillus soyae* and *Saccharomyces spp.*, respectively. Fermentation can also improve the nutritional value of food through the synthesis of glycosidases, such as β-galactosidases, which catalyse the hydrolysis of lactose. Naturally occurring phytases in plant ingredients may also catalyse the hydrolysis of phytic acid.

Fermentation of wheat by *Rhizopus spp.* to produce a wheat-based tempeh has been attempted and this is claimed to have resulted in a 30 per cent increase in available tryptophan. Further, the digestibility of the wheat proteins was improved which indicates again that prior fermentation may aid digestion, presumably as a result of the action of mould proteinases on the cereal proteins. Other products of enhanced nutritional value from different cereals, such as oats, barley or rye, theoretically may also be manufactured by the use of moulds or the isolated proteinases. However, full toxicological testing would be required before these products could be used for human food (App. IX).

Enzymatic reactions in fermented foods fulfil an important role for the formation of desirable flavour and texture characteristics. Irrespective of the initial pathway for lactose catabolism, the important intermediary products formed by microbial glycolysis of glucose or galactose are pyruvate and acetyl coenzyme A or acetyl phosphate. Acetyl CoA can also be formed by degradation of fatty acids. The short chain aldehydes, alcohols and ketones are formed by enzyme-catalysed reductions. For *Saccharomyces spp.* the decarboxylation of pyruvate is catalysed by pyruvate decarboxylase (EC 4.1.1.1) to form ethanal which is reduced to ethanol.

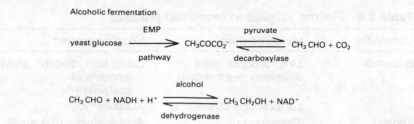

Alcoholic fermentation

$$\text{yeast glucose} \xrightarrow[\text{pathway}]{\text{EMP}} CH_3COCO_2^- \underset{\text{decarboxylase}}{\overset{\text{pyruvate}}{\rightleftharpoons}} CH_3CHO + CO_2$$

$$CH_3CHO + NADH + H^+ \underset{\text{dehydrogenase}}{\overset{\text{alcohol}}{\rightleftharpoons}} CH_3CH_2OH + NAD^+$$

For certain bacteria (e.g. *Zymomonas*), acetyl CoA is reduced to ethanol.

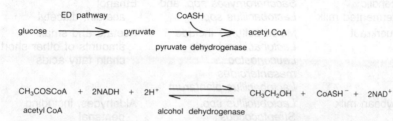

$$\text{glucose} \xrightarrow{\text{ED pathway}} \text{pyruvate} \xrightarrow[\text{pyruvate dehydrogenase}]{\text{CoASH}} \text{acetyl CoA}$$

$$\underset{\text{acetyl CoA}}{CH_3COSCoA} + 2NADH + 2H^+ \underset{\text{alcohol dehydrogenase}}{\rightleftharpoons} CH_3CH_2OH + CoASH^- + 2NAD^+$$

Other volatile substances such as sulphur compounds, esters and lactones may arise from the enzyme-catalysed hydrolysis, thermal degradation and oxidation of proteins and lipids during pasteurisation or cooking. Ethanol is a desirable component in plain yoghurt, whereas diacetyl is responsible for the butter-type flavour of butter-milks (Table 9.6). As various microorganisms used are endowed with different enzymes for the metabolism of pyruvate, acetyl CoA or acetyl phosphate, the chemical composition of the final product clearly depends on the microorganism present. In microbial cultures which generate substantial amounts of NADH, pyruvate is readily reduced to lactate (Fig. 9.19). In yoghurts, *Streptococcus thermophilus* produces L-lactic acid while *Lactobacillus bulgaricus* produces D-lactic acid. However, when the concentration of NADH is depleted, pyruvate may be converted (Fig. 9.20) to acetyl CoA from which diacetyl, acetoin or ethanol may be formed (Marshall 1984). In the absence of alcohol dehydrogenase the aldehyde, ethanal, accumulates in cultures of *Lactobacillus bulgaricus* and *Streptococcus thermophilus* used for the manufacture of yoghurt. Furthermore, the concentration of ethanal can be increased by the action of lactic acid bacteria on added thre-onine. However, the formation of ethanal varies according to the strains of bacteria used, with *Lactobacillus bulgaricus* species forming large amounts directly from threonine through the action of threonine aldolase (EC 4.1.2.5).

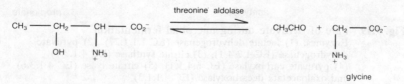

$$CH_3 - CH_2 - \underset{OH}{\overset{|}{C}}H - \underset{\underset{+}{NH_3}}{\overset{|}{C}}H - CO_2^- \xrightarrow{\text{threonine aldolase}} CH_3CHO + \underset{\underset{+}{NH_3}}{\overset{|}{C}}H_2 - CO_2^-$$

glycine

Table 9.6 Flavour volatiles in fermented products

Commodity	Microorganisms	Volatiles present
Buttermilk	*Streptococcus lactis* *Streptococcus cremoris*	Lactic acid, diacetyl, small amounts of acetaldehyde
	Lactobacillus bulgaricus	Acetaldehyde
Yoghurt	*Streptococcus thermophilus* and *Lactobacillus bulgaricus*	Acetaldehyde, plus small amounts of diacetyl, acetoin
Alcoholic fermented milk	*Saccharomyces spp.* and *Lactobacillus spp.*	Ethanol acetoin, diacetyl
Sauerkraut	Mixed cultures include *Lactobacillus brevis* *Leuconostoc mesenteroides* *Lactobacillus plantarum*	Acetate and small amounts of other short chain fatty acids
Soybean milk	*Lactobacillus spp.* *Streptococcus thermophilus*	Aldehydes, including pentanal
Soy sauce	*Aspergillus oryzae* *Lactobacillus spp.* *Saccharomyces rouxi*	Organic acids alkyl phenols pyrazines, esters
Tempeh	*Rhizopus spp.*	Fatty acids
Cocoa	*Saccharomyces spp.,* *Lactobacillus spp.* and *Acetobacter spp.*	Fatty acids and aromatic acids

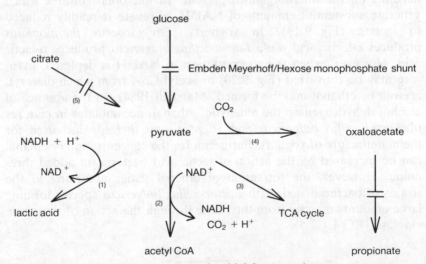

Fig. 9.19 Fate of pyruvate during microbial fermentation
Enzymes: (1) lactate dehydrogenase (EC 1.1.1.27), (2) pyruvate
dehydrogenase (EC 1.2.4.1), (3) citrate synthase (EC 4.1.3.7),
(4) pyruvate carboxylase (EC 6.4.1.1), (5) citrate lyase (EC 4.1.3.6)
and oxaloacetate decarboxylase (EC 4.1.1.3)

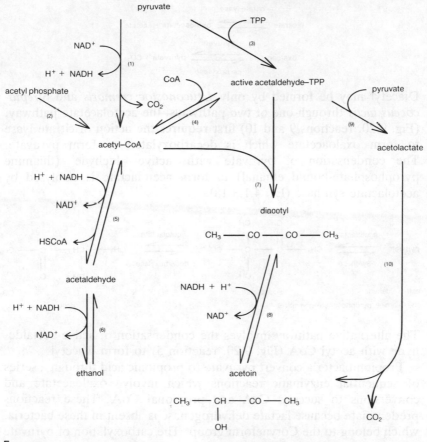

Enzymes
(1) pyruvate dehydrogenase (EC 1.2.4.1) (2) phosphate acetyl transferase (EC 2.3.1.8) (3) pyruvate decarboxylase (EC 4.1.1.1) (4) acetaldehyde dehydrogenase (EC 1.2.1.10) (5) acetaldehyde dehydrogenase (EC 1.2.1.10) (6) alcohol dehydrogenase (EC 1.1.1.1) (7) diacetyl synthase (8) acetoin dehydrogenase (EC 1.1.1.5) (9) acetolactate synthase (EC 4.1.3.18) (10) acetolactate decarboxylase (EC 4.1.1.5)

Fig. 9.20 Alternative pathways for volatile compounds formed during fermentation from pyruvate, acetyl CoA and acetyl phosphate

The addition of pyruvate to buttermilk cultures increases the concentration of diacetyl and possibly acetoin. In alcoholic milk products such as kefir, alcohol dehydrogenase is provided by yeasts which catalyse the reduction of ethanal to ethanol.

Addition of citrate to some cultures (e.g. *Streptococcus lactis* subsp. *diacetylactis*) may also increase the concentration of diacetyl (Marshall 1984) through a series of reactions starting with the direct conversion of citrate to oxaloacetate catalysed by citrate lyase (EC 4.1.3.6).

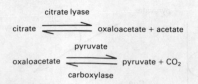

Diacetyl may be formed by only *Leuconostoc cremoris* and *Streptococcus lactis* through one of two pathways: the acetolacetate pathway, (Fig. 9.20, reactions 9 and 10) first requires the action of citrate lyase to form oxaloacetate which is decarboxylated to form pyruvate. The condensation of pyruvate with 'active aldehyde' (thiamine pyrophosphate-bound ethanal) to form acetolactate is catalysed by acetolactate synthase (EC 4.1.3.18).

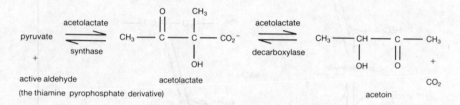

The alternative pathway involves the condensation of active acetaldehyde with acetyl CoA (Fig. 9.20, reaction 5) to form diacetyl.

Propionibacteria convert pyruvate to propionic acid through a series of sequential enzymatic reactions which involve oxaloacetate and conversions to succinyl CoA and propional CoA. These reactions predominate because lactate dehydrogenase is absent in these bacteria, which belong to the Coryneform group. The carboxylation of pyruvate is catalysed by transcarboxylase (EC 2.1.3.1): pyruvate receives a carboxyl group from methylmalonyl CoA to form oxaloacetate thus leaving propionyl CoA.

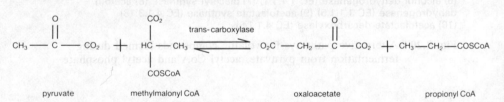

Propionibacterium shermanii is deliberately added to Swiss cheeses where the carbon dioxide produced is responsible for the formation of the 'eyes'. *Propionibacterium shermanii* is inhibited by penicillin and therefore Emmental cheese manufactured from milk contaminated with this antibiotic may not develop the eye holes or the appropriate flavour. The overall reaction is:

$$3\text{ glucose} \rightarrow 4\text{ propionate} + 2\text{ acetate} + 2\,CO_2 + 4\,H_2O$$

KEY FACTS

1.   The cellular control of enzymatic activity diminishes in post-harvest foods. Changes in colour, flavour, texture and nutrient content are catalysed by indigenous enzymes.

2.   Post-mortem enzymatic changes in meat triggered by cytoplasmic Ca^{2+} cause the conversion of glycogen to lactic acid, the loss of ATP and rigor mortis. Adenine and guanine nucleotides are degraded. Inosinemonophosphate acts as a meat flavour enhancer and is produced by the oxidative deamination of AMP.

3.   Amines in foods of animal origin are formed by decarboxylation of amino acids. Trimethylamine is responsible for fish odours and is formed by the reduction of trimethylamine oxide.

4.   In foods of plant origin, fatty acid hydroperoxides are degraded to form volatile aliphatic aldehydes and ketones by the action of hydroperoxide lyase. The nature of the predominant aldehyde present is determined by the specificity of indigenous enzymes towards different hydroperoxides.

5.   Volatile sulphur compounds in *Allium spp.* are formed by the action of first a lyase enzyme on S-substituted sulphoxides, and secondly through rearrangement of the liberated sulphenic acids.

6.   In *Brassica spp.*, isothiocyanates, thiocyanates and nitriles are liberated by the action of glucosinolases followed by a Lossen rearrangement. Goitrin (5-vinyloxazolidine-2-thione) acts by blocking the biosynthesis of thyroxine.

7.   Limonin and nomilin are triterpenes responsible for bitterness in citrus fruits. Nomilin acetyllyase and limonoate dehydrogenase can be used to remove bitter compounds or their precursors.

8.   During the ripening of fruits ethene is formed from methionine, via 5'-methylthioadenosine. The sulphur atom is recovered through a salvage cycle.

9.   In fermented foods, simple sugars like glucose and lactose are readily used for growth by selected microorganisms. Lactic, acetic and other simple organic acids as well as vitamins and volatile flavour compounds are synthesised by the microorganisms. Various glycolytic pathways are used by different microorganisms. The nature of the volatile compounds produced is also influenced by the composition of the growth medium.

REFERENCES

Astwood, E. B., Greer, M. A. and Ettlinger, M. G. (1949) 'L-5-Vinyl-2-thiooxazolidone, an antithyroid compound from yellow turnip and *Brassica* seeds', *J. Biol. Chem.*, **181**, 121–30.

Bergmeyer, H. U. (1984) *Methods of Enzymatic Analysis*, vol. 6, 3rd edn. *Metabolites* 1. *Carbohyrates*. Verlag Chemie, Weinheim.

Cohen, P. (1976) *The Control of Enzyme Activity*. Chapman and Hall, London.

Fabiansson, S. and Reuterswärd, A. L. (1985) 'Low voltage electrical stimulation and post-mortem energy metabolism in beef', *Meat Sci.* **12**, 205–23.

Fenwick, G. R. and Hanley, A. B. (1985) 'The genus *Allium* Part 2', *CRC Crit. Revs. Food Sci. Nutr.* **22**, 273–377.

Grossman, S., Bergman, M. and Sofer, Y. (1983) 'Purification and partial characterisation of eggplant linoleate hydroperoxide isomerase', *Biochim. Biophys. Acta*, **752**, 65–72.

Hasegawa, S., Vandercook, G. E., Choi, G. Y., Herman, Z. and Ou, P. (1985) 'Liminoid debittering of citrus sera by immobilised cells of *Corynebacterium fasciens*', *J. Food Sci.*, **50**, 330–2.

Herman, Z., Hasegawa, S. and Ou, P. (1985) 'Nomilin acetyllyase bacterial enzyme for nomilin debittering of citrus juices', *J. Food Sci.*, **50**, 118–20.

Horgan, D. J. and Kuypers, R. (1985) 'Post-mortem glycolysis in rabbit, *Longissimus dorsi*, muscles following electrical stimulation', *Meat Sci.* **12**, 225–41.

Jacober, L. F. and Rand, A. G. Jr. (1984) 'Biochemical evaluation of seafood', in *Chemistry and Biochemistry of Marine Food Products* (ed. Martin, R. E.), AVI Publishing Co., Westport, Connecticut.

Jeacocke, R. (1982) 'Does the sarcoplasmic reticulum achieve a chemiosmotic equilibrium in relaxed muscle?' *FEBS Lett.*, **147**, 225–30.

Lancaster, J. E. and Kelly, K. E. (1983) 'Quantitative analysis of the S-alk(en)yl-L-cysteine sulphoxides in onion (*Allium capa* L.)', *J. Sci. Food Agric.* **34**, 1229–35.

Large, P. J. and McDougall, H. (1975) 'An enzymic method for the micro-estimation of trimethylamine', *Anal. Biochem.*, **64**, 304–10.

Marshall, V. M. E. (1984) 'Flavour development in fermented milks', in *Advances in the Microbiology and Biochemistry of Cheese and Fermented Milk* (eds. Davies, F. L. and Law, B. A.). Elsevier Applied Science Publishers, London.

Schwimmer, S. (1981) *Source Book of Food Enzymology*. AVI Publishing Co. Westport, Connecticut.

Sekiya, J., Satoru, T. Kajiwara, T. and Hatanaka, A. (1984) 'Fatty acid hydroperoxide lyase in tobacco cells cultured *in vitro*', *Phytochemistry*, **23**, 2439–243.

Sones, K., Heaney, R. K. and Fenwick, G. R. (1984) 'An estimate of the mean daily intake of glucosinolates from cruciferus vegetables in the U.K.', *J. Sci. Food Agric.*, **35**, 712–20.

Storey, R. M., Davis, H. K., Owen, D. and Moore, L. (1984) 'Rapid approximate estimation of volatile amines in fish', *J. Food Technol.*, **19**, 1–10.

Stryer, L. (1981) *Biochemistry*, 2nd edn. Freeman and Co., San Francisco, California.

Vick, B. A. and Zimmerman, D. C. (1981) 'Lipoxygenase, hydroperoxide isomerase and hydroperoxide cyclase in young cotton seedlings', *Plant Physiol.* **67**, 92–7.

Whitaker, J. R. (1976) 'Development of flavour, odor and pungency in onion and garlic', *Adv. in Food Res.*, **22**, 73–133.

Wilkinson, A. P., Rhodes, M. J. C. and Fenwick, R. G. (1984) 'Myrosinase activity of cruciferus vegetables', *J. Sci. Food Agric.*, **35**, 543–2.
Yang, S. F. and Adams, D. O. (1980) 'Biosynthesis of ethylene', in *Biochemistry of Plants, A Comprehensive Treatise*, vol. 4 *Lipids: Structure and Function* (ed. Stumpf, P. K.). Academic Press, New York.
Yang, S. F. and Hoffman, N. E. (1984) 'Ethylene biosynthesis and its regulation in higher plants', *Ann. Rev. Plant Physiol.*, **35**, 155–89.

ADDITIONAL READING

Davies, F. L. and Law, B. A. (1984) *Advances in the Microbiology and Biochemistry of Cheese and Fermented Milk*. Elsevier Applied Science Publishers, London.
Fenwick, R. G., Heaney, R. K. and Mullin, W. J. (1983) 'Glucosinolates and their breakdown products in food and food plants', *CRC Revs. Food Sci. Nutr.* **18**, 123–201.
Galliard, T. and Chan, H. W. -S. (1980) 'Lipoxygenases', in *The Biochemistry of Plants, A Comprehensive Treatise*, vol. 4 *Lipids: Structure and Function* (ed. Stumpf, P. K.). Academic Press, New York.
Maier, V. P., Hasegawa, S., Bennett, R. D. and Echols, L. C. (1980) 'Limonin and limonoids: chemistry, biochemistry and juice bitterness', in *Citrus Nutrition and Quality* (eds. Nagy, S. and Attaway, J. A.). ACS Symposium series 143. American Chemical Society, Washington DC.
Martin, R. E. (1984) *Chemistry and Biochemistry of Marine Food Products*. AVI Publishing Co., Westport, Connecticut.
Stephens, E. M. and Grisham, C. M. (1982) 'The structure and mechanism of the sarcoplasmic reticulum Ca^{2+}-ATPase: A bio-inorganic perspective', in *Advances in Inorganic Biochemistry* (eds. Eichhorn, G. L. and Marzilli, L. G.). Elsevier, Amsterdam.
Whitaker, J. R. (1976) 'Development of flavour, odor and pungency in onion and garlic', *Adv. in Food Res.*, **22**, 73–133.

CHAPTER 10

Oxygen-dependent enzymatic reactions in post-harvest foods

The sequential reduction of both oxygen (O_2) by one, two and four electrons and activated oxygen species (H_2O_2) is catalysed by oxidases. Whereas oxygenases catalyse the incorporation of the one or two oxygen atoms from oxygen into organic molecules. For oxidases, electron abstraction by the enzyme is directly from the substrate without addition of oxygen to the substrate.

$$AH_2 + \tfrac{1}{2}O_2 \rightleftharpoons A + H_2O$$

Molecular oxygen acts as the electron acceptor.

For oxygenases, there is direct incorporation of either one or both atoms of oxygen into the substrate.

$$AH + O_2 \rightleftharpoons AOOH,$$

$$AH + \tfrac{1}{2}O_2 \rightleftharpoons AOH$$

REACTIVITY OF OXYGEN AND REDUCED OXYGEN SPECIES

Enzymes are required to catalyse biological oxidations because oxygen (O_2) is less reactive with organic compounds than is first expected from its electronegativity: oxygen is adjacent to fluorine and diagonal to chlorine, in the periodic table. The slow oxygenation, as opposed to chlorination, of organic compounds is reflected in the high activation energy required to activate ground state triplet oxygen. In the triplet state of oxygen two electrons are unpaired with parallel spins, such that spin restriction hinders the divalent reduction of the O_2 molecule, and hence permits the existence in atmospheric oxygen of many organic substances. The presence of two unpaired electrons in the molecule O_2 arises from the existence of only six valence electrons in each oxygen atom with the requirement for one electron to be placed in the $2p\pi$ orbitals of equal energy. However, the spin restriction of ground state molecular oxygen can be overcome in one of three ways: first, by stepwise addition of single electrons, one at a time, secondly, by coordination to transition metals,

$$\text{e.g. } Cu^{2+} + O_2 \rightleftharpoons Cu^{2+} \leftarrow : O_2$$

and thirdly, by movement of one of the unpaired oxygen electrons $(2\pi^*_g)$ to a higher energy orbital with reversal of spin to produce singlet oxygen ($'\Delta_g$).

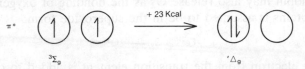

Singlet oxygen is not a free radical but is a highly electrophilic species containing two vacant molecular orbitals. Therefore singlet oxygen readily reacts with electron-dense groups such as double bonds present in carotenoids and unsaturated fatty acids.

In biological materials the univalent pathway for the reduction of O_2 is commonplace:

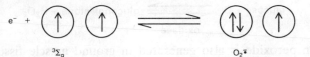

The stepwise univalent reduction of triplet oxygen results in the formation of a superoxide radical anion, the peroxide anion and subsequently the oxide anions of water.

$$
\begin{array}{ccccccc}
 & +1e & & +1e & & +2e & \\
O_2 & \rightarrow & O_2^{\cdot -} & \rightarrow & O_2^{2-} & \rightarrow & 2.O^{2-} \\
 & & \text{superoxide} & & \text{peroxide} & & \text{oxide} \\
 & & \text{radical} & & \text{anion} & & \text{anions}
\end{array}
$$

The redox potentials for the formation of the various reduced forms of oxygen are given in Table 10.1.

Due to the extra electrons the reduced oxygen species can also theoretically act as reductants. For example the superoxide radical

Table 10.1 Redox potentials for reduction of oxygen

$O_2 + e^- \rightleftharpoons O_2^{\bar{\cdot}}$	$E_0' = -0.45$ V
$O_2^{\bar{\cdot}} + 2H^+ + e^- \rightleftharpoons H_2O_2$	$E_0' = +0.98$ V
$H_2O_2 + H^+ + e^- \rightleftharpoons H_2O_2 + HO^{\cdot}$	$E_0' = +0.38$ V
$HO^{\cdot} + H^+ + e^- \rightleftharpoons H_2O$	$E_0' = +2.33$ V

(George 1965).

rapidly reduces ferricytochrome-c, nitroblue tetrazolium or tetranitro-methane. Alternatively, $O_2^{\overline{\cdot}}$ is also a powerful oxidising agent and oxidises ascorbate, vitamin E, phenols and sulphite. Thus the latter substances, which are used as antioxidants in foods, are chemical scavengers for $O_2^{\overline{\cdot}}$. However in biological tissues, the single electron reduced intermediate ($O_2^{\overline{\cdot}}$) of oxygen is not often liberated and is held firmly to the redox centres of the enzymes; oxygen radicals are bound at the active sites of the enzymes. However, for single electron catalysed oxidations by xanthine oxidase, and membrane-bound NADPH oxidases, the superoxide radical is liberated. Oxyhaemoglobin and oxymyoglobin may also release $O_2^{\overline{\cdot}}$ as the bonding of oxygen to these haem proteins is assumed to be in the superoxide form:

$$Fe^{II} \rightarrow O \ \text{---} \ O^{\overline{\cdot}}$$

where an electron from the transition element is added to one of the unpaired orbitals of oxygen. The liberated radical can be detected as a reducing agent with ferricytochrome-c or nitroblue tetrazolium salts.

Hydrogen peroxide is produced from either flavin or copper-containing enzymes such as glucose, galactose and amino acid oxidases by a two-electron reduction of the O_2 molecule.

$$glucose + O_2 \ \underset{\text{oxidase}}{\overset{\text{glucose}}{\rightleftharpoons}} \ gluconolactone + H_2O_2.$$

Hydrogen peroxide is also generated in ground muscle tissue (Harel and Kanner 1985). In rat liver it is estimated that up to 5 per cent of the oxygen consumed is reduced to $O_2^{\overline{\cdot}}$ and subsequently hydrogen peroxide. Superoxide radical and hydrogen peroxide can act as either reducing or oxidising agents (Table 10.1) and may arise from a number of natural sources (Table 10.2). Additionally, in foods small amounts of hydrogen peroxide may arise from its use as a sterilising agent for packaging materials and surfaces.

The superoxide radical has been claimed to have a novel role in the development of bread dough through a redox scheme involving O_2 copper and manganese and disulphide bonds. Both a Cu/Mn complex and a hydroquinone have been detected (Graveland et al. 1984), and it has been known for a long time that air or an oxygen atmosphere is required for dough development. Additionally, xanthine oxidase, a generator or $O_2^{\overline{\cdot}}$, and lipoxygenase – which is capable of forming activated oxygen species – can both act independently as dough improvers. However, further work is required to elucidate the mechanism of the reducing system for the disulphide bonds of wheat gluten (see p. 227), as there are other types of enzymes present in flour which may catalyse the rearrangement of gluten disulphide bonds. The other reactive species of oxygen which may arise from $O_2^{\overline{\cdot}}$ and H_2O_2 are the hydroxyl radical and singlet oxygen. The hydroxyl radical (HO$^\bullet$) is a

Table 10.2   Systems for the generation of active oxygen species in biological fluids

Reducing reactions	Activated oxygen species
Transition metals	$O_2^{\bar{\cdot}}$
Photosensitised oxidation of riboflavin	$O_2^{\bar{\cdot}}$
Leucoflavins	$O_2^{\bar{\cdot}}$
Hydroquinones	$O_2^{\bar{\cdot}}$
Iron–sulphur proteins	$O_2^{\bar{\cdot}}$
Xanthine oxidase	$O_2^{\bar{\cdot}}$
Glycolate oxidase	H_2O_2
Amino acid oxidases	H_2O_2
Amine oxidases	H_2O_2
Sulphite oxidase	H_2O_2
Flavin dehydrogenases	$O_2^{\bar{\cdot}}$
Ubiquinone cytochrome-c reductase	$O_2^{\bar{\cdot}}$
Peroxidases	$O_2^{\bar{\cdot}}$
Mitochondrial cytochrome P-450	$RO^{\cdot}$
Radical reactions $O_2 + R$	$ROO^{\cdot}$
Fenton reaction $Fe^{2+} + H_2O_2$	$Fe^{3+} + {}^{\cdot}OH + OH^-$
$Ce^{IV} + H_2O_2$	$O_2^{\bar{\cdot}}$

(Cadenas *et al*. 1983).

strong oxidising agent ($E_o' = +2.33$ V, Table 10.1) and represents the reactive oxygen species produced after the hypothetical three-electron reduction of diatomic oxygen. It is readily formed either from hydrogen peroxide, or the superoxide radical in the presence of catalytic amounts of transition metals by the well known Fenton reaction (2).

$$M^{n+1} + O_2^{\bar{\cdot}} \rightleftharpoons M^{n+} + O_2 \qquad (1)$$

$$M^{n+} + H_2O_2 \rightleftharpoons M^{n+1} + HO^{\bullet} + OH^- \quad (2)$$

Reductants other than $O_2^{\bar{\cdot}}$ could also be responsible for reformation of the reduced metal ion.

In post-harvest and post-mortem foods, where the cellular structure of the tissue breaks down, mechanical disruption may lead to an uncoupling of oxidase-catalysed reactions and liberation of different reactive oxygen species. In some instances singlet oxygen ($'O_2$) might be formed from light-sensitised (S^*) chlorophyll haemoglobin or myoglobin, whereas in other circumstances. $'O_2$ may arise by dismutation of $O_2^{\bar{\cdot}}$.

$$S^* + O_2 \rightarrow {}'O_2 + \text{light sensitive compound (Gs)}$$

Singlet oxygen may be responsible for the oxidation of unsaturated lipids and other constituents containing single and conjugated bonds

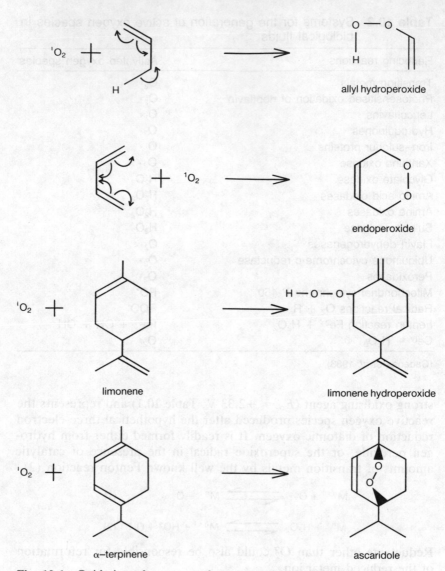

allyl hydroperoxide

endoperoxide

limonene

limonene hydroperoxide

α–terpinene

ascaridole

Fig. 10.1 Oxidation of unsaturated structures by singlet oxygen

to form allyl- and endoperoxides (Fig. 10.1). Singlet oxygen can yield hydroperoxide directly from unsaturated fatty acids. In essential oils, terpenes may be oxidised. However, owing to its high reactivity the hydroxyl radical (HO·) is regarded as the most destructive reduced oxygen species and can be partly blamed for loss of colour, flavour and formation of taints in foods:

The radical easily adds to double bonds and may also abstract hydrogen atoms from saturated compounds to form organic radicals.

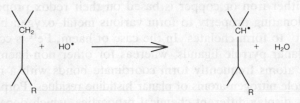

The hydroxyl radical also reacts with methional to form ethene which can influence the ripening of fruit, as ethene acting like a plant hormone accelerates ripening. The gas chromatographic detection of ethene offers a reliable method for assay of the hydroxyl radical.

$$CH_3-S-CH_2-CH_2-CHO + HO^\bullet \rightarrow CH_2 = CH_2 + HCO_2H + \tfrac{1}{2}CH_3-S-S-CH_3$$

$$\underset{\text{methional}}{} \qquad\qquad\qquad \underset{\text{ethene}}{}$$

Hydrogen peroxide is the most stable of the partially reduced oxygen species and is therefore detected easily. Either chemical assays using vanadic acid or titanium salts, and biochemical methods – based on the use of peroxidases and hydrogen donors – can be used to estimate hydrogen peroxide. Methods used for the detection of singlet oxygen, superoxide and hydroxyl radicals are given in Table 10.3, although in many cases the reagents are not entirely specific for the different species of reduced oxygen.

For the enzyme-catalysed transfer of electrons to oxygen or peroxides many of the enzymes involved are metallo-enzymes (Table 10.4).

Table 10.3 Reagents for the detection of reactive oxygen species in biological materials

Oxygen species	Reagents	Reaction
$O_2^{\overline{\bullet}}$	Ferricytochrome-c	Reduction to ferrocytochrome-c
	Nitroblue tetrazolium salt	Reduction to formazan
	Superoxide dismutase	Inhibitor of reactions requiring $O_2^{\overline{\bullet}}$
$HO^\bullet$	Methionine	Formation of ethene
	4-Methylthio-2-oxobutanoate, phenol	Hydroxylation
	Mannitol, ethanol or isopropanol	Hydrogen abstraction
H_2O_2	Peroxidase with 4-aminoantipyrine and phenol	Oxidation of hydrogen donors
$'O_2$	Radiolabelled cholesterol	Forms a 5α-hydroperoxide of cholesterol

(Green and Hill 1984)

Many enzymes contain several redox-active centres, while others like peroxidase contain only one well defined active site. The cofactor function for either iron or copper is based on their redox property, their electron-donating property to form various metal–oxygen bonds, and their ability to form chelates. In the case of haem, Fe^{II} is coordinated to four planar pyrrole ligands, whereas for other non-haem enzymes the metal atoms frequently form coordinate bonds with a number of the imidazole nitrogen atoms of planar histidine residues. Porphyrin–iron complexes display different chemical properties, which depend on the localised molecular environment in which the complex is located. Most of the metallo-active sites which contain either iron or copper, function by transfer of single electrons, because of the limited number of stable valency states for these metals. However, for molybdenum and probably manganese-dependent enzymes, together with the flavin-containing redox enzymes, a single step involving the transfer of two electrons is also possible. Enzymes, such as xanthine oxidase, which possess multiple redox centres containing molybdenum, flavin and two Fe–S groups require six electrons for full reduction although various intermediate oxidation states may exist during the acceptance and donation of electrons by the enzyme.

Recently the accumulation of information from spectroscopic studies (Eichhorn and Marzilli 1980) on purified metallo-enzymes, enzyme–substrate and inhibitor complexes and model compounds coupled to X-ray crystallographic analysis, has enabled a timely understanding of the way in which electron transfer processes can be catalysed by purified enzymes at a molecular level. Some examples of the occurrence of transition metals in redox enzymes is given in Table 10.4.

Table 10.4 Metals as active-site components of terminal oxidases and oxygenases

Fe haem groups	Fe atoms	Cu atoms
Peroxidases	Lipoxygenases	Superoxide dismutases, binuclear with Zn
Catalases	Prostaglandin cyclooxygenase	Phenolases – binuclear
Cytochromes	Superoxide dismutases	Ascorbate oxidase } metal
Sulphite oxidase		Laccases } clusters
		Cytochrome oxidase – binuclear with Fe

OXIDATION OF MYOGLOBIN AND MEAT COLOUR

The most striking effects of oxygen is on the colour of meat. Higher concentrations of oxygen give meat a bright red appearance, whereas anaerobic conditions give a meat a purple colour. Cut meat, aged at room temperature, is brown due to oxidation of myoglobin (Mb) to metmyoglobin (Met Mb).

At atmospheric concentrations of 30 per cent or more the preferred red meat pigment myoglobin is maintained in the oxygen-bound state:

$$Mb + O_2 \rightleftharpoons MbO_2$$

For myoglobin, haemoglobin and other haem proteins the porphyrin group is the protoporphyrin IX isomer (Fig. 10.2). Four of the coordinate positions of each iron atom are occupied by pyrolle nitrogens which are linked by methene bridges. The ionised propionate substituents aid non-covalent bonding, through electrostatic bonds, with the associated proteins. In haemoglobin and myoglobin, an axial imidazole nitrogen bond is formed with the iron atom, whereas for some haem-dependent enzymes, the axial bond is the sulphur of cysteine or methionine.

The packaging of meat, either minced or as slices in oxygen-enriched retail packs, is now widely practised by the industry: thus, the iron atom is maintained in the Fe^{2+}/O_2 state. However, this technology was only possible with the manufacture of oxygen-impermeable plastic wrappings. In the absence of added oxygen meat turns brown due to the slow oxidation by small amounts of oxygen of the haem iron atom to Fe^{3+} to form metmyoglobin:

$$MbFe^{2+} - O_2 \rightleftharpoons MetMbFe^{3+} + O_2^{-\bullet}$$

The rate of the above reaction is maximal at oxygen pressures of from 1 to 1.4 mm Hg and occurs more rapidly at low pH values.

Mn atoms	Mo	Se
Superoxide dismutases	Xanthine oxidase	Glutathione peroxidase
	Sulphite oxidase	
	Aldehyde oxidases	
	Nitrogenase	

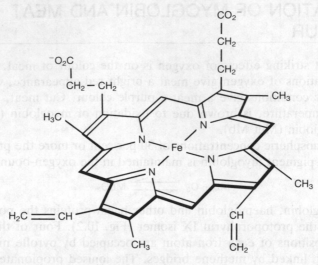

Haem (iron protoporphyrin IX)

Fig. 10.2 Haem (iron protoporphyrin IX)

In fresh meat metmyoglobin may be reduced back to Mb by metmyoglobin reductases which use reduced ferrocytochromes or NADH. However, in aged meat the reductive enzymes presumably become denatured, or hydrolysed by proteinases and are no longer capable of reducing the undesirable brown MetMb.

Other discoloration, mainly green, in meat can arise from a reaction with hydrogen sulphide produced by *Altermonas putrefaciens*, to form sulphmyoglobin. Green colours in cured meats are due to the oxidation of the haem pigments by peroxide when naturally present catalase has been denatured.

The pink pigment of nitrate-cured meats is believed to be nitric oxide myoglobin. Nitric oxide is thought to be formed by the reduction of nitrate catalysed by mammalian enzymes. Metmyoglobin–nitric oxide is believed to be reduced to the Fe^{2+} form by mitochondrial enzymes using NADH to form nitric oxide myoglobin.

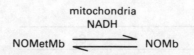

THE FORMATION OF SUPEROXIDE AND HYDROGEN PEROXIDE

As an illustration of the mechanism for the direct reduction of oxygen to hydrogen peroxide, the actions of xanthine, amine and sulphite oxidases are cited below.

Xanthine oxidase (EC 1.2.3.22)

Xanthine oxidase (xanthine : O_2 oxidoreductase) is widely distributed in animals, plants and microorganisms. 'Free' xanthine oxidase in milk catalyses the formation of H_2O_2 and O_2^- during the oxidation of purines (Fig. 10.3), whereas a bound form of the enzyme to the milk fat globule membrane seems less harmful as in the bound state the enzyme acts as a NAD-dependent dehydrogenase (xanthine dehydrogenase EC 1.1.1.204). Xanthine oxidase is one of only a small number of enzymes which contain molybdenum in the active site. The enzyme is also a flavoprotein, contains iron–sulphur centres and characteristically catalyses the hydroxylation of a wide range of substances, including purines. All fully functional molybdenum-type oxidases are now known to contain two Mo atoms, two FAD groups and eight Fe–S centres per mole (Coughlan 1980). For the purified enzyme the ratio A_{280}/A_{450} should be close to 4.8. The specificity with regard to electron acceptors is very broad and these include, in addition to oxygen, NAD$^+$, iodine, dichlorophenolindophenol, quinones, ferricyanide, cytochrome-c, phenazine methosulphate and methylene blue.

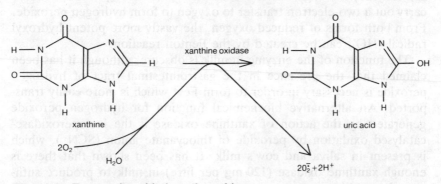

Fig. 10.3 Enzymatic oxidation of xanthine

Although considerable variation is seen for the means by which enzymes from different species use the various electron acceptors, for the human enzyme the order is generally ferricyanide $>O_2>$NAD$^+$. The molybdenum, flavin and iron–sulphur centres all participate in the catalytic reaction where:

$$Mo(VI) \rightleftharpoons Mo(V) \rightleftharpoons Mo(IV);$$

$$FAD \rightleftharpoons FADH \rightleftharpoons FADH_2, \text{ and Fe/S}_{ox}$$

$$Fe/S_{ox} \rightarrow Fe/S_{red} - \text{(Coughlan 1980)}.$$

The general reaction catalysed by xanthine oxidase is:

$$H\text{–}OH + RH \rightleftharpoons ROH + 2H^+ + 2e^-$$

where RH is the substrate and the oxygen introduced is derived from water. Where oxygen is the electron acceptor, either sequential single-electron or two-electron transfers can occur to form superoxide $(O_2^{\bar{}})$ and hydrogen peroxide, respectively.

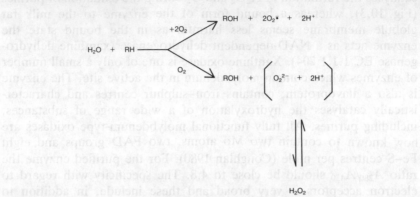

The superoxide radical is believed to be produced at the flavin site in the enzyme, although either reduced flavin ($FADH_2$) or Mo^{IV} could carry out a two-electron transfer to oxygen to form hydrogen peroxide. From both forms of reduced oxygen, the vastly more potent hydroxyl radical ($HO^{\cdot}$) can be created by the Fenton reaction.

The function of the enzyme in milk is obscure, although it has been claimed that the presence in the gastrointestinal tract of hydrogen peroxide is necessary in order to form Fe^{3+} which is more easily transported. An alternative biochemical function for hydrogen peroxide generated by the action of xanthine oxidase is the lactoperoxidase-catalysed oxidation by peroxide of thiocyanate anion (SCN^-), which is present in saliva and cow's milk. It has been shown that there is enough xanthine oxidase (120 mg per litre) in milk to produce sufficient hypothiocyanate to act as an antibacterial agent.

$$HSCN + H_2O_2 \xrightleftharpoons{\text{lactoperoxidase}} HOSCN + H_2O$$

Support for this proposal is strengthened by the knowledge that xanthine oxidase does remain active in the upper digestive tract. Thus it is possible that the salivary secreted thiocyanate and the action of lactoperoxidase or peroxidases in general may help to reduce the numbers of microorganisms in the upper digestive tract of mammals.

Amine oxidases

Amine oxidases degrade biogenic amines and catalyse the formation of aldehyde compounds associated with aromas in food. The enzymes are of two types: those which contain flavin (FAD) and the copper-containing enzymes. The enzymes occur widely in plant and animal tissues, the flavin enzymes being present in the cytosol and mitochondria. Monoamine oxidase (EC 1.4.3.4) is an FAD-dependent enzyme and catalyses the oxidation of primary, secondary and tertiary amines. During such oxidation, FAD (App. I) accepts electrons from the substrate and then passes these directly to diatomic oxygen. As like xanthine oxidase, which is also a flavin-dependent enzyme, hydrogen peroxide is formed, but for the amine oxidases O_2^- is not liberated.

The copper-dependent amine oxidases (EC 1.4.3.6) catalyse the oxidative deamination of diamines (Table 9.2) and primary and secondary amines. The enzymes have been found in a large number of plant and animal sources and are considered to be histamine scavengers in animals. The plant enzymes are more active towards diamines and are found mainly in seedlings, where a fast metabolism of polyamines would seem to be required for rapid growth. Diaminobutane is often used as a test substrate. The enzymes are now known to contain two atoms of copper and 1 mole of the unusual prosthetic group pyrroloquinoline, PQQ (Mondovì and Riccio 1984). The PQQ coenzyme (Fig. 10.4) contains a carbonyl group which is believed to form a Schiff base with the amino group of the substrate – analogous to the reaction of amino groups with the aldehyde group of pyridoxal phosphate. A scheme (Fig. 10.5) has been proposed for the mode of action of the Cu–PQQ-dependent enzyme that requires electron migration of the double bond of the Schiff base, and expulsion of the substituted α-carbon of the substrate. The oxidation of the enzyme–amine intermediate together with the reduction of oxygen, is likely to involve the copper atoms of the enzyme as electron carriers. The overall reaction produces stoichiometric amounts of hydrogen peroxide:

$$R.CH_2 - NH_3^+ + H_2O + O_2 \underset{\text{oxidase}}{\overset{\text{amine}}{\rightleftharpoons}} R.CHO + H_2O_2 + NH_4^+$$

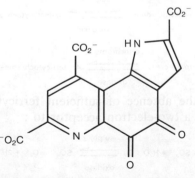

Fig. 10.4 Structure of pyrroloquinoline quinone (PQQ) (Mondovi and Riccio 1984)

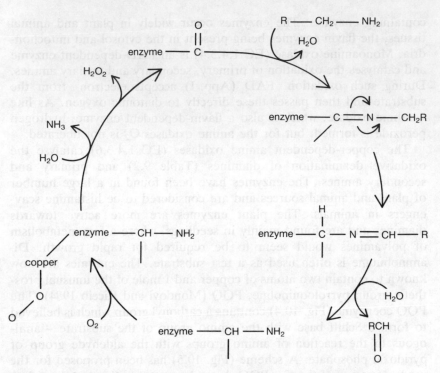

Fig. 10.5 Cyclic scheme for oxidative deamination by copper–PQQ dependent amine oxidase (after Mondovi and Riccio 1984)

Sulphite oxidase (Sulphite : ferricytochrome-c oxidoreductase EC 1.8.2.1 and sulphite : oxygen oxidoreductase EC 1.8.3.1).

Sulphite oxidase can catalyse the oxidation of sulphite to sulphate where either ferricytochrome ($E_0' = 0.26$ V) or ferricyanide ($E_0' = 0.41$ V) are single electron acceptors:

$$2SO_3^{2-} + 2H_2O + 4\,\text{ferricytochrome-c} \underset{\text{oxidase}}{\overset{\text{sulphite}}{\rightleftharpoons}} 4\text{--ferrocytochrome-c} + 2SO_4^{2-} + 4H^+$$

$$4H^+ + 4\,\text{ferrocytochrome-c} + O_2 \underset{\text{oxidase}}{\overset{\text{cytochrome-c}}{\rightleftharpoons}} 4\ \text{ferricytochrome-c} + 2H_2O$$

Alternatively, in the absence of sufficient ferricytochrome-c oxygen can act directly as a two-electron acceptor to :

$$SO_3^{2-} + H_2O + O_2 \underset{\text{oxidase}}{\overset{\text{sulphite}}{\rightleftharpoons}} SO_4^{2-} + O_2^{2-} + 2H^+$$

Sulphite oxidase is found in many plants, animals and microorganisms, and is essential in animals for the detoxification of sulphite formed from the catabolism of the sulphur amino acids, cysteine and methionine. Studies have been carried out mainly with the animal liver enzymes which contain non-covalent protoporphyrin IX (1 mole per subunit) and molybdenum (Rajagopalan 1980). The K_m values (Wedzicha 1984), for ferricytochrome-c (2 μM) and diatomic oxygen (580 μM) indicate that in living tissues the preferential reductive pathway will be by electron transfer to ferricytochrome-c to produce water and sulphate as final products. However, in post-harvest foods, and in particular for homogenised products where considerable cellular disruption has occurred, it is possible that some hydrogen peroxide might be produced by the alternative oxygen-dependent reaction. The ferricytochrome-c reductive pathway is inhibited by anions commonly present in foods and also the protein domain containing the haem group of the enzyme associated with ferricytochrome-c reduction is quite sensitive to proteolysis. The larger polypeptide fragments of sulphite oxidase containing molybdenum, but no haem, do retain the sulphite : oxygen oxidoreductase activity (Johnson and Rajagopalan 1977). The K_m value for SO_3^{2-} is 140 μm when oxygen is the electron acceptor for the bovine liver enzyme.

Sulphite oxidation is believed to take place at the molybdenum centre and ferricytochrome-c reduction at the haem site. During the enzymatic reaction Mo^{IV} is formed from Mo^{VI} by reduction with sulphite.

$$Mo(VI) + SO_3^{2-} + H_2O \rightleftharpoons Mo(IV) + SO_4^{2-} + 2H^+$$

For the formation of hydrogen peroxide the two electrons are thought to be transferred to oxygen directly from Mo^{IV}. A cyclic scheme has been proposed for the mode of action of sulphite oxidase which incorporates the two mechanisms for reoxidation of the reduced enzyme (Mo^{IV}–Fe^{III}) by either molecular oxygen or ferricytochrome-c. For a one-electron transfer to ferricytochrome-c, haem iron is reduced to Fe^{2+} – reactions (3) and (5) – and after the two separate sequential transfers – reactions (4) and (6) – to ferricytochrome-c, the native enzyme (Mo^{VI}–F^{III}) is reformed (reaction (6)). For the direct reoxidation of the Mo^{IV} form of the enzyme by oxygen, as indicated below in Fig. 10.6 the haem iron is not required (reaction (2)). The presence of Mo^V species in sulphite oxidase, has been demonstrated for the reduced enzyme by electron paramagnetic resonance spectroscopy.

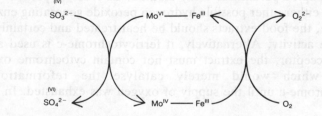

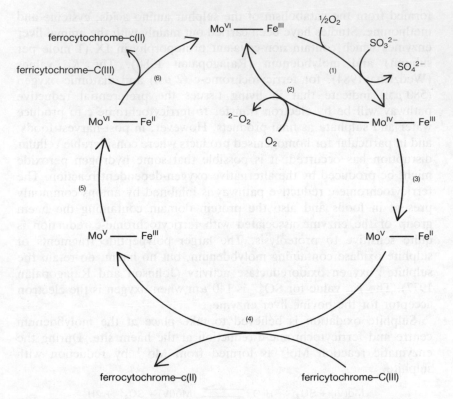

Fig. 10.6 Scheme for oxidation of sulphite by sulphite oxidase (adapted from Rajagopalan 1980)

Thus the electrons may be transferred singly via Mo^V. The EPR signal for Mo^V is unique and provides a means for observing the reduced enzyme in whole tissues and complex products.

One potentially important application for sulphite oxidase is for the analysis of sulphite in foods. Sulphur dioxide and sodium hydrogen sulphite are frequently used as preservatives. For the enzymatic analysis of sulphite when oxygen is used as the oxidising agent, then other electron acceptors such as ferricytochrome-c should be absent so that they do not interfere with the transfer of electrons directly to oxygen. The hydrogen peroxide formed can be detected through the use of a coupled peroxidase assay method. In order to prevent interference by either other possible hydrogen peroxide generating enzymes or catalase, the food extracts should be heat-treated and certainly free of catalase activity. Alternatively, if ferricytochrome-c is used as the electron acceptor, the extract must not contain cytochrome oxidase activity, which would merely catalyse the reformation of ferricytochrome-c until the supply of oxygen was exhausted. In order to test the efficacy of the assay further, the presence of other reducing agents which may act on ferricytochrome-c can be detected before the final addition of the sulphite-oxidising enzyme.

SCAVENGING ENZYMES AND CATALASES

In living tissues the levels of O_2^- are reduced by superoxide dismutases. The amounts of H_2O_2 are reduced by haem-type catalases, peroxidases and glutathione peroxidase (an unusual selenium-containing enzyme). In living cells, the presence of substantial amounts of these scavenging enzymes indicates that they may act frequently in concert with each other, such that hydrogen peroxide formed by the catalytic action of superoxide dismutase may be used to form either other oxidised products, or be decomposed to water or oxygen and water. In living tissues, a logical defence mechanism includes a scavenging of O_2^- and the peroxide anion O^{2-}. However, in post-harvest foods the compartmentalisation of enzymes is disrupted, and the stability of the various scavenging enzymes is likely to decline differentially during storage and food processing. Whereas in the living cell H_2O_2 is degraded by catalase to water and oxygen, in comminuted foods the effects of O_2^-, associated radicals and H_2O_2 are likely to be different and the oxidative reactions may account for loss of food quality, in terms of flavour, nutritional value and colour (von Elbe and Attoe 1985). For example, catalase is generally thermolabile, and therefore any accumulation in heat-treated foods of H_2O_2 in the presence of Fe^{2+} is likely to produce the highly reactive hydroxyl radical (HO·) (Table 10.2). Although O_2^- may not itself be very reactive, it can give rise in the presence of Fe^{2+} ions, through Fenton chemistry, to the highly destructive hydroxyl radical (HO·).

$$O_2^{-\bullet} + Fe^{3+} \rightleftharpoons Fe^{2+} + O_2 \quad \triangle E_o' = 1.22V$$

$$Fe^{2+} + H_2O_2 \rightleftharpoons HO^{\bullet} + OH^- + Fe^{3+} \quad \triangle E_o' = -0.39V$$

The hydroxyl radical (HO·) will attack many organic molecules and thus deactivate enzymes and oxidise nutrients like vitamins C and E which also function as chemical scavengers for free radicals. The toxicity of oxygen in biological tissues has been reviewed extensively by Halliwell (1984). Single electron donors, other than Fe^{2+}, such as Cu^+, coordinated transitional elements and even the hydrogen sulphite radical (HSO_3^-) might also produce the hydroxyl radical from hydrogen peroxide:

$$HSO_3^{-\bullet} + H_2O_2 \rightleftharpoons HO^{\bullet} + OH^- + HSO_3$$

Superoxide dismutase (EC 1.15.1.1)

Superoxide dismutases (superoxide : superoxide oxidoreductase) are found universally in all aerobic-respiring cells. They are responsible for the removal of the superoxide radical by a dismutation reaction:

$$2H^+ + O_2^{\overline{\cdot}} + O_2^{\overline{\cdot}} \rightleftharpoons H_2O_2 + O_2, \; \Delta E_o' = +1.27v$$

Superoxide dismutase occurs naturally in milk and has been detected in seeds, citrus fruits and vegetables. Separate additions to foods of superoxide dismutase may serve as a natural antioxidant.

The discovery of superoxide dismutase is relatively recent (1969). Although its role is dedicated to the destruction of superoxide free radicals, both the occurrence of different types of enzymes and the presence of the enzyme in strictly anaerobic bacteria which do not reduce oxygen is puzzling. Throughout living organisms, the enzyme occurs in three forms: Cu–Zn–SOD, Mn–SOD and Fe–SOD. The enzymes have a transition metal at the active centre which is either Cu, Fe or Mn. Prokaryotes contain the Fe and Mn enzymes, whereas the higher eukaryotes contain both the Mn–SOD and the Cu–Zn enzymes. The lowest forms of living organisms to contain the Cu–Zn enzymes are the green algae. In yeast, liver and heart tissue, the Cu–Zn superoxide dismutase has been claimed to occur in the cytosol, while the Mn enzyme is mitochondrial. The bovine erythrocyte Cu–Zn superoxide dismutase is relatively thermostable with a half-life of 30 min. at 70 °C (Walker *et al.* 1987). The bovine milk enzyme can withstand pasteurisation temperatures up to 80 °C, whereas the unidentified superoxide dismutases present in aqueous extracts of cabbage have a short half-life at 70 °C ($t_{\frac{1}{2}}$ 0.25 min). In crude extracts of oats and corn, superoxide dismutases are claimed to be more stable to heat than the cereal peroxidases. Generally, plant mitochondria contain the Mn enzyme, while the chloroplasts contain the Cu–Zn enzyme. Structurally the apoproteins of the Cu–Zn and Mn and Fe enzymes are completely unrelated, whereas there is extensive homology in the amino acid sequences for the Cu–Zn superoxide dismutases obtained from various sources.

Although the superoxide radical ($O_2^{\overline{\cdot}}$) is itself relatively unstable and in aqueous solutions undergoes a chemical dismutation reaction to form oxygen and hydrogen peroxide, the function of the enzyme is to accelerate the dismutation reaction. At neutral pH values the radical exists mainly as $O_2^{\overline{\cdot}}$, the anion of the weak acid HO_2 (pK_a. 4.8). At pH 7, the dismutation reaction, which is bimolecular, is relatively slow ($k = 0.3 \text{ M}^{-1}\text{s}^{-1}$), due to the electrostatic repulsion between the negatively charged radicals. Whereas at lower pH values the rate of reaction increases very substantially:

$$HO_2 + HO_2 \rightleftharpoons H_2O_2 + O_2, \; k = 8 \times 10^5 \text{ M}^{-1}\text{S}^{-1}$$

The equilibrium lies very favourably thermodynamically in the direction of dismutation $\Delta G^{0\prime} = -29$ kcal. A very fast rate of reaction ($k = 2 \times 10^9$ $\text{M}^{-1}\,\text{s}^{-1}$) has been reported for the enzymatic catalysis, which suggests that the rate of reaction is mainly limited by diffusion of the superoxide radical to the active site of the enzyme. The enzymatic dismutation by Cu–Zn enzyme is believed to proceed by reduction and oxidation of an essential atom of copper which acts as an electron carrier (Fridovich 1979). A decrease in the absorption at 680 nm, which is due to the Cu^{II} centre of the enzyme, occurs in the presence of $O_2^{\overline{\cdot}}$ and thus indicates the reduction of Cu^{II} to Cu^{I}. For all the superoxide dismutase enzymes the general dismutation reaction is:

(1) $E–M^{n+1} + O_2^{\overline{\cdot}} \rightleftharpoons E–M^n + O_2$ and

(2) $E–M^n + O_2^{\overline{\cdot}} + 2H^+ \rightleftharpoons E–M^{n+1} + H_2O_2$

Thus the enzyme undergoes cycles of reduction and reoxidation by $O_2^{\overline{\cdot}}$. By this means the enzyme circumvents the electrostatic repulsion between the two superoxide radicals, and simultaneously acts as an electron carrier between these two radicals to produce peroxide anion and diatomic oxygen.

For assay of superoxide dismutase, special and unusual difficulties arise because of the instability of superoxide anion as the substrate, which is self-reactive and has only a short life: thus stable stock solutions cannot easily be prepared. For the generation of $O_2^{\overline{\cdot}}$, the aerobic oxidation of xanthine by xanthine oxidase is the most frequent method used (Fig. 10.3). As ferricytochrome-c is reduced by superoxide, it can be used as the detecting agent to determine quantitatively the rate of formation of $O_2^{\overline{\cdot}}$.

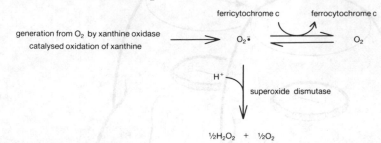

The presence of superoxide dismutase which accelerates the dismutation of $O_2^{\overline{\cdot}}$, thus decreases the rate of reduction of ferricytochrome-c and hence the amount of the enzyme is measured indirectly. Unfortunately, interference with this indirect enzymatic assay method may arise from inhibition by metal ions of xanthine oxidase, separate chemical catalysis of the dismutation reactions by metal ions, and the reoxidation of the reduced ferrocytochrome-c by peroxidases. Therefore control reactions using dialysed samples, additions of EDTA and 10^{-5}M cyanide ion (to inhibit haem peroxidases) coupled to measurements at 295 nm for uric acid formation are necessary, in order to establish the validity of enzymatic assays for superoxide dismutase in complex extracts of foods or plant tissues. However, the superoxide dismutase enzymes, after electrophoresis on polyacrylamide gels, can be detected as discrete bands with a riboflavin-sensitized photo-production of O_2^- with nitroblue tetrazolium (NBT) as scavenger. In this reaction the presence of superoxide dismutases is shown by prevention of the reduction of NBT to the formazan, and therefore the isoenzymes are revealed as clear zones against a purple formazan background. The Cu–Zn enzyme can be distinguished by inhibition with cyanide (1×10^{-3}M). However, copper can be removed with diethyldithiocarbamate and tests for restoration of activity by either Cu, Mn or Fe to the inactive apoenzymes affords a more reliable method for classification of SOD enzymes, as substitutions by other metals cannot be made. The bovine erythrocyte Cu–Zn enzyme is thought to be a dimer (MW approximately 32,000) composed of two identical subunits. Each subunit has a β-barrel type structure and the active site containing Cu^{II} and Zn^{II} is exposed to solvent (Fig. 10.7). The bovine enzyme uniquely requires Cu, although the zinc atom can be replaced by Co^{2+} or Hg^{2+} without loss of enzymatic activity. Crystallographic analysis and spectroscopic techniques have shown that four histidine residues are arranged tetrahedrally around the Zn atom and likewise for the Cu atom where only one residue (His-61) is

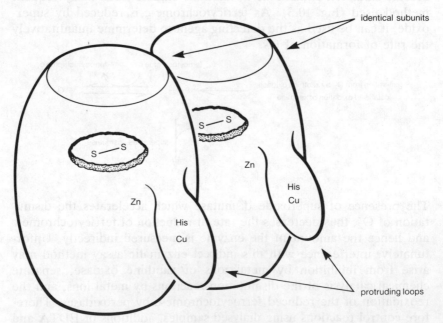

Fig. 10.7 Schematic diagram of the quaternary structure of Cu–Zn superoxide dismutase subunits

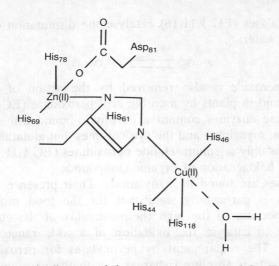

Fig. 10.8 Schematic diagram of the active site groups of Cu–Zn superoxide dismutase (Fielden and Rotilio 1984)

common to both Zn and Cu, which thus acts as a bridging imidazolate ligand (Fig. 10.8). It has been suggested that during enzymatic catalysis $O_2^{\bar{\;}}$ is bound to the Cu atom and thus reduces Cu^{2+} to Cu^+ with the simultaneous cleavage of the imidazole $N-Cu^{2+}$ bond.

$$—N—Cu^{2+} + O_2^{\bar{\;}} \rightleftharpoons —NH + Cu^+ + O_2 - - - - - (1)$$

$$—NH + Cu^+ + O_2^{\bar{\;}} \rightleftharpoons —N—Cu^{2+} + HO_2^{-} - - - - - (2)$$

hydroperoxide anion

The liberated protonated imidazole group can then act as a proton source to stabilise a peroxide (O_2^{2-}) anion generated from the second molecule of $O_2^{\bar{\;}}$ to form the hydroperoxy anion. For erythrocyte superoxide dismutase a K_m value for $O_2^{\bar{\;}}$ of 0.36 M has been reported. Positively charged amino groups of the protein may help to funnel $O_2^{\bar{\;}}$ to the active site.

Peroxidases and catalases

Peroxidases and catalases are enzymes which catalyse the decomposition of hydrogen peroxide. Peroxidases (donor: H_2O_2 oxidoreductase, EC 1.11.1.7) catalyse oxidative reactions by peroxides:

$$2RH + H_2O_2 \rightleftharpoons 2H_2O + 2R$$

whereas catalases (EC 1.11.16) catalyse the dismutation of H_2O_2 to oxygen and water:

$$2H_2O_2 \rightleftharpoons 2H_2O + O_2$$

Hydrogen peroxide is also removed by the action of glutathione peroxidase and in plants by ascorbic acid peroxidase (EC 1.11.1.11). Most of these enzymes contain a porphyrin-bound iron atom as in haemoglobin, myoglobin and the cytochromes, but glutathione peroxidase contains only selenium. Halide peroxidases (EC 1.11.1.8 and 10) catalyse the halogenation of organic compounds.

Peroxidases are found in many foods. Their presence in foods of plant origin is particularly significant for the food processor and consumer, because of the high thermostability of the enzymes and their ability to catalyse the oxidation of a wide range of organic compounds. The requirement by peroxidases for peroxides as the oxidising agents is absolute, whereas – with the exception of gluta-thione peroxidase – the specificity of the enzymes for a wide range of H-donors, which include phenols, ascorbate and amines is low. However, peroxidases occur as isoenzymes and therefore it is possible that individual isoenzymes specifically catalyse the oxidation of different hydrogen donors in homogenised food products. The ther-mostability of haem peroxidases has been investigated for green beans, *Brassica spp.*, citrus fruits and a range of plant products, where the peroxidase activity is correlated to the loss of flavour, colour and texture (Burnette 1977 and Haard 1977). Unfortunately, the high-temperature short-time treatments commonly used commercially in fruit and vegetable processing for the destruction of bacteria, are less effective for the inactivation of peroxidases. Also for some peroxi-dases, in addition to their high thermostability, regeneration after heat-treatment occurs. Both soluble and particulate-bound isoenzymes with different thermostabilities have been found in peroxidase prep-arations obtained from fruits and vegetables, like tomatoes and green beans and cabbage (McLellan and Robinson 1981 and 1983). For oranges a high level of peroxidase activity is associated with the albedo, which might influence adversely the quality of whole fruit products (McLellan and Robinson 1984).

The peroxidases of higher plants are glycoproteins containing vari-able amounts of carbohydrate. An understanding of the mode of action of peroxidases has been gained from substantial investigations with mainly horseradish peroxidase. Horseradish peroxidase (MW approximately 42,000) contains 18 per cent carbohydrate and two Ca^{2+} ions per mole. There are eight oligosaccharide groups, which lie on the surface of the molecule attached through glycosylamine bonds with asparagine residues. Horseradish peroxidases also contain four disul-phide bonds to maintain the tertiary structure of the monomeric protein molecule. Conversely, catalase exists as a tetrameric molecule with a molecular weight in excess of 100,000. The purity of peroxidases, as for cytochromes and catalase, is determined by ratio of absorption (the *RZ* value) at 403 and 280 nm which should approach 3.55. The haem group of peroxidases, as in haemoglobin, myoglobin and many other haem compounds, is iron protoporphyrin IX. For enzymatically active peroxidases the metal atom is Fe^{3+}, whereas in native myoglobins and haemoglobins Fe^{2+} is responsible for the binding of molecular oxygen. The coordination number of Fe^{3+} of native peroxidase is five, which therefore differs from myoglobin where the sixth coordinate position of the iron atom (Fe^{2+} above and perpendicular to the porphyrin ring) is occupied by a molecule of water. Otherwise, the prosthetic groups are identical with the fifth coordinate position occupied by the imidazole group of a histidine residue. The sixth coordinate position in peroxidases is the binding site for peroxide and the characteristic Soret band and visible spectra changes markedly on the binding of substrate. For peroxidases a spectrally distinct peroxidase–H_2O_2 substrate is formed (Fig. 10.9). Other spectrally distinct compounds with characteristic absorption are formed

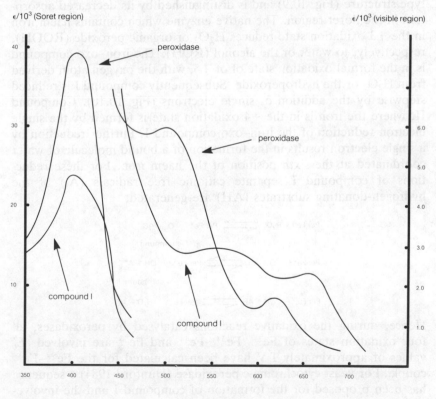

Fig. 10.9 The Soret and visible spectra of peroxidase and compound I

with either fluoride or pyridine. Six-coordinated ferric protoporphyrins IX–fluoride complexes have a mean molar absorption of 138 ± 7 mм$^{-1}$cm^{-1} between 403 and 411 nm. For the pyridine haemochromogen complex of peroxidase the mean molar absorption value between 403 and 411 nm is 102 mм$^{-1}$cm^{-1}. The haem group is not rigid: the iron atom can move slightly in the perpendicular plane and thus influence sterically the access of substrates to the sixth coordinate position. The planar position of the double bonds in the vinyl substituents of the protoporphyrin group can result in greater basicity of the pyrolle nitrogens leading to an increase in the affinity for oxygen atom binding. Furthermore, the protein may influence the spatial direction of the vinyl substituents and thus the precise position of the iron atom differs for the various protoporphyrin IX enzymes. The measured midpoint redox potentials at pH 7 for various peroxidases have ranged from -0.109 to -0.27 V for the turnip and horseradish enzymes, respectively.

Peroxidases catalyse the oxidation of a diverse number of substrates, by the reduction of compound I which is the common first-stage for all peroxidase-catalysed oxidations. Compound I has a ferryl-type structure (Fig. 10.9) and is distinguished by its decreased absorption in the Soret region. The native enzyme which contains haem iron in the $+3$ oxidation state reduces H_2O_2 or organic peroxide (ROOH), respectively, to water or the alcohol (ROH). The iron–oxo compound is in the formal oxidation state of of $+5$, with the oxygen atom derived from H_2O_2 or the hydroperoxide. Subsequently compound I is reduced stepwise by the addition of single electrons (Fig. 10.10). Compound II, where the iron is in the $+4$ oxidation state is formed by the single electron reduction of the iron–oxo compound I. Further reduction by a single electron results in the formation of a bound molecule of water coordinated at the sixth position of the haem iron. For these reductions of compound I separate cationic free radicals (A$^{\cdot}$) of the hydrogen-donating substrates (AH) are generated:

$$\text{Per Fe}^{III} + H_2O_2 \rightleftharpoons \text{Per Fe}^{V} = O + H_2O$$

compound I

$$\text{Per Fe}^{V} = O + AH \rightleftharpoons \text{Per Fe}^{IV} - OH + A^{\bullet}$$

compound II

$$\text{Per Fe}^{IV} - OH + AH \rightleftharpoons \text{Per Fe}^{III} - H_2O + A^{\bullet}$$

Hence, during the oxidative reactions catalysed by peroxidases, all four oxidation states of Fe^{2+}, Fe^{3+}, Fe^{4+} and Fe^{5+} are involved. E_0' values of approximately 1 V have been calculated for the Fe^{5+}–Fe^{4+} couple. For yeast cytochrome-c peroxidase (Dunford 1984) a sequence has been proposed for the formation of compound I and the involvement of a proximal imidazole ligand, acting as first a proton acceptor and then a proton donor to form a molecule of water (Fig. 10.10). The

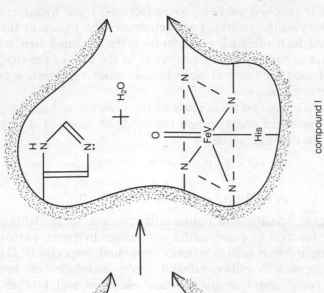

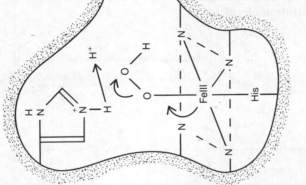

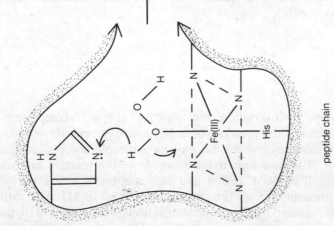

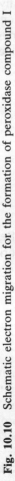

Fig. 10.10 Schematic electron migration for the formation of peroxidase compound I

haem iron is oxidised to Fe^{5+} on reduction of the hydroperoxide. The chemistry of the radicals $(A^{\bullet})$ determines the nature of the final products. At high substrate concentration the liberated free radicals $(A^{\bullet})$ interact to form polymers $(A-A)$ as in the case of the oxidation of guaiacol used for assay of peroxidases, which represents a typical peroxidatic reaction.

The catalatic reaction takes place in the presence of higher concentrations of hydrogen peroxide and the mode of action of the enzyme is identical to that of catalase.

$$Per-Fe^V = O + H_2O_2 \rightarrow HO^{\bullet}_2 + Per-Fe^{IV}-OH$$

$$Per-Fe^{IV}-OH + HO^{\bullet}_2 \rightarrow Per-Fe^{III}-H_2O + O_2$$

The divergent catalatic and peroxidatic reactions of peroxidases are due to the reaction of compound I with either hydrogen peroxide or other hydrogen donors such as hydroxy compounds respectively. Oxidatic reactions occur with either substrates like ascorbate, or hydroxyfumarate: compound I abstracts single electrons and protons from separate substrate molecules:

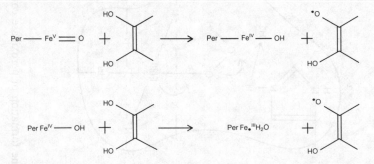

The free radicals may disproportionate to form one molecule of the original substrate (ascorbate) and the oxidised substrate (dehydroascorbate).

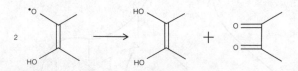

Alternatively, hydroxylation reactions of aromatic compounds are known to occur in the presence of either hydroxyfumarate or ascorbate radicals and oxygen, where the oxygen molecule accepts an electron and proton to form a superoxide anion from the reactive radicals.

The overall mode of action and reformation of native peroxidase can be represented by a cyclic mechanism (Fig. 10.11). The different peroxidatic, oxidatic and catalatic reactions with different hydrogen donor substrates are shown at (a), (b) and (c). The $O_2^{\overline{}}$ radical, possibly

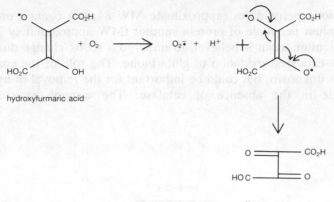

hydroxyfurmaric acid

diketosuccinic acid

through the Fenton reaction and generation of the reactive hydroxyl radical (HO˙), may ultimately cause the hydroxylation of aromatic phenols, such as tyrosine, to form an *o*-diphenol. Alternatively, for some peroxidase-catalysed reactions the oxygen atom of compound I and thus of the original peroxide may be transferred to an oxygen acceptor.

$$A + ROOH \rightleftharpoons ROH + AO$$

The presence of the different substrates like phenolics, hydroxyacids and ascorbate, together with the large number of isoperoxidases present in plant tissues, makes it probable that in post-harvest fruits and vegetables a whole series of oxidative reactions catalysed by peroxidases alone may take place. More than twenty compounds have been claimed for the oxidation of quercetin by peroxidases (Schreier and Miller 1985).

The biological function in the living plant of peroxidases is not fully understood, but in intact growing plants hydroxyl radicals (HO˙), formed as a result of peroxidase action, are believed to be required in order to complete the polymerisation of lignin and possibly initiate ethene production from methional. Peroxidase activity also increases either during the ripening of fruits and senescence in plants or as a result of physical and microbial damage to cellular tissues. Peroxidases occur in the antrocellular regions of plant cells and are not associated with mitochondria or peroxisomes. However, catalase enzymes are predominantly found in peroxisomes where they are required for the removal of hydrogen peroxide.

Glutathione peroxidases (EC 1.11.1.9.)

Living cells can also reduce hydrogen peroxide by using reduced glutathione acting as a specific hydrogen donor for glutathione peroxidase. In contrast to all other known peroxidases, tetrameric glutathione peroxidases (approximate MW 84,000) contain one atom of selenium per mole of protein subunit (MW approximately 24,000). The selenium atom is believed to undergo a redox change during the enzyme-catalysed oxidation of glutathione. The role of the enzyme in foods is unknown, but could be important for the removal of hydrogen peroxide in the absence of catalase. The enzyme may also be

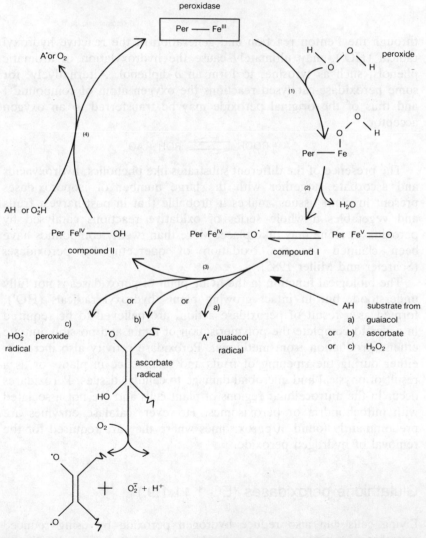

Fig. 10.11 Cyclic scheme for the formation of compound I and subsequent catalysed oxidation of electron-donating substrates

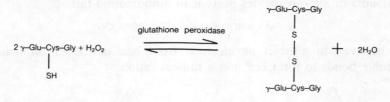

Action of glutathione peroxidase

important for bread dough development where excess reduced gluta-thione and any peroxide that arises during mechanical mixing may be simultaneously removed.

OXYGENASES

Enzymes which catalyse oxidation by the introduction of one oxygen atom into organic substrates are known as monooxygenases, whereas dioxygenases are responsible for catalysing the incorporation of both atoms of oxygen. From the triplet ground state oxygen will form complexes with transition metals:

$$Fe^{2+} \to O — O^{\bullet}$$

All oxygenases contain transition metals which form weak reversible coordination compounds with ligands and oxygen. Subsequently the way in which the metal–oxygen complex reacts with the substrate to incorporate either one or two atoms of oxygen, is influenced first, by the electron affinity of the active site ligands coordinated to the metal cation and secondly, by the electron-donating property of the substrate.

Although there are a large number of oxygenases specific for various aromatic substrates, only a small number of these enzymes are of obvious importance to the food industry. Of the dioxygenases only lipoxygenase, and possibly pyrocatechase, exert any significant oxida-tive effect in food products. From a biochemical point of view direct oxygenation of enoic acids is also important for prostaglandin synthesis.

Dioxygenases

LIPOXYGENASE (EC 1.13.11.12)

Lipoxygenases (linoleate : oxygen oxidoreductase) contain non-haem iron. Lipoxygenase catalyses the formation of stereospecific hydro-peroxides from polyunsaturated fatty acids containing the *cis,cis*-1,4-pentadiene unit (Ch. 6). Activated enzyme, containing high-spin ferric ion, Fe^{3+}, formed as a result of the oxidation of Fe^{2+} by only trace amounts of hydroperoxides present in autooxidised fats:

$$E–Fe^{2+} + ROOH \rightarrow E–Fe^{3+} + RO^{\bullet} + OH^{-}$$

is believed to abstract an electron from one of the unconjugated double bonds to form Fe^{II} and a radical cation:

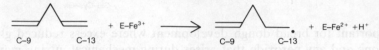

The involvement of oxygen is twofold: first, a metal oxygen complex ($Fe^{2+} \rightarrow O–O$) is formed and secondly, a subsequent oxygen radical formed by electron migration is directed on to the adjacent C-13 allylic radical to form a new carbon–oxygen bond.

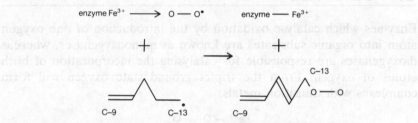

This mechanism assumes that the organic substrate is activated by the transition metal and not the ground state triplet oxygen. Such a mechanism overcomes the spin barrier between ground state triplet oxygen and the unsaturated fatty acid. However, as the transition metal and the activated oxygen molecules are in close proximity on the lipoxygenase enzyme, it seems likely (Jefford and Cadby 1981) that the dioxygenase enzyme, through the metal–oxygen complex, will bring together both the activated organic substrate and oxygen for the period of catalysis. The mechanism of action of lipoxygenases has been reviewed by Veldink and Vliegenthart (1984).

Although lipoxygenases are found in many plant tissues and particularly in cereal and legume seeds, their physiological function in living plants is not understood. However, in harvested fruits and vegetables, the hydroperoxides are degraded by hydroperoxide lyases to form unsaturated volatile carbonyl compounds which contribute to the characteristic flavour and aroma of many fruits. In living animals, dioxygenases, which include lipoxygenases and cyclooxygenase, convert polyunsaturated fatty acids present in cell membranes to hydroperoxides and prostaglandins. The mammalian lipoxygenases have been found mainly in various blood cells and several enzymes oxygenate polyunsaturated fatty acids at different positions. As in plant tissues small amounts of indigenous hydroperoxides convert Fe^{2+} to Fe^{3+}, the initial reaction in animal tissues likewise requires hydrogen abstraction from the substrate. Owing to a number of *cis*-double bonds in each molecule of the higher homologues, dioxygenation occurs at a number of different positions in the carbon chain. Thus mixtures of mono-hydroperoxy and dihydroperoxy fatty acids and endoperoxides are formed. Subsequent reduction of the conjugated hydroperoxides results in the formation of physiologically active compounds (see Ch. 6).

PYROCATECHASES (EC 1.13.11.1)

These are dioxygenases which catalyse the oxidative cleavage of ene-diols to form dicarboxylic acids. In most instances the substrates are aromatic diphenols. Chlorogenic acid and other diphenols present in plant tissues may afford suitable substrates for specific dioxygenases. The nutritional value of foods may also be affected by dioxygenases as ascorbate (a 1,2-diol) might be oxidised by ascorbate dioxygenase (EC 1.13.11.13), although the presence of this enzyme in foods has not yet been reported.

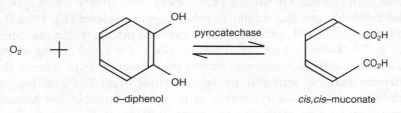

Fig. 10.12 Enzymatic action of pyrocatechase

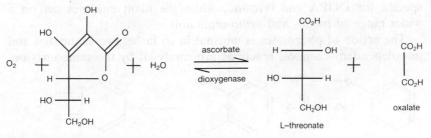

Fig. 10.13 Enzymatic action of ascorbate dioxygenase

Monooxygenases

PHENOLASES OR TYROSINASES (MONOPHENOL OXYGENASE EC 1.14.18.1 AND CATECHOL OXIDASE EC 1.10.3.1)

The most obvious non-microbiological deteriorative change in damaged fruit and vegetable products is browning caused by enzymatic oxidation. The enzymatic browning reaction is a result of a stepwise conversion of monophenol first to o-diphenol and secondly to quinone.

The carbonyl product then reacts non-enzymatically with other constituents, and in particular with amino compounds to form coloured pigments. Enzymatic browning is obvious in most peeled and cut fruits and occurs rapidly after cellular disruption. However, although excessive browning gives rise to undesirable products, advantage is sometimes taken of the reaction to produce a slightly yellow product as in pasteurised apple purée. Enzymatic browning is also responsible for the desirable colour of cocoa, coffee, tea products and dried fruits. Although substituted phenols comprise a large group of compounds, the substrates for enzymatic browning are in some cases simple substituted phenols or the more complex chlorogenic acid (Fig. 10.14) catechin and flavonyl glycosides. For tea, cocoa and coffee beans where enzymatic browning is beneficial, all the above biochemical parameters as well as the concentration of substrates are likely to vary between cultivars and depend on growing conditions. The affinity for the substrates by the plant phenolases is relatively low; the K_m values are high, usually of approximately 1 mM (although K_m values of 1.0 μM have been claimed for banana phenolases). The affinity for oxygen is also relatively low and similar to other copper oxidases (K_m from 0.1 to 0.5 mM). The pH optima for the enzymes is usually within the range 5.0 to 7.0. Damage to plant tissues results in the rapid mixing of the substrates and monophenol oxygenases (phenolases), where the enzymes may be activated by release from organelles and loss of inhibitors. In animals 'tyrosinase activity' is responsible for melanin formation by first catalysing the hydroxylation of tyrosine to form dihydroxyphenylalanine (DOPA) and subsequently catalysing the oxidation to form DOPA quinone. The animal enzymes are relatively specific for DOPA and tyrosine, while the plant enzymes act on a wider range of mono- and *ortho*-diphenols.

The action of phenolases is unusual in so far as two sequential and interdependent chemical reactions are catalysed by the same enzyme.

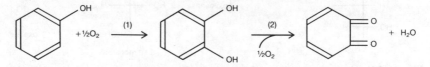

First an *o*-diphenol is formed by hydroxylation of monophenol and secondly *o*-quinone is formed by dehydrogenation of the diphenol. The overall reaction is a simplified representation of the phenolase-catalysed reactions. For hydroxylation a reducing agent is required to provide two electrons to reduce one atom of oxygen to water:

$$AH + O_2 + 2H^+ + 2e \rightleftharpoons H_2O + AOH$$

This is a typical reaction of monoxygenases where a separate reducing agent, which is the *o*-diphenol (Fig. 10.15), is required. The reaction is overall thermodynamically favourable due to the energy released by

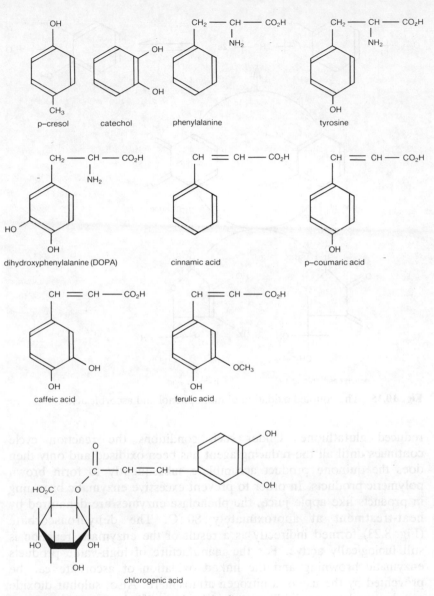

Fig. 10.14 Possible substrates for phenolase

the formation of water. The incorporation of the oxygen atoms into both water and the *o*-diphenol is verified by the use of $^{18}O_2$. The requirement of *o*-diphenol as the reducing agent is demonstrated by its ability to reduce a characteristic lag phase for the reaction. During enzymatic browning in whole fresh fruit products, the formed quinone is first recycled as it is reduced back to *o*-diphenol by reducing agents naturally present, such as ascorbate and possibly NADH, NADPH and

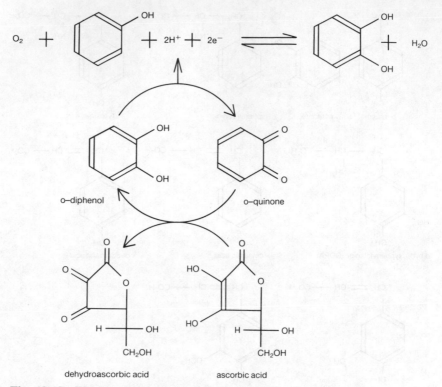

Fig. 10.15 The coupled oxidation of monophenol and ascorbic acid

reduced glutathione. Under such conditions the reaction cycle continues until all the reducing agent has been oxidised and only then does the quinone product accumulate subsequently to form brown polymeric products. In order to prevent excessive enzymatic browning in products like apple juice, the phenolase enzymes are denatured by heat-treatment at approximately 80 °C. The dehydroascorbate (Fig. 8.23) formed indirectly as a result of the enzymatic reaction is still biologically active. For the manufacture of high-value products enzymatic browning and the linked oxidation of ascorbate can be prevented by the use of a nitrogen atmosphere. Also, sulphur dioxide can be used as an inhibitor of phenolase (Wedzicha 1984). Small amounts of hydroxamic acids (10 nM) can be used as inhibitors (K_i 50 nM) as well as amino acids like cysteine (Kahn 1985).

For the laboratory preparation of phenolases, it is important to prevent the browning reactions which also involve deactivation of the phenolase enzyme itself by quinone products. Normally either excess ascorbate, or polyvinyl pyrrolidone are used to remove the quinone, while the enzyme is quickly separated from the substrates. Protamine sulphate has also been used to remove unwanted inactive protein. For purification of isoenzymes, hydrophobic chromatography using phenyl sepharose has proved useful because of the hydrophobic character of the enzymes. Enzymatic assays are based on the use of either p-cresol or catechol as mono- and diphenol substrates, with coupled measurements of either oxygen uptake, or the simultaneous formation of coloured addition products between the enzymatically generated quinone and amino acids like proline. Phenolases from different sources show a wide range of molecular sizes; some exist as monomers and others as dimers and tetramers. However, a characteristic of phenolases is the presence of two atoms of copper per active site which exists as a binuclear copper complex, $E(Cu^{2+})_2$. The distance between the copper atoms is calculated to be 0.6 nm. Spectral measurements indicate that the unpaired electrons of the two copper atoms interact in an antiferromagnetically coupled state and that a peroxy complex (Fig. 10.16) is formed in the presence of oxygen (Robb 1984). Both atoms of Cu^{2+} are reduced by transfer of electrons from o-diphenol to Cu^+ which are then used to reduce oxygen to water with coupled acceptance of $2H^+$ from the oxidised substrate. Cyanide acts as a competitive inhibitor to oxygen. For hydroxylation reactions with monophenol substrates, the O–O bond must undergo distortion and cleavage – a reaction which is thought to be influenced by the substituent ligands of the enzyme and the electrophilic nature of the substrate.

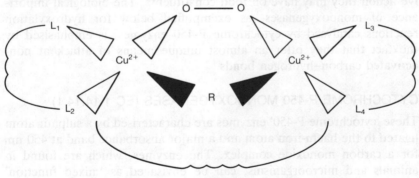

L = ligand

Fig. 10.16 A molecular structure for the oxygenated active site of tyrosinase (Robb 1984)

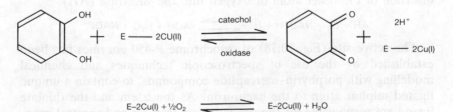

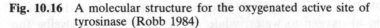

Fig. 10.17 The redox role of copper in catechol oxidase

Table 10.5 Some monooxygenase-catalysed reactions

Enzyme	Co-factors	Chemical changes
Phenylalanine monooxygenase	Dihydropterin	Phe→Try
Tyrosine monooxygenase	Tetrahydropterin	Tyr→DOPA
Proline monooxygenase	Fe, ascorbate and α-ketoglutarate	Pro→OHPro
Lysine monooxygenase	Fe, ascorbate and α-ketoglutarate	Lys→OHLys
Bacterial cytochrome P-450 (haem–thiolate proteins).	NADH/NADPH and flavins	Alkyl chains→alcohols
Liver microsome cytochrome P-450	NADPH and flavins	Aliphatic and aromatic hydroxylations as in drugs and steroids

There are many other monooxygenases present in foods of both animal and plant origin (Table 10.5). The significance of these enzymes in post-harvest and post-mortem foods remains largely unknown and attention can only be drawn to their presence and the possible oxidative action they may have on food constituents. The biological importance of monooxygenases, as exemplified below for hydroxylation reactions catalysed by cytochrome P-450 enzymes, is emphasised by the fact that they offer an almost unique means of attack at non-activated carbon–hydrogen bonds.

CYTOCHROME P-450 MONOOXYGENASES (EC 1.14.14.1)

These 'cytochrome P-450' enzymes are characterised by a sulphur atom ligated to the haem-iron atom and a major absorbance band at 450 nm for a carbon monoxide complex. The enzymes, which are found in animals and microorganisms, can be envisaged as 'mixed function' monooxygenases as these enzymes use a reducing agent, like $FADH_2$ or NADPH, as a source of two electrons to catalyse the reduction of one atom of oxygen to water, while at the same time catalysing the insertion of the other atom of oxygen into the substrate (AH).

$$AH + O_2 + NADPH + H^+ \rightleftharpoons AOH + H_2O + NADP^+$$

The active site (Fig. 10.18) of cytochrome P-450 enzymes has been established by the use of spectroscopic techniques and chemical modelling with porphyrin–mercaptide compounds, to contain a unique ligated sulphur atom to the haem-iron. As the haem and the thiolate ligand are responsible for the oxygen atom transfer and spectral properties, it has been suggested that these enzymes are renamed

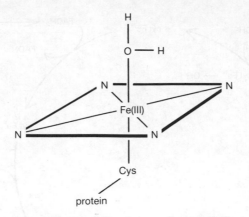

Fig. 10.18 Schematic diagram of the six coordinated Fe^{III} atom in cytochrome P-450 enzymes

haem–thiolate proteins (Enzyme Nomenclature 1984). The term 'cytochrome' is also inappropriate as the enzymes catalyse the transfer of oxygen atoms and not electrons. It seems likely that the sulphur atom plays a significant part as an electron donor to the iron atom to aid the cleavage of the diatomic oxygen molecule. The cytochrome P-450 monooxygenases also require flavins as a cofactor, because the overall cyclic scheme for the mode of action of the monooxygenase, requires reduction of Fe^{3+} to Fe^{2+} by a one-electron transfer step. The ferrous state serves to bind oxygen (Fig. 10.19) to form an iron peroxide after the transfer of two electrons from 2 moles of $FADH_2$. Support for the peroxide intermediate lies in the observations that first, peroxide may be released during the reaction at low substrate concentration and secondly, that hydrogen peroxide and other peroxides can replace the need for the FADH electron donor. The mechanism is similar to the mode of action of peroxidase, but in the latter case the radical A˙ is released. Whereas for hydroxylations catalysed by cytochrome P-450 type enzymes the radical cation A˙ is retained to combine with HO˙ to form AOH.

As for the many other enzyme catalysed reactions which occur in foods, the extent of catalysed oxidations depends substantially on the availability of substrate, the reaction rate constants and K_m values for the various enzymes.

ASCORBIC ACID OXIDATION

In fresh foods of plant origin, ascorbate can be oxidised by four separate mechanisms: ascorbate can be oxidised in the presence of transition metals; ascorbate is oxidised by a chemically coupled reac-

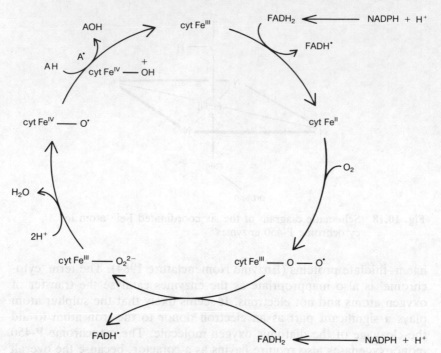

Fig. 10.19 A proposed scheme for hydroxylation of substrate (AH) by cytochrome P-450 (from White and Coon 1980)

tion with quinones which arise from the action of phenolase; ascorbate is dehydrogenated by ascorbate oxidase and Wedzicha (1984) has also described how ascorbate is degraded chemically during non-enzymic browning reactions.

In solution, in the presence of Cu^{2+} or Fe^{3+}, ascorbate is oxidised over a wide range of pH values, although the redox potential is pH dependent.

$$\text{dehydroascorbate} + 2H^+ + 2e^- \rightleftharpoons \text{ascorbate } E_o' = 0.08V$$

Therefore the overall coupled oxidative reaction with Fe^{3+} as oxidant

$$(Fe^{3+} \rightarrow Fe^{2+} \; E_o' = 0.77V)$$

is thermodynamically highly favourable at pH 7.0.

$$2Fe^{3+} + \text{ascorbate} \rightleftharpoons 2Fe^{2+} + \text{dehydroascorbate} + 2H^+ \; \triangle E_o' = 1.46V$$

Such a thermodynamically favourable reaction is obviously of major importance and accounts for the instability of ascorbate in processed foods as well as in fresh comminuted plant products. Indeed, the frequent occurrence of the autooxidative reaction for a long time prevented confirmation of the presence of ascorbate oxidase in plants until highly purified preparations of the enzyme were obtained.

Ascorbic acid oxidase (EC 1.10.3.3)

The enzyme is not an oxygenase, as oxygen is not incorporated into the oxidised substrate during the enzyme-catalysed reaction. However, it is convenient to describe its action here first, because of its effect during post-harvest changes in fruits and vegetables, secondly, because the enzyme is copper-dependent and thirdly, the enzyme catalyses a four-electron reduction of oxygen to water. Ascorbic acid oxidase has not been found in animals, but is very widespread in vegetables and fruits, where it is often associated with particulate cell wall material. In homogenised plant foods, such as fruit juices, it seems likely that as a result of the catalytic action of the enzyme that dehydroascorbate, will accumulate. K_m values for ascorbate of 0.2 mM have been quoted (Mondovi and Avigliano 1984). The enzyme-catalysed reaction results in the oxidation of 2 moles of ascorbate for the reduction of 1 mole of oxygen (Fig. 8.23). However, the biological function of ascorbate in plant tissues is largely unknown and only small amounts of dehydroascorbate ($< 5\%$ of the total vitamin C) are found in living plant cells. This equilibrium position may arise partly due to the action of glutathione dehydrogenase (EC 1.8.5.1) which catalyses the oxidation of reduced glutathione and the reduction of dehydroascorbate.

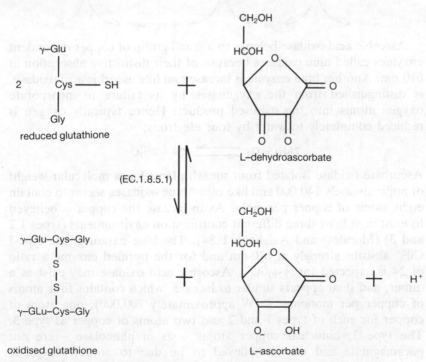

Fig. 10.20 The coupled oxidation of reduced glutathione and oxidation of dehydroascorbate

The reaction is thermodynamically favourable and a moderate affinity of the enzyme for dehydroascorbate (K_m, 0.3 mM) has been reported. Consequently, it has been suggested that dehydroascorbate (Mapson and Moustafa 1956) may be part of an indirect redox system for the reoxidation of NADPH – without coupled ATP synthesis (Butt 1980) – during lignin synthesis when extensive oxidation of carbon compounds takes place. A similar oxidative mechanism may also explain how ascorbate acts as an improver during the accelerated development of dough for bread manufacture. In this case it is postulated that the wheat flour ascorbate oxidase catalyses the formation of dehydroascorbate which then in turn oxidises reduced glutathione (GSH), either chemically or by an enzyme-catalysed reaction, so that reduced glutathione does not disrupt the required disulphide network of gluten proteins. Ascorbic acid oxidase is highly specific for the vicinial enediol adjacent to a carbonyl group, and therefore the enzyme might also catalyse the oxidation of naturally occurring o-diphenols which include catechols and flavonoids.

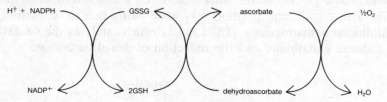

Ascorbic acid oxidase belongs to a small group of copper-dependent enzymes called blue oxidases because of their distinctive absorption at 610 nm. Another blue enzyme is laccase and like ascorbic acid oxidase, is distinguished from the oxygenases by its failure to incorporate oxygen atoms into the oxidised product. Hence typically oxygen is reduced completely to water by four electrons:

$$2AH_2 + O_2 \rightleftharpoons 2A + 2H_2O$$

Ascorbate oxidase isolated from squash plants has a molecular weight of approximately 140,000 and like other blue oxidases seems to contain eight atoms of copper per mole. As in laccase the copper is believed to exist in at least three different coordination environments (types 1,2 and 3) (Mondovì and Avigliano 1984). The blue paramagnetic type-I Cu^{2+} absorbs strongly at 610 nm and for the purified enzyme a ratio of 24 is expected for A_{280}/A_{610}. Ascorbic acid oxidase may exist as a dimer, and if so appears similar to laccase, which contains four atoms of copper per monomer (MW approximately 700,000); one atom of copper for each of types 1 and 2 and two atoms of copper as type 3. The type 3, binuclear copper atoms – as in phenolase – are not paramagnetic and this is believed to be due to antiferromagnetic coupling between closely positioned copper atoms. The four atoms per monomer would correspond with four different redox centres required to effect the reduction of O_2 to water.

For laccase[†] it has been proposed that single-electron single-electron reductions of the enzyme occur through type 1 (Cu^{2+}) and are transferred to type 3 ($Cu^{2+}-Cu^{2+}$). The type 1 (Cu^{2+}) site seems to be the ascorbate binding site while the type 3 binuclear site may represent the O_2 binding site as in phenolase. Redox titrations have given E_0 values of approximately 350 mV for the type 1 and type 3 sites. The removal of one electron from ascorbate by the type 1 (Cu^{2+}) atom generates an ascorbate free radical, which may permit further oxidation to proceed by non-enzymatic disproportionation.

KEY FACTS

1.   The stepwise univalent enzyme-catalysed reduction of oxygen results in the formation of superoxide radical, peroxide and oxide anions. Superoxide can act as either a reducing or oxidising agent towards other cellular constituents.

2.   Foods contain a large number of enzyme systems able both to regenerate and remove reduced oxygen species. In living tissues, superoxide dismutase and catalase protect cellular constituents by catalysing the removal of O_2^- and H_2O_2.

3.   In post-harvest foods both the cellular control of enzymatic activity and compartmentalisation of substrates may diminish, so that new substrates become available for oxidation. In heat-processed foods the activity of different enzymes is differentially affected by heat: some plant peroxidases are particularly thermostable.

4.   Many oxidative enzymes contain atoms of Fe or Cu for coordination of oxygen and the catalysis of redox reactions.

5.   Oxygenases active in foods include lipoxygenases, phenolases, cytochrome P-450 monoxygenases and ascorbic acid oxidase.

6.   Lipoxygenases catalyse the oxidation of polyunsaturated fatty acids to form hydroperoxides. They are responsible for oxidative rancidity and some loss of colour in plant foods.

7.   Phenolases catalyse the hydroxylation of phenolic compounds and the coupled oxidation of o-diphenols to form quinones. The quinones are responsible for enzymatic browning in fruits and vegetables. The quinones may also oxidise ascorbate to dehydro-ascorbate. Cytochrome P-450 (haem–thiolate proteins) enzymes can also catalyse hydroxylation of organic compounds.

[†] Laccase is not an enzyme significantly associated with food, although it has been found in peaches. Laccase (EC 1.10.3.2) is distinguished from phenolase by its oxidation of paradiphenols.

8.   Ascorbic acid oxidase catalyses the oxidation of ascorbate to dehydroascorbate in homogenised fruit products.
9.   During the development of wheat flour dough dehydroascorbate may oxidise reduced glutathione (GSH).

REFERENCES

Burnette, F. S. (1977) 'Peroxide and its relationship to food flavour and quality: A review', *J. Food Sci.*, **42**, 1–6.

Butt, V. S. (1980) 'Direct oxidases and related enzymes', in *The Biochemistry of Plants, A Comprehensive Treatise*, vol. 2 *Metabolism and Respiration* (ed. Davies, D. D.). Academic Press, New York.

Cadenas, E., Brigelius, R., Akerboom, T. and Sies, H. (1983) 'Oxygen radicals and hydroperoxides in mammalian organs: aspects of redox cycling and hydrogen peroxide metabolism', in *Biological Oxidations* 34. *Colloquium der Gesellschaft fur Biologische Chemie* (eds. Sund, H. and Ullrich, V.). Springer-Verlag, Berlin and Heidelberg.

Coughlan, M. P. (1980) 'Aldehyde oxidase, xanthine oxidase and xanthine dehydrogenase : hydroxylases containing molybdenum, iron–sulphur and flavin', in *Molybdenum and Molybdenum-containing Enzymes* (ed. Coughlan, M. P.). Pergamon Press, Oxford.

Dunford, H. B. (1984) 'Peroxidases', in *Advances in Inorganic Biochemistry*, vol. 4 (eds. Eichhorn, G. C. and Marzilli, L. G.). Elsevier Biomedical, Amsterdam.

Eichhorn, G. L. and Marzilli, L. G. (1980) 'Method for determining metal ion environments in proteins: structure and function of metalloproteins', *Advances in Inorganic Biochemistry*, vol. 2 (eds. Eichhorn, G. L. and Marzilli, L. G.). Elsevier North Holland, New York.

Elbe, J. H. von and Attoe, E. L. (1985) 'Oxygen involvement in betanine degradation – measurement of active oxygen species and oxidation reduction potentials', *Food Chem.*, **16**, 49–67.

Enzyme Nomenclature (1984) *Recommendations of the Nomenclature Committee of the International Union of Biochemistry on the Nomenclature and Classification of Enzyme-catalysed Reactions*. Academic Press, Orlando, Florida.

Fielden, E. M. and Rotilio, G. (1984) 'Structure and mechanism of Cu/Zn superoxide dismutase', in *Copper Proteins and Copper Enzymes*, vol. II (ed. Lontie, R.). CRC Press, Boca Raton, Florida.

Fridovich, I. (1979) 'Superoxide and superoxide dismutases', in *Advances in Inorganic Biochemistry*, vol. I (eds. Eichhorn, G. L. and Marzilli, L. G.). Elsevier North Holland, New York.

George, P. (1965) *Oxidases and Related Redox Systems*, vol. 1 (eds. King, T. E., Mason, H. S. and Morrison, M.). John Wiley and Sons, New York.

Graveland, A., Bosveld, P., Lichtendonk, W. J. and Moonen, J. H. E. (1984). 'Isolation and characterisation of (3-methoxy-4-hydroxyphenyl)-β-cellotrioside from wheat flour: a substance involved in the reduction of disulphide-linked glutenin aggregates', *J. Cer. Sci.*, **2**, 65–72.

Green, M. J. and Hill, H. A. O. (1984) 'Chemistry of dioxygen', in *Methods in Enzymology*, vol. 105 *Oxygen Radicals in Biological Systems* (ed. Packer, L.). Academic Press, Orlando, Florida.

Haard, N. F. (1977) 'Physiological roles of peroxidase in post-harvest fruits and vegetables', in *Enzymes in Food and Beverage Processing* (eds. Ory, R. L. and St Angelo, A. T.), American Chemical Society Symposium series 47. American Chemical Society, Washington DC.

Halliwell, B. (1984) 'Superoxide dismutase and the superoxide theory of oxygen toxicity. A critical appraisal', in *Copper Proteins and Copper Enzymes*, vol. II (ed. Lontie, R.). CRC Press, Boca Raton, Florida.

Harel, S. and Kanner, J. (1985) 'Hydrogen peroxide generation in ground muscle tissues', *J. Agric. Food Chem.*, **33**, 1186–88.

Jefford, C. W. and Cadby, P. A. (1981) 'Molecular mechanisms of enzyme-catalysed deoxygenation (an interdisciplinary review)', in *Fortschritte der Chemie organischer Naturstaffe (Progress in the Chemistry of Organic Natural Products)*, vol. 40 (eds. Herz, W., Grisebach, H. and Kirby, G. W.). Springer-Verlag, Vienna and New York.

Johnson, J. L. and Rajagopalan, K. V. (1977) 'Tryptic cleavage of rat liver sulphite oxidase. Isolation and characterisation of molybdenum and heme domains', *J. Biol. Chem.*, **252**, 2017–25.

Kahn, V. (1985). 'Effect of proteins, protein hydrolysates and amino acids on *o*-dihydroxyphenolase activity of polyphenol oxidase of mushrooms, avocado and banana', *J. Food Sci.*, **50**, 111–15.

McLellan, K. M. and Robinson, D. S. (1981) 'The effect of heat on cabbage and Brussels sprout peroxidase enzymes', *Food Chem.*, **7**, 257–66

McLellan, K. M. and Robinson, D. S. (1983), 'Cabbage and Brussels sprout peroxidase isoenzymes separated by isoelectric focussing', *Phytochem.*, **22**, 645–7.

McLellan, K. M. and Robinson, D. S. (1984) 'Heat stability of peroxidases from orange', *Food Chem.*, **13** , 139–47

Mapson, L. W. and Moustafa, E. M. (1956) 'Ascorbic acid and glutathione as respiratory carriers in the respiration of pea seedlings', *Biochem. J.*, **62**, 248–59.

Mondovì, B. and Avigliano, L. (1984) 'Ascorbate oxidase', in *Copper Proteins and Copper Enzymes*, vol. III (ed. Lontie, R.). CRC Press, Boca Raton, Florida.

Mondovì, B. and Riccio, P. (1984) 'Copper amino oxidases: structure and function', in *Advances in Inorganic Biochemistry*, vol. **6**, PP. 225–44 (eds. Eichhorn, G. L. and Marzilli, L. G). Elsevier, Amsterdam.

Rajagopalan, K. V. (1980) 'Sulphite oxidase', in *Molybdenum and Molybdenum-containing Enzymes* (ed. Coughlan, M. P.). Pergamon Press, Oxford.

Robb, D. A. (1984) *Tyrosinase* in *Copper Proteins and Copper Enzymes*, vol. II (ed. Lontie, R.). CRC Press, Boca Raton, Florida.

Schreier, P. and Miller, E. (1985) 'Studies on flavanol degradation by peroxidase (donor : H_2O_2-oxidoreductase, EC 1.11.1.7): part 2 – quercetin', *Food Chem.*, **18**, 301–17.

Veldink, G. A. and Vliegenthart, J. F. G. (1984) 'Lipoxygenases, nonheme iron-containing enzymes', in *Advances in Inorganic Biochemistry*, vol. 6 (eds. Eichhorn, G. L. and Marzilli, L. G.). Elsevier, Amsterdam.

Walker, J. L., McLellan, K. M. and Robinson, D. S. (1987) 'Heat stability of superoxide dismutase in cabbage', *Food Chem*, **23**, 245–56.
Wedzicha, B. L. (1984) *Chemistry of Sulphur Dioxide in Foods*. Elsevier Applied Science Publishers, London.
White, R. E. and Coon, M. J. (1980) 'Oxygen activation by cytochrome P-450', *Ann. Rev. Biochem.*, **49**, 315–56.

ADDITIONAL READING

Dunford, H. B. (1982) 'Peroxidases', in *Advances in Inorganic Biochemistry*, vol. 4 (eds. Eichhorn, G. L. and Marzilli, L. G.). Elsevier Biomedical, Amsterdam.
Fielden, E. M. and Rotilio, G. (1984) 'The structure and mechanism of Cu/Zn-superoxide dismutase', in *Copper Proteins and Copper Enzymes*, vol. 2. (ed. Lontie, R.). CRC Press, Boca Raton, Florida.
Groves, J. T. (1979), Cytochrome P-450 and other heme-containing oxygenases', in *Advances in Inorganic Biochemistry*, vol. 1 (eds. Eichhorn, G. L. and Marzilli, L. G.). Elsevier Biomedical, Amsterdam.
Hayaishi, O. and Asada, K. (1976) *Biochemical and Medical Aspects of Active Oxygen*. University Park Press, London.
Korycha-Dahl, M. B. and Richardson, T. (1978) 'Activated oxygen species and oxidation of food constituents', *CRC Crit. Revs. Food Sci. Nutr.*, **10** 209–41.
Ledward, D. A. (1984) 'Haemoproteins in meat and meat products', in *Developments in Food Proteins*, vol. 3 (ed. Hudson, B. J. B.). Elsevier Applied Science Publishers, London.
Mondovì, B. and Avigliano, L. (1984) 'Ascorbate oxidase', in *Copper Proteins and Copper Enzymes*, vol. III (ed. Lontie, R.). CRC Press, Boca Raton.
Mondovì, B. and Riccio, P. (1984) 'Copper amine oxidases: structure and function', in *Advances in Inorganic Biochemistry*, vol. 6 (eds. Eichhorn, G. L. and Marzilli, L. G.). Elsevier, Amsterdam.
Oberley, L. W. (1982) *Superoxide Dismutase*, vol. 1. CRC Press, Boca Raton, Florida.
Packer, L. (1984) 'Oxygen radicals in biological systems', in *Methods in Enzymology*, vol. 105 (ed. Packer, L.). Academic Press, Orlando, Florida.
Que, L. (1980) 'Non-heme iron dioxygenases. structure and mechanism', in *Structure and Bonding* vol. 40 (eds. Dunitz, J. D., Goodenough, J. B., Hemmerich, K., Ibers, J. A., Jorgensen, C. K., Nielands, J. B., Reinen, D. and Williams, R. J. P.). Springer-Verlag, Berlin and Heidelberg.
Robb, D. A. (1984) 'Tyrosinase', in *Copper Proteins and Copper Enzymes*, vol. II (ed. Lontie, R.). CRC Press, Boca Raton, Florida.
Spiro, T. G. (1985) *Molybdenum Enzymes*. John Wiley and Sons, New York.
Vámos-Vgyázó, L. (1981) 'Polyphenol oxidase and peroxidase in fruits and vegetables', *CRC Revs. Food Sci. Nutr.* **15**, 49–127.
Veldink, G. A. and Vliegenthart, J. F. G. (1984) 'Lipoxygenases nonheme iron-containing enzymes', in: *Advances in Inorganic Biochemistry*, vol. 6 (eds. Eichhorn, G. L. and Marzilli, L. G.) vol. 6. Elsevier, Amsterdam.

Vleingenthart, J. F. G., Veldink, G.A., Verhagen, J. and Slappendel, S. (1983). 'Lipoxygenases from plant and animal origin', in *Biological Oxidations*, vol. 34, *Colloquium der Gesellschaft fur Biologische Chemie* (eds. Sund, H. and Ullrich, V.). Springer-Verlag, Berlin and Heidelberg.

White, R. E. and Coon, M. J. (1980) 'Oxygen activation by cytochrome P-450', *Ann. Rev. Biochem.*, **49**, 315–56.

Appendices

INTRODUCTION

This main text describes catabolic processes relevant to food materials. The food scientist is chiefly concerned with the stability and manipulation of raw materials, like wheat flour, milk, meat, fish or fruits. The fundamental metabolic processes for all biological materials that take place are well understood and fully documented widely in other texts. Here the appendices provide quick reference to the basic concepts and metabolic pathways.

APPENDIX I   STANDARD REDOX POTENTIALS

NAD, FMN and FAD as electron acceptors

The transfer of pairs of electrons from the powerful reductants, e.g. acetaldehyde, hydrogen or NADH, directly to either triplet oxygen or

Table A.1   Standard oxidation–reduction potentials of some reactions[†]

Oxidant	Reductant	n	E_0' (V)
α-Ketoglutarate	Succinate + CO_2	2	−0.67
Acetate	Acetaldehyde	2	−0.60
Ferredoxin (oxidised)	Ferredoxin (reduced)	1	−0.43
$2H^+$	H_2	2	−0.42
O_2	$O_2^{\bar{}}$	1	−0.33
NAD^+	$NADH + H^+$	2	−0.32
$NADP^+$	$NADPH + H^+$	2	−0.32
Lipoate (oxidised)	Lipoate (reduced)	2	−0.29
Glutathione (oxidised)	Glutathione (reduced)	2	−0.23
Acetaldehyde	Ethanol	2	−0.20
Pyruvate	Lactate	2	−0.19
Flavoproteins	Reduced flavoproteins	1	−0.1 to 0.1

Table A.1 (Cont'd)

Oxidant	Reductant	n	E_0' (V)
Fumarate	Succinate	2	0.03
Cytochrome-b (+3)	Cytochrome-b (+2)	1	0.07
Dehydroascorbate	Ascorbate	2	0.08
Ubiquinone (oxidised)	Ubiquinone (reduced)	2	0.10
Cytochrome-c (+3)	Cytochrome-c (+2)	1	0.22
2,6-dichlorophenolindophenol (DCPIP)	Reduced DCPIP	2	0.26
Cu^{II}	Cu^{I}	1	0.34
Ferricyanide	Ferrocyanide	1	0.41
Fe^{3+}	Fe^{2+}	1	0.77
$\frac{1}{2}O_2 + 2 H^+$	H_2O	2	0.82
$O_2^{-} + 2 H^+$	H_2O_2	1	0.94

† After Lubert Stryer, *Biochemistry*, 2nd edn. Copyright © 1975, 1981 Lubert Stryer. Used by permission of W. H. Freeman and Company.

E_0' = standard oxidation – reduction potential (pH 7.0, 23 °C), n = number of electrons. A positive E_0' value signifies an exergonic reaction.

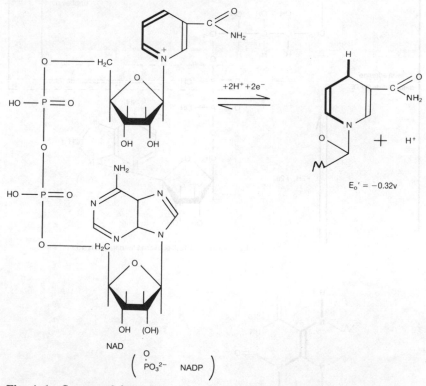

Fig. A.1 Structural formulae of electron carriers. NADHP is mainly used for synthetic reactions and is distinguished for this purpose by the phosphoryl group on the C-2 atom of ribose

Fe^{3+} does not occur. The energy change would be large ($\Delta G^{0\prime} = -n.\,F.\Delta E_0{}'$), harmful to the cell and wasteful. The series of electron carriers, NAD, FAD and cytochromes trickle electrons from low to high redox couples in the form of a cascade that allows the chemical trapping of energy at each step. For flavoprotein oxidases and dehydrogenases the variable redox potentials of protein-bound flavin chromophores determine whether O_2 or NAD^+ is used as an electron acceptor.

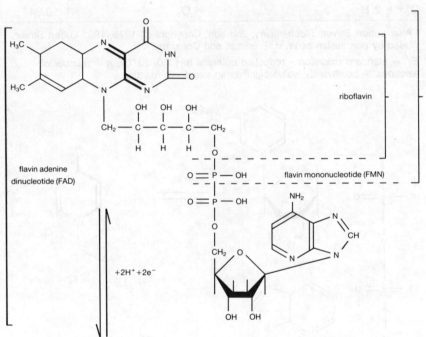

$E_o{}'$ = approx −0.15V, but varies for different flavoproteins

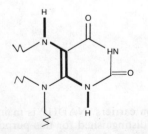

Fig. A.2 Flavin adenine nucleotides

APPENDIX II   ADENOSINE TRIPHOSPHATE AND OTHER ENERGY-RICH INTERMEDIATES

The free energy change ($\Delta G^{0\prime}$ at pH 7.0) of oxidative reactions can be trapped as chemical energy in the form of ATP. The biosynthesis of ATP is achieved by transfer of phosphate anions to either AMP or ADP. ATP is an energy-rich molecule because it contains negatively charged phosphate groups as anhydrides in a tetra-anionic form. On hydrolysis a large amount of free energy is released. ATP is the immediate source of energy in living tissues. The amounts of ATP are depleted in foods, as the energy released is used to fuel catabolic reactions.

$$ATP + H_2O \rightarrow ADP + PO_3^{2-} \quad \triangle G^{\circ\prime} = -7.6 \, Kcal$$

$$ATP + H_2O \rightarrow AMP + Pyrophosphate \quad \triangle G^{\circ\prime} = -8.8 \, Kcal$$

$$Pyrophosphate + H_2O \rightarrow 2PO_4^{2-} + 2H^+ \quad \triangle G^{\circ\prime} = -8.0 \, Kcal$$

In living tissues other high-energy phosphate (UTP and GTP) compounds provide the energy for biosynthetic reactions. UTP is synthesised from UMP by the transfer of a phosphate group from ATP catalysed by UMP kinase.

$$UMP + ATP \rightleftharpoons UDP + ADP$$

$$UDP + ATP \rightleftharpoons UTP + ADP$$

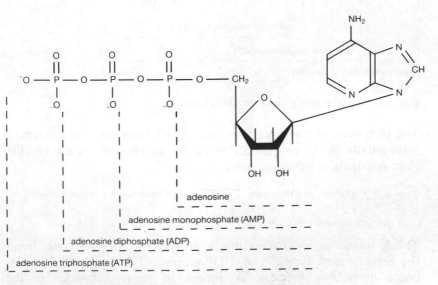

Fig. A.3   Adenosine phosphates

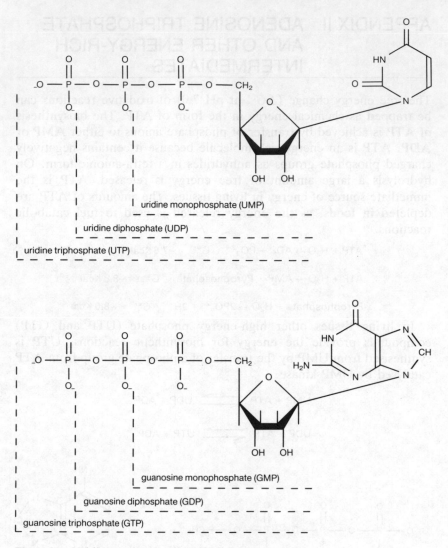

Fig. A.4 Uridine and guanosine phosphates

The directions of these reactions are evenly balanced and influenced substantially by the concentrations of the metabolites, as the equilibrium constants are close to unity.

$$\text{UTP} + \text{glucose-1-phosphate} \rightleftharpoons \text{UDP-glucose} + \text{pyrophosphate}$$

$$\text{pyrophosphate} + H_2O \rightarrow 2PO_4^{2-} + 2H^+ \quad \triangle G^{\circ\prime} = -8.0 \, \text{Kcal}$$

The spontaneous and irreversible hydrolysis of pyrophosphate drives the reaction and synthesis of UDP-glucose. The nucleoside diphosphate derivatives function as donors of monosaccharides in the synthesis of starch, glycogen, cellulose and oligosaccharides.

Table A.2 Energy-rich compounds formed by substrate level phosphorylation[†]

Compound	$\Delta G^{0'}$[‡] (kcal)
Glucose-1-phosphate	5.0
Glucose-6-phosphate	3.3
Glycerol-3-phosphate	2.2
Phosphoenolpyruvate	−14.8
Acetyl phosphate	−10.1
Acetyl CoA	−7.5

([†] Bridger and Henderson 1983).

[‡] $\Delta G^{0'}$ is the calculated free energy change on hydrolysis under physiological conditions at pH 7.0.

Phosphorylation of substrates provides a means of trapping energy. As end products of glycolysis, phosphoenolpyruvate and acetyl phosphate are very high energy compounds and readily transfer their phosphate group to either AMP, or ADP to form ATP.

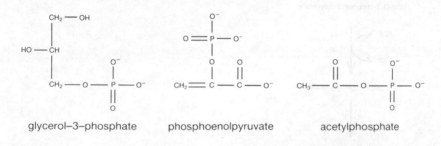

glycerol–3–phosphate   phosphoenolpyruvate   acetylphosphate

APPENDIX III   GLYCOLYTIC PATHWAYS

Glucose can be utilised chiefly for the production of reducing power (NADH) and ATP by four different pathways. The Embden–Meyerhoff–Parnas (EMP) and hexose monophospate (HMP) glycolytic pathways are used by mammals, plants, yeast and bacteria. Two other glycolytic pathways, the Entner–Doudoroff and phosphoketolase pathways are used by some bacteria. Glycolysis is the breakdown of glucose to pyruvate.

(a)   Embden–Meyerhoff–Parnas pathway

The EMP pathway is described as homofermentative because it gives rise to only one product, while the other pathways are heterofermentative.

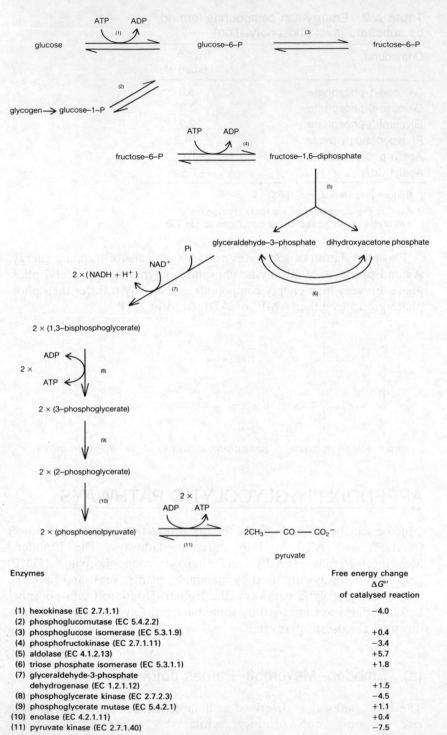

Enzymes	Free energy change $\Delta G^{o'}$ of catalysed reaction
(1) hexokinase (EC 2.7.1.1)	−4.0
(2) phosphoglucomutase (EC 5.4.2.2)	
(3) phosphoglucose isomerase (EC 5.3.1.9)	+0.4
(4) phosphofructokinase (EC 2.7.1.11)	−3.4
(5) aldolase (EC 4.1.2.13)	+5.7
(6) triose phosphate isomerase (EC 5.3.1.1)	+1.8
(7) glyceraldehyde-3-phosphate dehydrogenase (EC 1.2.1.12)	+1.5
(8) phosphoglycerate kinase (EC 2.7.2.3)	−4.5
(9) phosphoglycerate mutase (EC 5.4.2.1)	+1.1
(10) enolase (EC 4.2.1.11)	+0.4
(11) pyruvate kinase (EC 2.7.1.40)	−7.5

Fig. A.5 Embden–Meyerhoff–Parnas pathway

In the EMP pathway phosphorylation of fructose-6-phosphate to produce the hexose diphosphate is the control point. The enzyme, phosphofructokinase is inhibited by a lowering (allosterically by ATP) of its affinity for the substrate: thus glycolysis is inhibited when the energy content and the level of cellular ATP is high. The allosteric effect of ATP can also be amplified by citrate, which therefore also reduces glycolysis when ample supplies of citrate are available. The transfer of free energy from phosphoenolpyruvate is also inhibited allosterically by ATP.

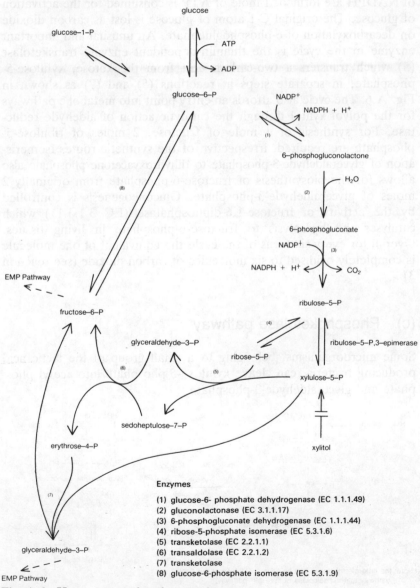

Enzymes

(1) glucose-6- phosphate dehydrogenase (EC 1.1.1.49)
(2) gluconolactonase (EC 3.1.1.17)
(3) 6-phosphogluconate dehydrogenase (EC 1.1.1.44)
(4) ribose-5-phosphate isomerase (EC 5.3.1.6)
(5) transketolase (EC 2.2.1.1)
(6) transaldolase (EC 2.2.1.2)
(7) transketolase
(8) glucose-6-phosphate isomerase (EC 5.3.1.9)

Fig. A.6 Hexose monophosphate pathway

(b) Hexose monophosphate pathway (pentose phosphate cycle)

This is an alternative pathway for the oxidation of glucose. The HMP pathway is important for the synthesis of pentoses as precursors of nucleotides. Although the pathway is principally cyclic and contains the pentose phosphate cycle, there are two separate links to the EMP pathway, through fructose-6-phosphate and glyceraldehyde-3-phosphate.

During the formation from glucose of ribulose-5-phosphate 2 moles of NADPH are formed, 1 mole of ATP is consumed for the activation of glucose. The original C-1 atom of glucose is lost as carbon dioxide on decarboxylation of 6-phosphogluconate. An unusual and important enzyme in the cycle is the thiamin-dependent enzyme transketolase (5) which transfers a two-carbon unit from the ketose, xylulose-5-phosphate, in separate steps at reactions (5) and (7) as shown in Fig. A.6. The cycle also affords an entry point into metabolic pathways for the polyol xylitol through the catalytic action of aldehyde reductase. For synthesis of 1 mole of fructose, 2 moles of ribulose-5-phosphate are required, irrespective of the synthetic route. Isomerisation of glyceraldehyde-3-phosphate to dihydroxyacetone phosphate also allows for the biosynthesis of fructose-6-phosphate from originally 2 moles of glyceraldehyde-3-phosphate. Gluconeogenesis is controlled by the activity of fructose-1,6-diphosphatase (EC 3.1.3.11) which catalyses the hydrolysis to fructose-6-phosphate in living tissues. Overall for every six turns of the cycle the equivalent of one molecule is completely oxidised to six molecules of carbon dioxide (see reaction 3).

(c) Phosphoketolase pathway

Some microorganisms, belonging to a small group of the lactic acid producing bacteria, can cleave xylulose-5-phosphate into acetyl phosphate and glyceraldehyde-3-phosphate.

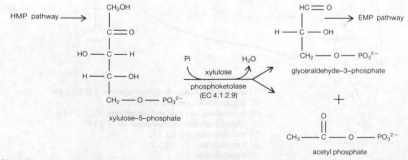

Note: the heterofermentative lactobacilli lack aldolase of the EMP pathway and transaldolase of the HMP pathway.

The glyceraldehyde-3-phosphate produced enters the EMP pathway and is oxidised to yield pyruvate and 2 moles of ATP. Acetyl phosphate obtained by substrate phosphorylation is an energy-rich compound able to supply 1 mole of ATP. Therefore overall, only 3 moles of ATP are synthesised per mole of glucose oxidised by the transketolase pathway. The overall reaction is:

$$ATP + glucose \rightarrow pyruvate + acetate + CO_2 + 3ATP + 2NADPH + NADH$$

(d) Entner–Doudoroff pathway

This pathway for glycolysis functions in strongly aerobic microorganisms such as pseudomonads. As with the HMP pathway, 6-phosphogluconate is produced alongside 1 mole of NADPH. However, the phosphogluconate is not decarboxylated but dehydrated.

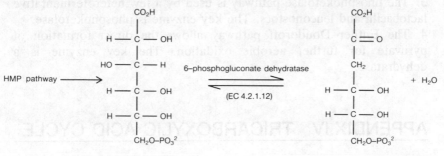

6-phosphogluconate   2 Keto-3-deoxy-6-phosphogluconate

The 2-ketose is cleaved by a specific aldolase (EC 4.2.1.14) to form pyruvate and triose.

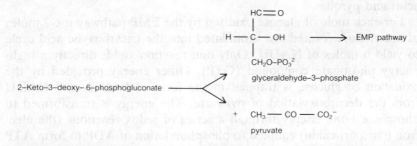

2 moles of ATP and 1 mole of NADH are formed if glyceraldehyde-3-phosphate enters the EMP pathway. The overall reaction is:

$$ATP + glucose \rightarrow 2\text{–pyruvate} + 2ATP + NADPH + NADH$$

Alternatively, by reversal of reaction (7) in the HMP pathway, transketolase may catalyse the biosynthesis of xylulose-5-phosphate from glyceraldehyde-3-phosphate and fructose-6-phosphate. Xylulose-5-phosphate can then provide pentoses for the biosynthesis of nucleotides.

Other monosaccharides such as galactose and fructose are isomerised and epimerised by enzyme-catalysed reactions in mammals to glucose phosphates. Sucrose and lactose are hydrolysed to yield monosaccharides. In some bacteria, and in particular those using milk as a growth medium, lactose can be phosphorylated and metabolised as galactose-6-phosphate (Tagatose pathway, Thompson 1978).

Summary

1. The EMP pathway provides the greatest yield of energy in the form of ATP. The key enzymes are phosphofructokinase and aldolase.
2. The HMP pathway provides less ATP but yields precursors for the biosynthesis of purines and pyrimidines. The key enzymes are 6-phosphogluconate dehydrogenase, transketolase and transaldolase.
3. The phosphoketolase pathway is used by a few heterofermentative lactobacilli and leuconostocs. The key enzyme is phosphoketolase.
4. The Entner–Doudoroff pathway allows the direct formation of pyruvate for further aerobic oxidation. The key enzyme is a dehydratase.

APPENDIX IV   TRICARBOXYLIC ACID CYCLE

The tricarboxylic acid cycle used by mammals, plants and microorganisms provides mainly NADH. Also three-, four- and five-carbon compounds are provided as precursors for the biosynthesis of amino acids and pyrolles.

For each mole of glucose oxidised by the EMP pathway the 2 moles of acetyl CoA formed are assimilated into the tricarboxylic acid cycle to yield 6 moles of NADH. Only one reaction yields directly a high-energy phosphate compound (GTP). Other energy provided by the oxidation of glucose is trapped in the form of $FADH_2$ and NADH from the decarboxylation of pyruvate. The energy is transformed to phosphate bond energy through a series of redox reactions (the electron transport chain) coupled to phosphorylation of ADP to form ATP and the reduction of oxygen to water: 1 mole NADH + H^+ yields 3 moles of ATP. The complete oxidation of glucose yields 36 moles of ATP. Without regeneration of NAD and FAD the tricarboxylic acid cycle fails to operate and therefore its use is confined to aerobic metabolism. An accumulation of reduced nucleotides causes product inhibition of pyruvate dehydrogenase (EC 1.2.4.1) and hence blocks the supply of acetyl CoA into the tricarboxylic acid cycle. In living tissues the accumulation of ATP inhibits isocitrate and α-ketoglutarate dehydrogenases.

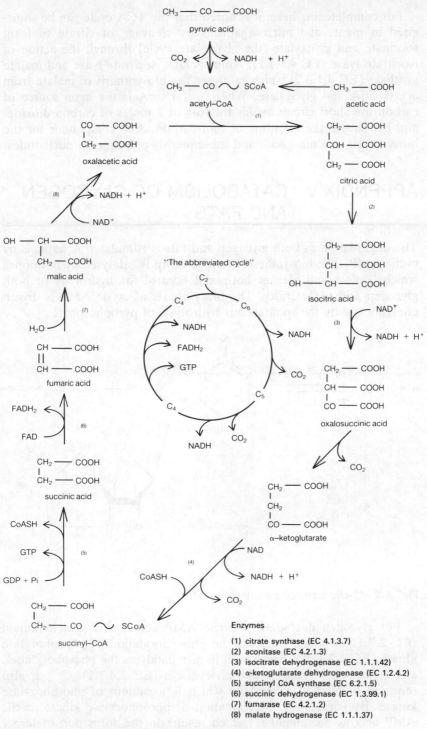

Fig. A.7 The tricarboxylic acid (TCA) cycle

For completeness here, it is noted that the TCA cycle can be short-ened in plants and microorganisms by cleavage of citrate to form succinate and glyoxylate (the glyoxylate cycle) through the action of isocitrate lyase (EC 4.1.3.1). Animals lack isocitrate lyase and malate synthase (EC 4.1.3.2) which catalyses the biosynthesis of malate from acetyl CoA and glyoxalate. When acetyl CoA is the main source of carbon the short circuit avoids the loss of 2 moles of carbon dioxide, and hence aids the retention of four-carbon atom compounds for the biosynthesis of amino acids and subsequently pentoses for nucleotides.

APPENDIX V   CATABOLISM OF GLYCOGEN AND FATS

The degradation of both glycogen and fats is stimulated in animals by cyclic AMP. The biosynthesis of cyclic AMP is catalysed by hormones which leads to an elegant hormonal control for hydrolysis of both glycogen and triglycerides. The biosynthesis of cyclic AMP is driven energetically by the spontaneous hydrolysis of pyrophosphate.

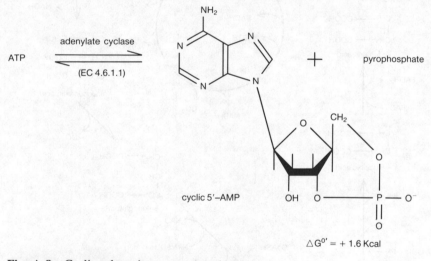

Fig. A.8   Cyclic adenosine monophosphate

For glycogen degradation, cyclic AMP activates a protein kinase (EC 2.7.1.37) which catalyses the phosphorylation of phosphorylase kinase (EC 2.7.1.38), which then in turn catalyses the phosphorylation and formation of (active) phosphorylase-a (EC 2.4.1.1). Ca^{2+} is also required to bind to calmodulin which is a subunit of phosphorylase kinase. By stimulating the formation of phosphorylase kinase, cyclic AMP acts as an 'amplifier' which results in the formation of larger amounts of active phosphorylase. Approximately 5 per cent of soluble muscle protein is phosphorylase, which in the active form catalyses the hydrolysis of glycogen to glucose-1-phosphate.

$$PO_4^{2-} + glycogen \xrightleftharpoons[]{\text{phosphorylase a}} glucose\text{–}1\text{–}phosphate$$

For the degradation of fats in animals cyclic AMP again stimulates the formation of a protein kinase which catalyses the phosphorylation of lipases. The liberated fatty acids are transported from adipose tissue via albumin–fatty acid complexes by the plasma to cells where they are degraded for the production of energy. The glycerol liberated by lipolysis diffuses into the plasma and as in other tissues such as liver and kidney is phosphorylated and reduced to dihydroxyacetone phosphate. This compound is an intermediate in the EMP pathway and can therefore be used either to form pyruvate, or alternatively for synthesis of fructose-1,6-diphosphate by the reverse EMP pathway.

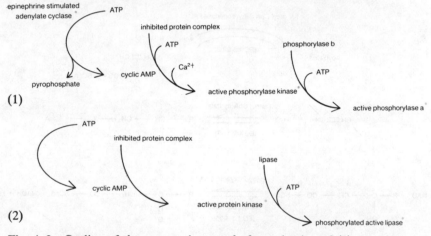

Fig. A.9   Outline of the enzymatic cascade for activation of (1) phosphorylase (2) lipases

Fatty acids are oxidised in mitochondria by β-oxidation to liberate sequentially the two-carbon units of acetyl CoA. The initial step requires activation of the fatty acid to the acyl CoA derivative before entry into the mitochondria. The overall reaction is irreversible due to spontaneous hydrolysis of pyrophosphate. An acyl-AMP derivative is formed as an intermediate.

Long-chain fatty acids (greater than C-10) are transferred across the mitochondrial membrane by carnitine as an acyl carnitine derivative.

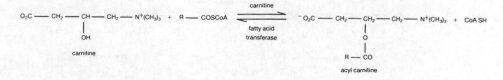

Inside the mitochondrion the reverse reaction results in the formation of free carnitine and an acyl CoA derivative, which is then degraded

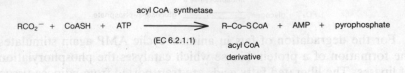

completely to produce acetyl CoA by sequential removal of two-carbon units.

For the β-oxidation of fatty acids two separate dehydrogenases are required with NAD and enzyme-linked FAD as hydrogen acceptors. A β-hydroxyacyl CoA derivative formed by hydration of the *trans*-enoyl CoA compound is the L-isomer. Carbon–carbon bond cleavage is catalysed by β-ketoacylthiolase.

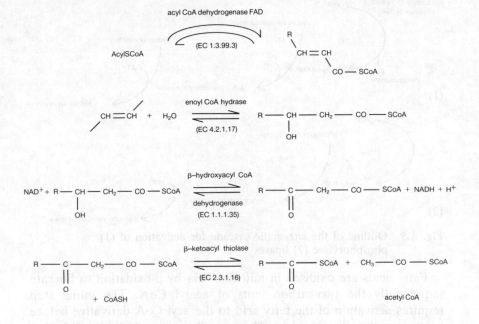

For natural unsaturated fatty acids the double bond of a 3-enoic acid of the *cis*-configuration is first isomerised to facilitate the formation of the L-3-hydroxyacyl CoA derivative.

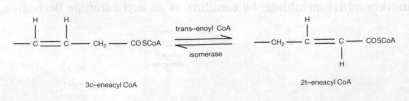

APPENDIX VI   CLASSIFICATION OF ENZYMES

The SI unit of activity is the Katal, which is the amount of enzyme required to convert 1 mole of substrate to product in 1 sec. *Specific activity of an enzyme* is the catalytic activity per milligram of protein.

Nomenclature (after Enzyme Nomenclature 1984)

Enzymes are classified as described by the IUPAC–IUB Commission on Biochemical Nomenclature–revised Enzyme Nomenclature 1984 under six headings according to the nature of the chemical reactions they catalyse. The main divisions are:

1. *Oxidoreductases*: this class of enzymes includes all those which catalyse oxidation–reduction reactions by either the transfer of hydrogen or the incorporation of oxygen into the substrate.
2. *Transferases*: these are enzymes which transfer chemical groups such as methyl, glycosyl and amino groups.
3. *Hydrolases*: these enzymes catalyse hydrolytic reactions, for example, the hydrolysis of glycosides and phosphate esters.
4. *Lyases*: these enzymes catalyse the cleavage of carbon–carbon bonds, carbon–oxygen bonds, and carbon–nitrogen bonds, by reactions other than hydrolysis. For example, the β-elimination reaction for pectin lyase.
5. *Isomerases*: these enzymes catalyse intramolecular rearrangements. These may include isomerisation and mutarotation.
6. *Ligases*: these enzymes catalyse biomolecular synthetic reactions which require ATP for a source of energy. They are coupled to the hydrolysis of the pyrophosphate bond or similar triphosphate.

Each enzyme is given a four-digit number which indicates its main features as a catalyst. Name of enzyme, A, B, C, D.
A. indicates the class of enzyme, e.g. oxidoreductase.
B. indicates the nature of the general substrate of the group involved.
C. indicates the specific coenzyme or substrate.
D. indicates the numerical or serial number of the enzyme.

Further details of the key to numbering the classification of the enzymes, and a full enzyme list is given in Enzyme Nomenclature (1984).

APPENDIX VII   ENZYME KINETICS

The catalytic activity of enzymes is frequently expressed in the terms of K_m values, rate constants or turnover number. The derivatisation of these constants is given in specialist texts of enzymology with elements of this reproduced in numerous other texts. A suitable standard treatment of kinetics is given by Holme and Peck (1983). Given in this appendix is a summary of the conceptual meaning of the various constants.

Turnover number

This is the rate of catalysis per molecule of enzyme so that:

$$k_{cat} = V_{max}/e \tag{1}$$

where e is the total concentration of enzyme. Therefore

$$V_{max} = k_{cat} \cdot e$$

For industrial processes where the substrate is present in large excess, V_{max} can be estimated simply from the enzyme concentration. However, frequently the precise concentration of pure enzyme is unknown. Only for very pure enzymes can the concentration be related to protein concentration. For impure enzymes, sometimes titration of an active site group, such as a thiol group, can be carried out separately to determine the real concentration of enzyme.

Michaelis constant K_m

It follows from the classical well known Michaelis–Menten equation for a single substrate reaction at intermediate concentrations of substrate:

$$V_i = \frac{V_{max} \; [S]}{K_m + [S]} \tag{2}$$

$V_i = V_{max}/2$, when $K_m = [S]$ (substrate concentration).
The numerical value of K_m is the concentration of substrate, expressed in molar quantities required to achieve half the maximum velocity for an enzyme-catalysed reaction. K_m, is essentially the dissociation constant for an enzyme–substrate complex

$$E + S \underset{k_2}{\overset{k_1}{\rightleftharpoons}} ES \underset{k_4}{\overset{k_3}{\rightleftharpoons}} E + P$$

So that

$$K_m = \frac{k_2 + k_3}{k_1 + k_4}$$

but k_4 is negligible, therefore

$$K_m = \frac{k_2 + k_3}{k_1}$$

The K_m value, which varies from 10^{-1} to 10^{-6}M is a particularly useful measurable parameter to determine the behaviour of an enzyme towards different substrates. The K_m value measures the equilibrium constant of the enzyme–substrate complex. It is an indicator of the affinity of the enzyme for substrate, and is used to identify the concentration of substrate required for fast reactions. However, it does not provide a measure of the maximum velocity at which enzyme-catalysed reactions take place when an enzyme is fully saturated with a substrate present in excess. Under these conditions $V_{max} = k_3[e]$, which is zero-order with respect to substrate as given in equation (1).

For intermediate levels of substrates the relative importance of enzyme-catalysed reactions in living cells, or homogenates, can only be assessed if both V_{max} and K_m values are known. The ratio V_{max}/K_m is the best value to indicate the relative effectiveness of an enzyme towards various substrates. The numerator includes both k_{cat} and e. Thus the ratio incorporates the key parameters that determine the speed of enzyme-catalysed reactions in either homogenates or cell organelles. For many enzymes the ratio V_{max}/K_m is 10^9, and therefore the rate of reaction (V_i) is only limited by diffusion of substrates and products.

The food scientist, for practical purposes, is mainly concerned with the use of enzyme-catalysed reactions for both the detection of enzymes in foods (e.g. lipase activity in milk) and the analysis of food constituents (e.g. glucose in honey using the glucose oxidase assay). For both these purposes the initial velocity of the catalysed reaction is frequently the measurement preferred.

For the detection of enzymes, the substrate is required in excess, so that $V_i \propto k_{cat}[e]$, (or $k_3.e$). The K_m value should be low, so that the rate of formation of ES is maximised and $V_i = k_3[e]$. The concentration of the substrate should be at least five times the K_m value. From

$$V_i = \frac{V_{max}\ [S]}{K_m + [S]}$$

the initial velocity of the reaction at various substrate concentrations can be calculated as below:

[S]	V_i
$5 \times K_m$	83.3 % V_{max}
$10 \times K_m$	90.9 % V_{max}
$100 \times K_m$	99.0 % V_{max}

However, the requirement for a high concentration of substrate may be limited in some cases by either the solubility of the substrate, or possible substrate inhibition of the enzymatic reaction.

For the assay of substrates, excess enzyme is required to be present in the assay solution so that $V_i = k_1[S]$, and is first order with respect to substrate concentration. Therefore for both types of application,

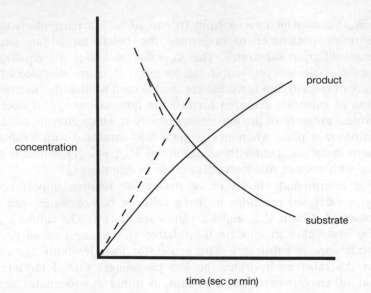

Fig. A.10 Characteristic reaction curves for enzyme-catalysed reactions

knowledge of the V_{max}/K_m ratio is useful for the preliminary selection of the most appropriate enzymes and substrates.

For measurement of the initial velocity (V_i) of an enzymatic reaction, the tangent is drawn to a progress curve (Fig. A.10). The initial rate phase of an enzymatic reaction may last for a few seconds or up to several minutes. For measurement of the changing concentrations of reactants and products, spectrophotometric, or pH stat methods may be used for continuous assay, as opposed to sampling methods based on longer time periods, where the rates of reactions are no longer linear. Generally the initial rate will persist until approximately 5 to 10 per cent of the substrate has been used, where for thermodynamically favourable reactions, the system is not approaching equilibrium. The most common assays involve NAD$^+$-linked dehydrogenases, where the high molar extinction value for NADH is beneficial ($\epsilon_m = 6.22 \times 10^3$ M^{-1} cm^{-1}). In some systems the inhibition constants for a particular product are quite low, whereas for others the product formed is frequently a potent inhibitor. For the dehydrogenases the rate of the forward and reverse reactions are often substantially affected by hydrogen ion concentration and therefore the appropriate pH value should be selected for the direction of the reaction which is going to be used.

Alternative methods for enzymatic assays using end-point methods have been frequently used for quantifying substrates. The reactions do not go to completion nor reach equilibrium; the extent of which may be variable between samples. The equilibrium position may be changed by the use of trapping agents for one of the products or by changing the pH value. Numerous methods have been devised and experimental details are given in the series by Bergmeyer.

Coupled enzymatic assays for substrates

One example of many coupled assays is the estimation of glucose with either hexokinase and glucose-6-phosphate dehydrogenase, or with glucose oxidase coupled to peroxidase. Many other examples of coupled assays have been tabulated by Allison and Purich (1979).

Generally a large excess of the second enzyme (E_2) is used to ensure that the second reaction is first order with respect to (I) as the substrate for the second indicator reaction.

$$S \xrightarrow{E_1} P(I) \xrightarrow{E_2} P(II)$$

Normally the concentration of [P(I)] is small, hence

$$V_i \simeq \frac{V_{max} \cdot [P(I)]}{K_m} \text{ for } E_2$$

The ratio V_{max}/K_m for E_2 is adjusted to 100 times that for E_1, by increasing the amount of enzyme (E_2). The only rate-limiting factor in a coupled assay should be the concentration of the initial test substrate for the enzyme (E_1); and all other substrates used should be present in excess and be saturating with respect to the enzymes E_1 and E_2. For example, for the estimation of glucose, E_1 (hexokinase) should be saturated with ATP and Mg.

E_2 (glucose-6-phosphate dehydrogenase) should be saturated with NAD$^+$. For assay of the enzyme hexokinase, then V_i for E_1 should be zero order with respect to both glucose and ATP, so that all substrates are saturating for E_2.

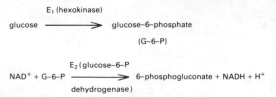

However, in practice too high a concentration of ATP inhibits the glucose-6-phosphate dehydrogenase (E_2). For economical use the required amounts of coupled enzymes should be calculated using a procedure outlined by Allison and Purich (1979).

Determination of K_m and V_{max} values

The most popular method has been the double reciprocal plot of

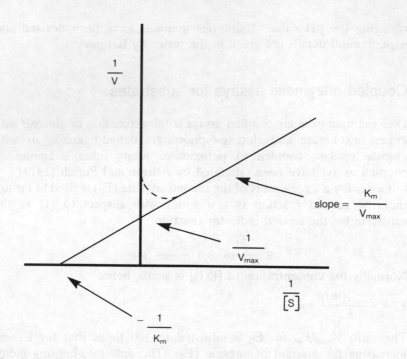

Fig. A.11 Typical Lineweaver–Burk plot for $1/V$ versus $1/[S]$

$1/V$ against $1/[S]$ (Fig. A.11) derived by rearrangement of the Michaelis–Menten equation for single substrate reactions:

$$\frac{1}{V_i} = \frac{K_m}{V_{max}} \cdot \frac{1}{[S]} + \frac{1}{V_{max}}.$$

Numerical values for V_{max} and K_m are determined from the intercept

$$\frac{1}{S} = -\frac{1}{K_m} \text{ at } \frac{1}{V_i} = 0$$

and

$$\frac{1}{V_i} = \frac{1}{V_{max}} \text{ at } \frac{1}{S} = 0$$

Unfortunately the experimental values obtained at very low substrate concentrations (high values of $1/V_i$) are the furthest from the origin of the graph and hence tend to exert the greatest influence on the extrapolated values for K_m and V_{max}. However, statistical analysis of results from a number of separate experiments coupled to computerised techniques minimises the incurred errors. K_m values of 10^{-6}M demonstrate a high affinity of the enzyme for the substrate, although even for such enzymes the rate of reaction may still be low as determined by V_{max}.

Two substrate (S_1 and S_2) reactions

There are mainly two ways in which enzymes catalyse the biomolecular reaction of two substrates. Further small modifications involving the ordering of reactants are given by Fromm (1979). Summarising either a ternary complex is formed:

$$E + S_1 + S_2 \rightleftharpoons ES_1S_2$$

or binary complexes are formed

$$E + S_1 \rightleftharpoons ES_1 \text{ and}$$

$$E(\text{modified}) + S_2 \rightleftharpoons E.S_2$$

The mechanisms are distinguished in the double reciprocal plots.

For the ternary complex, all substrates are present simultaneously at the enzyme active site before catalysis of the reaction can occur.

$$\text{For } S_1 + S_2 \rightarrow P_1 + P_2$$

The ternary complex is ES_1S_2 which gives EP_1P_2 before liberation of the products. The reaction may be ordered, as with many NAD(P)-dependent dehydrogenases where the coenzyme is the leading substrate (S_1) to form a non-catalytic S_1E complex, viz. the ordered BiBi mechanism (Fig. A.12(a)),

For these reactions, K_m values for S_2 can be obtained at high concentrations of S_1 (e.g. when S_1 is NAD$^+$), that are well in excess of the K_m value for NAD. However, separately from the above schematic mechanism ternary complexes can also be formed in a random manner.

For the binary mechanism S_1 is bound to the enzyme to form a modified enzyme.

$$E + S_1 \rightarrow ES_1 \rightarrow P_1 + F$$

$$F + S_2 \rightarrow FS_2 \rightarrow P_2 + E$$

When P_1 is liberated the enzyme is modified to F, which complexes with the second substrate (S_2); the mechanism is described as Binary Ping-Pong BiBi.

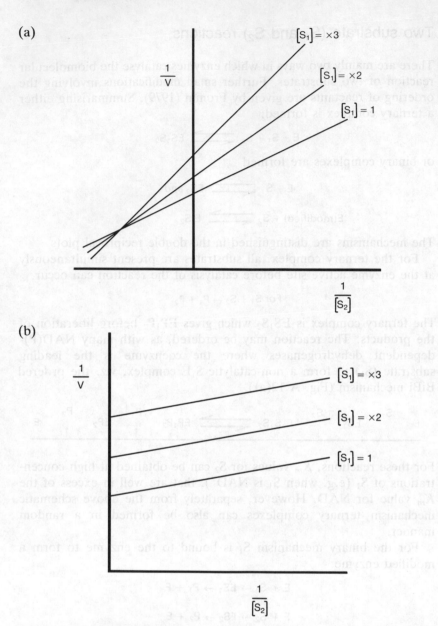

Fig. A.12 Reciprocal plots for two substrate reactions

For such a reaction the double reciprocal plot consists of series of parallel lines (Fig. A.12(b)) and is exemplified by transaminations where the enzyme–pyridoxamine complex carrying the $-NH_2$ group represents F. Reciprocal plots for glucose oxidase catalysed reactions show that the two substrates (oxygen and glucose) interact separately with the enzyme to form binary complexes.

Enzymatic inhibition

An inhibitor (I) decreases the rate of enzyme-catalysed reactions. The efficiency of an inhibitor is quantified by K_i, the dissociation constant of the enzyme inhibitor which can be determined as described below.

Competitive inhibition

$$E + I \rightleftharpoons EI$$

The effects are reversible and are reduced by high concentrations of substrate:

$$K_i = \frac{[E][I]}{[EI]}$$

The total enzyme concentration is the sum of three components, so substituting for [EI]:

$$\Sigma e = [E] + \frac{[E][I]}{K_i} + [ES]$$

$$= [E]\left(1 + \frac{[I]}{K_i}\right) + [ES]$$

As $\quad K_m = \frac{[E][S]}{[ES]}$

$$[E] = \frac{K_m[ES]}{[S]}$$

Therefore

$$\Sigma e = \frac{K_m \cdot [ES]}{[S]}\left(1 + \frac{[I]}{K_i}\right) + [ES]$$

$$\Sigma e = [ES]\left\{\frac{K_m}{[S]}\left(1 + \frac{[I]}{K_i}\right) + 1\right\}$$

$$[ES] = \frac{e\,[S]}{K_m\,(1 + [I_i]/K_i) + [S]}$$

substituting

$$V_i = k_3\,[ES]$$

$$V_i = \frac{e \cdot k_3\,[S]}{K_m\,(1 + [I]/K_i) + [S]}$$

Therefore

$$V_i = \frac{V_{max} \cdot [S]}{K_m\,(1 + [I]/K_i) + [S]}$$

Thus for the reciprocal plot of Michaelis–Menten equation (Fig. A.13(a)) the intercept on the abscissa is increased by $(I + [I]/K_i)$

(a)

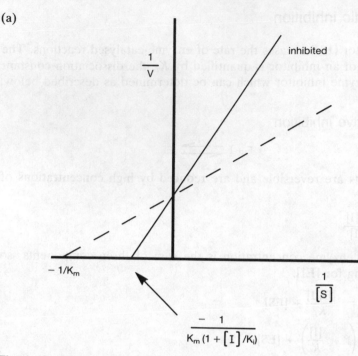

Fig. A.13   Reciprocal plots to determine K_i
(a) Competitive inhibition

and therefore a greater concentration of substrate is needed to saturate the enzyme:

$$\frac{1}{V_i} = \frac{K_m\,(1 + [I]/K_i)}{V_{max}[S]} + \frac{1}{V_{max}}$$

Competitive inhibitors are effective because the chemical structure of the inhibitor mimics that of the substrate. Examples are pepstatin and proteinase inhibitors, like trypsin inhibitors found in plant seeds. These inhibitors possess peptide bonds for which the enzyme's active site has a high affinity. For substrates the products are released, whereas for an inhibitor the enzyme–inhibitor complex remains.

Non-competitive inhibition

The process is not reduced by excess substrate and generally there is no chemical similarity between the inhibitor and the substrate. Thus the quantity of available active enzyme is less, and therefore the measurable V_{max} is reduced. The K_m value for the residual active enzyme remains unchanged. The substrate does not affect the binding of the inhibitor to the enzyme, and none of the inhibitor–enzyme complexes can yield products. The inhibited species are EI and EIS or ESI, where

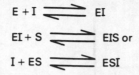

so e = E + ES + EI + EIS

and $K_i = \dfrac{[E][I]}{[EI]} = \dfrac{[EIS]}{[E][I]}$

For the reciprocal plot of the Michaelis–Menten equation (Fig. A.13(b)) the intercept on the ordinate is increased by $(I + [I]/K_i)$. Using a similar method of derivation as above:

$$V_i = \frac{[S].V_{max}/(1 + [I]/K_i)}{[S] + K_m}$$

$$\frac{1}{V_i} = \frac{K_m(1 + [I]/K_i)}{[S]\, V_{max}} + \frac{(1 + [I]/K_i)}{V_{max}}$$

Examples are the inhibition of haem- and copper-containing enzymes by cyanide and the inhibition of serine proteinases by diisopropylphospho-fluoridate which react irreversibly with the active sites to destroy a proportion of the enzyme. Inhibition by excess substrate is also a special example of non-competitive inhibition where,

e = E + ES + ESS

and $K_i = \dfrac{[ESS]}{[S][ES]}$

At high substrate concentration, the enzyme is thus present entirely as the unreactive complex, ESS.

Uncompetitive inhibition

Both K_m and V_{max} are changed by uncompetitive inhibitors. For both K_m and V_{max} to decrease less substrate is required to saturate the enzyme, but the amount of active enzyme–substrate complex present [ES] has fallen. Thus indicating that the effect of the inhibitor is to increase the stability of the enzyme–substrate complex (ESI), so that ESI does not yield product

$$\text{E + S} \rightleftharpoons \text{ES + I} \rightleftharpoons \text{ESI}$$

therefore e = E + ES + ESI

$$V_i = \frac{V_{max}\,[S]/(1 + [I]/K_i)}{[S] + K_m/(1 + [I]/K_i)}$$

$$1/V_i = \frac{K_m}{V_{max}.[S]} + \left(1 + \frac{[I]}{K_i}\right).\frac{1}{V_{max}}$$

(b)

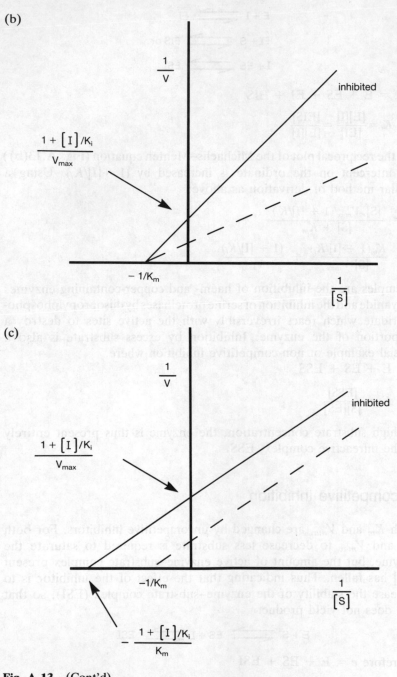

(c)

Fig. A.13 (Cont'd)
(b) Non-competitive inhibition
(c) Uncompetitive inhibition

The intercept on the ordinate is increased while the intercept on the abscissa is decreased (Fig. A.13 (c)).

ALLOSTERIC ENZYMES

The activity of some enzymes is controlled by the presence of allosteric inhibitors and activators. The term 'allosteric' means that there is not necessarily any stereochemical relationship between the inhibitors or activators and the substrate. Allosteric enzymes do not follow Michaelis–Menten kinetics, as the velocity substrate curve is of a sigmoidal shape (Fig. A.14). The allosteric inhibitors and activators control the activity of the enzyme, and hence the rate of the reaction, by changing the conformational structure of the enzyme. An allosteric inhibitor, like ATP, changes the conformation of an enzyme such that its substrate binding is reduced, or even prevented. Whereas an allosteric activator, like AMP, changes the conformation of the enzyme, so that the binding of the substrate to enzyme is enhanced. However, the sigmoidal nature of the curves is explained by assuming that the favoured conformation of the enzyme not only binds substrate, but also acts as an amplifier by affecting directly the conformation of other enzyme molecules. In this way the effect of a small amount of allosteric component is amplified throughout the enzyme molecules present in solution. By analogy haemoglobin is an allosteric protein;

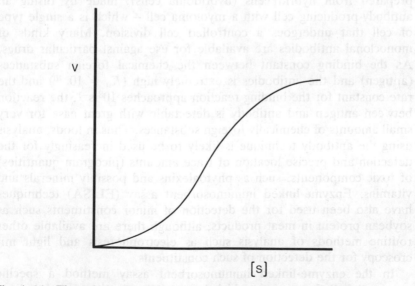

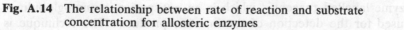

Fig. A.14 The relationship between rate of reaction and substrate concentration for allosteric enzymes

the binding of one molecule of oxygen to haemoglobin enhances the binding of additional oxygen molecules to the same haemoglobin molecule; a well known allosteric enzyme is 6-phosphofructokinase which is inhibited by ATP and citrate but is activated by AMP, ADP, inorganic phosphate and fructose-6-phosphate. Activation by AMP or ADP, changes the conformation of the enzyme such that it is converted to a more active form. Additionally this active form of the enzyme also generates further molecules of active enzyme. Allosteric enzymes contain separate sites in the enzyme molecule for the complexing of the allosteric activators and inhibitors. These sites are also different from the catalytic sites of the enzyme. Because of the cooperative effects, allosteric inhibitors are not regarded as competitive and non-competitive inhibitors.

APPENDIX VIII   ENZYME-LINKED IMMUNOSORBENT ASSAY

In animals, antibodies (immunoglobulins) are secreted by plasma cells in response to the presence of foreign macromolecules; small foreign molecules do not stimulate antibody formation. However, an immunological response can be elicited if the small molecules are attached to large macromolecules, which then act as carriers. Although antibodies produced by all animals are heterogenous, antibodies produced by single cells are homogenous. Monoclonal antibodies can now be prepared from hybrid cells (hybridoma cells), made by fusing an antibody-producing cell with a myoloma cell – which is a single type of cell that undergoes a controlled cell division. Many kinds of monoclonal antibodies are available for use against particular drugs. As the binding constant between the chemical foreign substances (antigen) and the antibodies is extremely high ($K_a = 10^{-10}$) and the rate constant for the binding reaction approaches 10^8 s^{-1}, the reaction between antigen and antibody is detectable with great ease for very small amounts of chemically foreign substances. Thus in foods, analysis using the antibody technique is likely to be used increasingly for the detection and precise location of trace amounts (picogram quantities) of toxic components, such as phytoalexins and possibly minerals and vitamins. Enzyme-linked immunosorbent assay (ELISA) techniques have also been used for the detection of minor constituents such as soybean protein in meat products, although there are available other routine methods of analysis such as electrophoresis and light microscopy for the detection of such constituents.

In the enzyme-linked immunosorbent assay method a specific enzyme labelled reagent – which is an antispecies immunoglobulin – is used for the detection of the immune products. The technique is analogous to the radioimmune assays. The presence of the enzyme

(E) on the antispecies immunoglobulin, permits the final visualisation of the total complex by means of a specific enzyme assay. For the enzyme labelled 'anti-immunoglobulin', the fraction of the catalytic activity of the bound enzyme is proportional to the antibody content of the sample. The anti-immunoglobulin enzyme conjugate is prepared by coupling the enzyme to the anti-immunoglobulin by means of glutaraldehyde or other coupling agents. In order to prevent non-specific interactions it is important that the soluble antibody and anti-immunoglobulin are raised in quite unrelated phyla species. The enzymes chosen for linking have included alkaline phosphatase, β-

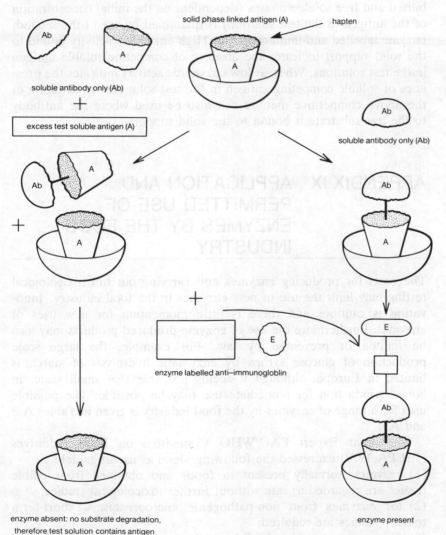

Fig. A.15 Competitive antigen ELISA technique

galactosidase and in particular horseradish peroxidase. The bound enzymatic activity is detected by spectrophotometric assay. For the ELISA technique a microplate consisting of ninety-six wells each of 0.4 cm³ volume is used.

There are a number of experimental modifications of the ELISA technique. Shown in Fig. A.15 is an indirect procedure which depends on the stoichiometric relationship between antibody and antigen. A competitive technique for ELISA is where the assay incorporates a competition between the specific antigen previously immobilised to a solid surface, and the test soluble antigen for antibodies specific to the antigen. The resulting distribution of antibodies between the immobilised and free soluble phases (dependent on the initial concentration of the antigen in the test solution) is quantified by use of the second, enzyme labelled anti-immunoglobin. High enzymatic activity bound to the solid support indicates the absence of competing soluble antigen in the test solutions. Whereas low enzymatic activity indicates the presence of soluble competing antigen in the test solutions. A variation of the above competitive method can also be used where the antibody to the test substrate is bound to the solid support.

APPENDIX IX   APPLICATION AND PERMITTED USE OF ENZYMES BY THE FOOD INDUSTRY

The costs for producing enzymes and carrying out full toxicological testing may limit the use of new enzymes in the food industry. Innovation is cautious and there is little momentum for new uses of enzymes. Furthermore the use of enzyme-produced products may also be limited or prevented by law. For example, the large scale production of glucose syrups by enzymatic hydrolysis of starch is limited in Europe, although it seems probable that small scale 'in house' production for immediate use may be possible. The possible uses for a range of enzymes by the food industry is given in Tables A.3 and A.4.

The Joint Expert FAO/WHO Committee on Food Additives (JECFA 1978) expressed the following views as useful guidelines:
(1) enzymes normally present in foods and obtained from edible tissues are regarded as safe without further toxicological studies;
(2) for enzymes from non-pathogenic microorganisms, short-term toxicity studies are required;
(3) for enzymes from less 'well known' sources extensive toxicological studies are required in rodent species.

Table A.3 Uses for range of enzymes in the food industry

Purpose analysis	Possible enzymes	Capital equipment	Comment
Glucose	Glucose oxidase: hexokinase, glucose-6-phosphate dehydrogenase	UV or visible spectrophotometer	A microelectrode incorporating glucose oxidase has been designed
	Glucose dehydrogenase	Visible spectrophotometer	A direct estimation using only one enzyme
Fructose	Hexokinase, glucose-6-phosphate isomerase, glucose-6-phosphate dehydrogenase	UV spectrophotometer	
	Fructose dehydrogenase linked $Fe(CN)_6^{3-}$	Visible spectrophotometer	A direct estimation using only one enzyme
Galactose	Galactose oxidase linked to peroxidase, galactose dehydrogenase linked to $Fe(CN)_6^{3-}$	Visible spectrophotometer	
Sucrose	Invertase and then as for glucose or fructose	UV spectrophotometer	No enzyme has been found for the direct oxidation or reduction of sucrose The free monosaccharides require separate estimation
Lactose	β-Galactosidase and then as for glucose or galactose using galactose dehydrogenase, cellobiose oxidase	UV spectrophotometer	The free monosaccharides require separate estimation A direct estimation using only one enzyme
Maltose	α-Glucosidase and then as for glucose	UV or visible spectrophotometer	The free monosaccharides require separate estimation
Raffinose and stachyose	α-Galactosidase and then as for galactose using galactose dehydrogenase	UV spectrophotometer	Other α-galactosides such as galactopinitols will be included

Table A.4 Possible uses for a range of enzymes in the food industry[†]

Purpose processing aids	Possible enzymes	Sources	Benefits[‡]
For Carbohydrates			
Starch	α-Amylase	Pancreatic tissues	Production of syrups, bread improvers
	β-Amylase	Fungi and bacteria	
	β-Glucoamylase		
	Pullulanase		
Cellulose	Cellulases	Fungi	Production of syrups, and coffee whiteners
	β-Glucanases		
	β-Glucosidases		
	Dextranases		
Hemicellulose	Hemicellulase	Bacteria	Reduce viscosity, removal of colloidal precipitates
Pectins	Pectinesterase	Fungi and bacteria	
	Pectin lyase		
	Polygalacturonase		
Alginates	Epimerase		Enhance gelation
Gums	Carbohydrases		Aid gelation
Pentosans	Pentosanase	Fungi and bacteria	Reduce viscosity
Dextrins	Dextrinases	Fungi	
Raffinose series	α-Galactosidase	Microorganism	Reduce flatulence factors
Lactose	β-Galactosidase	Fungi and yeasts	Removal of colloidal precipitates
Sucrose	Invertase	Yeast	Sweetening
Glucose	Glucose isomerase	Fungi and bacteria	Sweetening
	Glucose oxidase	Fungi	Reduce non-enzymic browning, oxygen removal.

For proteins

Enzyme	Source	Application
Rennin	Calf stomach	Cheese manufacture
Carboxyl proteinases	Fungi	Cheese manufacture
Pepsin	Stomach	
Papain	Papaya plant	Tenderisation of meat, solubilisation of proteins, for instant foods and concentrates
Bromelain	Pineapple	
Ficin	Fig	
Serine proteinase	Pancreas	Solubilisation of proteins and concentrates
Neutral proteinase	Fungi	

For fats and oils

Enzyme	Source	Application
Lipases	Stomach tissues	Transesterification of fats
	Fungi	
Lipoxygenase	Plant seeds	Bread flour improver

Other constituents

Constituent	Enzyme	Source	Application
Phenols	Phenolases	Plants	Possible colouring agents
Fatty acids	Esterases	Plants	Flavouring
Naringin	Naringinase	Fungi	Debittering
Anthocyanins	Glycosidases	Plants	Decolouring
Carotenoids	Lipoxygenases	Plants	Bleaching
Sulphur compounds	Allinases	Plants	
	Myrosinases	Plants	Flavouring

† The listing does not mean that any of the enzymes or their sources have been approved which varies between countries. In the United States GRAS (generally recognised as safe) status is given to some of the enzymes while elsewhere some enzymes may be included in permitted lists.

‡ The absorption to inert support material or encapsulation may influence subsequent proteolysis and thus affect the toxicological properties.

Such requirements are, in general terms, similar to those for the use of chemical additives, including colours, flavours, stabilisers and emulsifiers. During the last 30 years increased knowledge of toxins, carcinogens, mutagens and allergic substances has led to an awareness of potential hazards associated with all foods. It is now being increasingly realised that not all enzymes are harmless under all circumstances. The products of enzymatic action need to be safe and in at least one well known case, for the action of pectin esterase, both methanol and possibly formaldehyde are direct and indirect products which arise from the action of the enzyme. Peptides with neurological properties may also be produced by the action of proteinases (Zioudrou *et al.* 1979). For microbial enzymes the main fear is associated toxin production, the detection of which is largely dependent on efficient and rapid screening tests which in future may be based on immunological assay methods.

Enzymes may be classified as: analytical; pharmaceutical; food and technical. For the latter group, good analytical methods are also required for assignment of assay methods for the determination of essential purity of such enzymes to be used in food. As many enzymes contain metal cofactors, adventitious uptake of metals during large scale processing and preparation of enzymes is also a potential hazard, as of course it may also be with protein preparations in general. However, the new protein–mycoprotein (Edelman *et al.* 1983) has undergone nutritional and toxicological testing and received approval for marketing in the United Kingdom from the Ministry of Agriculture, Fisheries and Food. The principle and the protocol developed is likely to form the framework for future testing of new foods and maybe, if required, less common essential food products.

The reports for the evaluation of food enzymes are JECFA (1978, 1981), MAFF (1982) which includes a report of the Committee on Toxicity. For the United Kingdom, MAFF (1982) recommended that Group A and B enzymes be included in a permitted list (Table A5).

Table A.5 Recommended permitted list of enzymes by the Committee on Toxicity in the United Kingdom[†]

Source		Enzyme preparation
Group A	*Ananas comosus*	Bromelain
	Ananas bracteatus	Bromelain
	Carica papaya	Papain; chymopapain
	Edible oral or forestomach tissues of the calf, kid or lamb	Triacylglycerol lipase
	Porcine or bovine pancreatic tissues	Triacylglycerol lipase
		α-Amylase
		Trypsin

Table A.5   (Cont'd)

	Porcine gastric mucosa	Pepsin A, B and C
	Abdomasum of calf, kid or lamb	Chymosin (rennet)
	Adult bovine abdomasum	Bovine pepsin A and B
	Bovine liver	Catalase
Group B	*Aspergillus niger*	α-Amylase
		Immobilised and non-immobilised exo-1,4-α-D-glucosidase (glucoamylase)
		Cellulase
		β-D-Galactosidase (lactase)
		Endo-1,3(4)-β-D-glucanase
		Glucose oxidase
		Catalase
		Pectinesterase
		Pectin lyase
		Polygalacturonase
	Aspergillus oryzae	α-Amylase
		Neutral proteinase
	Bacillus coagulans	Immobilised and non-immobilised glucose isomerase
	Bacillus licheniformis	α-Amylase
		Serine proteinase
	Bacillus subtilis	α-Amylase
		Endo-1,3(4)-β-D-glucanase
		Neutral proteinase
	Endothia parasitica	Endothia carboxyl proteinase
	Klebsiella aerogenes	Pullulanase
	Mucor miehei	Acid proteinase
	Mucor pusillus	Acid proteinase
	Penicillium emersonii	Endo-1,3(4)-β-D-glucanase
	Penicillium funiculosum	Dextranase‡
	Penicillium lilacinum	Dextranase‡
	Saccharomyces cerevisiae	β-D-fructofuranosidase (invertase)
	Streptomyces fradiae	Serine proteinase
	Streptomyces olivaceous	Immobilised glucose isomerase
	Trichoderma viride	Cellulase

(† From MAFF 1982). Reproduced with permission from Report on the preview of enzyme preparations 1982 paragraph 25.

‡ In the case of dextranases from *Penicillium funiculosum* and *Penicillium lilacinum*, it is recommended that they should only be permitted in the early stages of sugar refining.

Group A: substances that the available evidence suggests are acceptable for use in food.

Group B: substances that on the available evidence may be regarded meanwhile as provisionally acceptable for use in food, but about which further information must be made available within a specified time for review. In the United States specifications for enzyme preparations have been given by the NAS/NRC (1981a,b). Enzyme preparations should be free of pathogenic bacteria and antibiotics and should be non-toxic. However, in the United States the position is less clear because of the designation of 'generally recognised as safe' (GRAS status) and GRAS status may be obtained by scientific assessment independent of the FDA.

APPENDIX X   BIOSYNTHESIS OF ISOPRENOID COMPOUNDS

Carotenoids, tocopherols, vitamin K, terpenes, the phytyl group of chlorophyll and steroids possess an isoprenoid structure derived biosynthetically from the mevalonic acid pathway. Mevalonic acid and the subsequent activated isopentenylpyrophosphate are synthesised from three molecules of acetyl CoA (Fig. A.16). The stereochemistry of the enzymatic reactions and the R S nomenclature describing the absolute configuration at a chiral centre is given by Goodwin (1974, 1979).

Isomerisation of isopentenylpyrophosphate to dimethylallylpyrophosphate catalysed by isopentenyldiphosphate isomerase (EC 5.3.3.2) followed by condensation with a molecule of the five-carbon isopentenyl pyrophosphate results in the formation of the ten-carbon compound (Fig. A.17).

Essential oils are complex mixtures, but frequently contain the volatile mono- and sesquiterpenes. Diterpenoids are contained in the oleoresins of conifers and triterpenoids are mainly polycyclic compounds. Oleoresins are the concentrated soluble residues which contain volatile substances obtained by solvent extraction.

For food aroma, terpenes and the biosynthetically related benzenoid compounds are of particular significance. Many of the monoterpenes also undergo ring closure to produce unsaturated cyclic acids. The main monoterpenes responsible for aroma are alcohols and aldehydes which are formed from geranyl pyrophosphate cyclisation by hydrolysis, oxidation and isomerisation (Fig. A.18). The monocyclic alkanes occur widely in plant tissue from which many of the oxygenated derivatives are formed. Interconversions catalysed by dehydrogenases seem likely. Further oxidation may arise through the action of oxygen

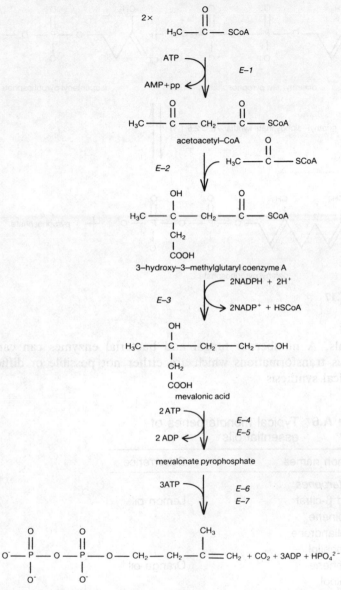

Fig. A.16 The pathway of conversion of acetyl CoA to 3-isopentenyl pyrophosphate

E–1   acetoacetyl-CoA synthase (EC 6.2.1.16)
E–2   3-hydroxy-3-methylglutaryl CoA synthase (EC 4.1.3.5)
E–3   3-hydroxy-3-methylglutaryl CoA reductase (EC 1.1.1.34)
E–4   mevalonate kinase (EC 2.7.1.36)
E–5   phosphomevalonate kinase (EC 2.7.4.2)
E–6   mevalonate kinase
E–7   mevalonate pyrophosphate decarboxylase

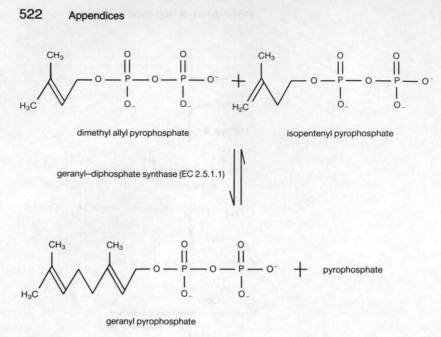

dimethyl allyl pyrophosphate

isopentenyl pyrophosphate

geranyl–diphosphate synthase (EC 2.5.1.1)

geranyl pyrophosphate   + pyrophosphate

Fig. A.17

radicals. A number of fungal and bacterial enzymes can carry out various transformations which are either not possible or difficult by chemical synthesis.

Table A.6 Typical monoterpenes of essential oils

Common names	Occurrence
Monoterpenes	
α- and β-citral	Lemon oil
γ-Terpinene	
α-Phellandrene	
δ-Citronellol	
δ-Limonene	Orange oil
δ-Linalool	
Menthol	Mint oil
Carvone	Carraway
Myrcene	Bay leaves
Thymol	Thyme
Sesquiterpenes	
Zingiberene	Ginger
Nootkatone	Grapefruit
Selinene	Celery oil
α-Eudesmol	Eucalyptus oil

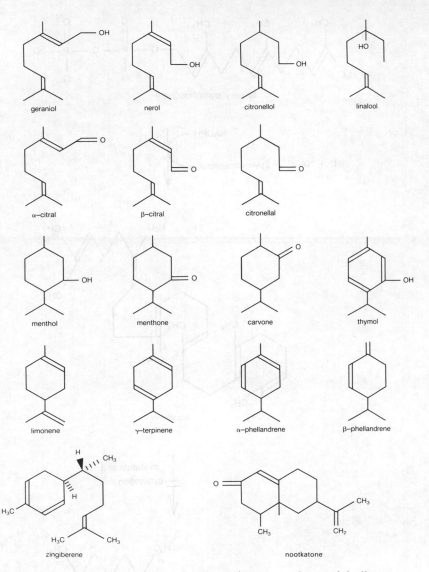

Fig. A.18 Typical monoterpenes and sesquiterpenes of essential oils

The classification of the terpenes is related to the number of isoprene units:

monoterpenes (C-10)   –2 isoprenyl units
sesquiterpenes (C-15)   –3 isoprenyl units
diterpenes (C-20)   –4 isoprenyl units
triterpenes (C-30)   –6 isoprenyl units
tetraterpenes (C-40)   –8 isoprenyl units

Geranyl pyrophosphate is also a precursor of the higher terpenes which include the liminoids, squalene, carotenoids and steroids which

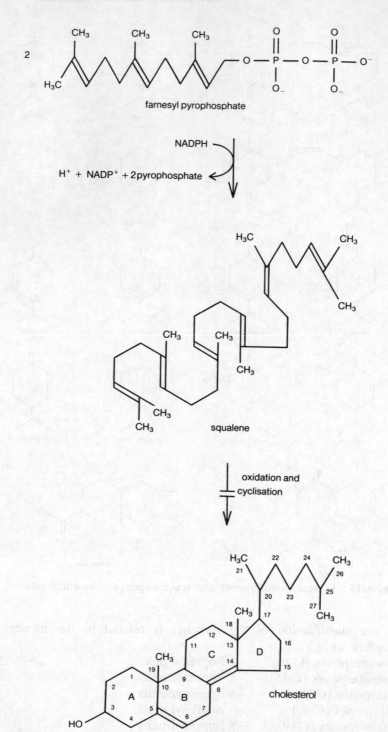

2

farnesyl pyrophosphate

NADPH

H⁺ + NADP⁺ + 2 pyrophosphate

squalene

oxidation and cyclisation

cholesterol

Fig. A.19 Biosynthesis of cholesterol

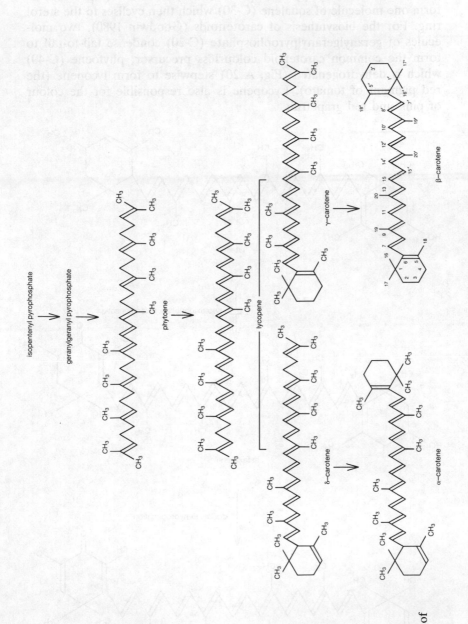

are all formed by consecutive addition of five-carbon isoprene units and condensation reactions. In the animal pathway to sterols two molecules of farnesyl pyrophosphate (C-15) condense (Fig. A.19) to form one molecule of squalene (C-30) which then cyclises to the sterol ring. For the biosynthesis of carotenoids (Goodwin 1980), two molecules of geranylgeranylpyrophosphate (C-20) condense tail-to-tail to form the common carotenoid colourless precursor, phytoene (C-40) which is dehydrogenated (Fig. A.20) stepwise to form lycopene (the red pigment of tomato). Lycopene is also responsible for the colour of pink and red grapefruit.

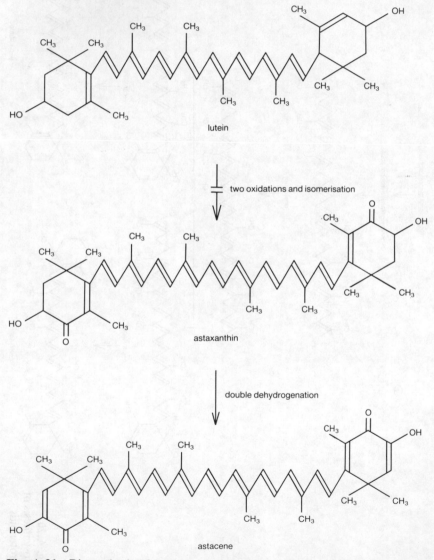

lutein

two oxidations and isomerisation

astaxanthin

double dehydrogenation

astacene

Fig. A.21 Biosynthesis of astacene

The cyclic carotenoids are formed by the action of cyclising enzymes. Oxygenated derivatives are xanthophylls which have no vitamin A activity. The characteristic colours are due to the presence of linear chains of conjugated double bonds. In α-carotene the double bond is displaced in the ionone ring, whereas in δ- and γ-carotene only one ionone ring is formed. All photosynthetic tissues contain carotenoids in the grana of the chloroplast. On ripening in fruits carotenoid biosynthesis is stimulated. Lutein, a yellow xanthophyll (the 3,3'-dihydroxy derivative of α-carotene) occurs extensively in fruits, vegetables and eggs. Higher animals are unable to carry out biosynthesis of carotenoids, but some fish can convert lutein to astaxanthin (Fig. A.21), a red pigment found in salmon, crab, lobster and other marine species. Retinol derivatives like 3,4-didehydroretinal are also formed from lutein by fish. In citrus fruits more than 100 different carotenoids have been claimed to be present. However, the most

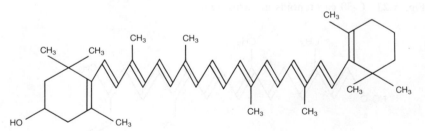

α—cryptoxanthin

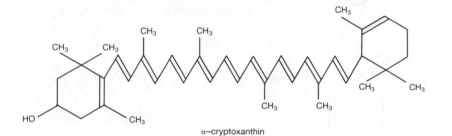

β—cryptoxanthin

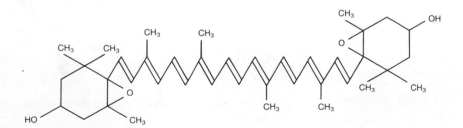

violaxanthin

Fig. A.22

important in orange juice are α- and β-carotenes, α-cryptoxanthin, β-cryptoxanthin, lutein and violaxanthin (Fig. A.22). Carotenoids containing thirty carbon atoms (the apocarotenes) are present in citrus peel and arise by the degradation of the C-40 carotenoids. The C-30 carotenoids, β-citraurin and β-apo-8'-carotenal (Fig. A.23) contain a carbonyl group conjugated with the polyene chain, which is responsible for the intense red-to-purple colour in the peels of citrus hybrids. The colour of annato which is used in margarine and cheese is due to

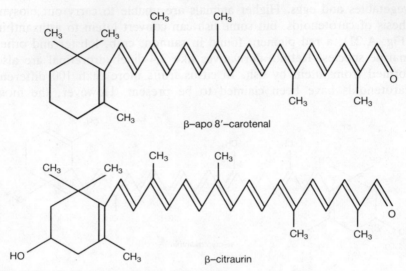

β–apo 8'–carotenal

β–citraurin

Fig. A.23   C-30 carotenoids in citrus peel

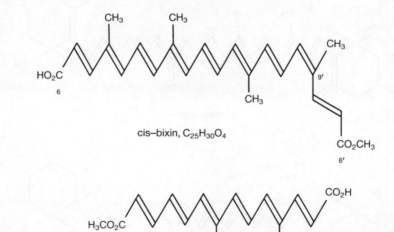

cis–bixin, $C_{25}H_{30}O_4$

C-17 yellow pigment

Fig. A.24

the presence of *cis*-bixin (a C-25 carotenoid) (Fig. A.24) and its degradation products obtained from the pericarp extract of *Bixa orellana*. During extraction at 130 °C red *cis*-bixin is partially isomerised to the *trans*-form and degraded to produce a C-17 yellow carotenoid derivative (Fig. A.24). The colour of the mixture of the C-25 and C-17 carotenoids matches the colour required for margarine.

Due to the high degree of unsaturation, carotenoids are easily oxidised and degraded by microorganisms and some of the products often contain oxidised derivatives of the ionone rings (Fig. A.25). β-Ionone possesses a violet aroma and may occur in incorrectly stored carrots.

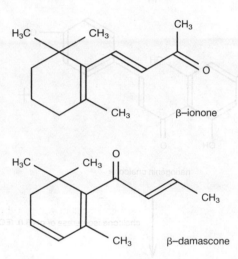

Fig. A.25

APPENDIX XI   FLAVONOIDS

The common molecular structure of the flavonoids is a C-15 skeleton of two benzene rings (A and B) joined together by a central three-carbon group, a chromane ring. Flavonoids have been reviewed by Hahlbrock (1981) and Rouseff (1980).

All the flavonoids have a common precursor which arises from phenylalanine or tyrosine by deamination catalysed by phenylalanine ammonia lyase to form cinnamic acid and then condensation of malonyl CoA and acetyl CoA units in a head-to-tail manner (Fig. A.26). Malonyl CoA is formed by the action of acetyl CoA carboxylase (EC 6.4.1.2).

$$CH_3-CO-SCoA + HCO_3^- + ATP \rightleftharpoons {}^-O_2C-CH_2-CO-SCoA + ADP + HPO_4^{2-}$$

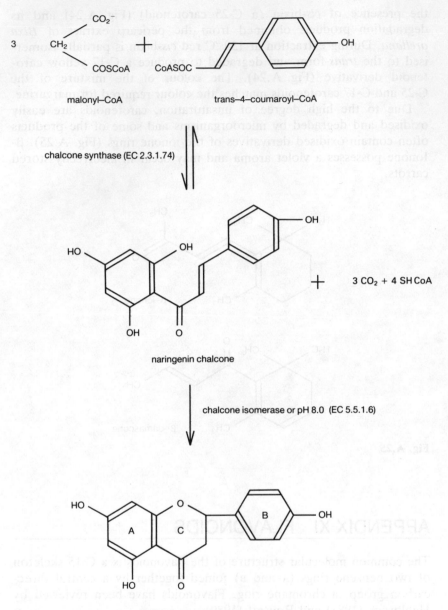

Fig. A.26 Scheme for the biosynthesis of naringenin

Glycosylation is from UDP-glucose and other UDP-sugars catalysed by specific transferases.

The flavonoids are prevalent in the higher plants and are found in roots, stems, flowers, fruit and seeds. They occur as *O*-glycosides so that the phenolic groups substituted in rings A and B are protected.

Most are derivatives substituted in the 5,7,-3' and 4' positions. For the isoflavanones and isoflavones the B-ring is at position 3.

The range of flavonoids is obtained by modification of the intermediate through dehydrogenation and hydroxylation reactions. The different types of flavonoids are classified by the level of oxidation of the chromane ring where catechins are the least oxidised forms of the chromane c-ring (Fig. A.27). The most frequent derivatives, the anthocyanins (glycosylated anthocyanidin bases), are the more highly oxidised flavonol glycosides. Not all the hydroxyl groups are glycosy-

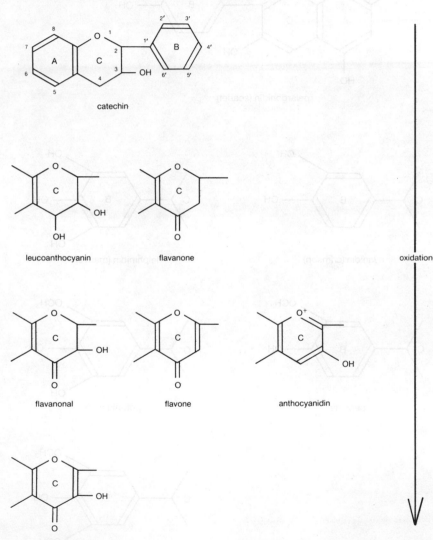

Fig. A.27 The various oxidation-states of the chromane c-ring in flavonoids (Rouseff 1980)

lated as some are protected by methylation. However, for antho-cyanins, glycosylation at position 3 is necessary to stabilise the ring structure as the aglycones (the anthocyanidines) rapidly decompose with loss of colour. There are basically six types of anthocyanidins which differ only in the number of hydroxyl groups present in the B-

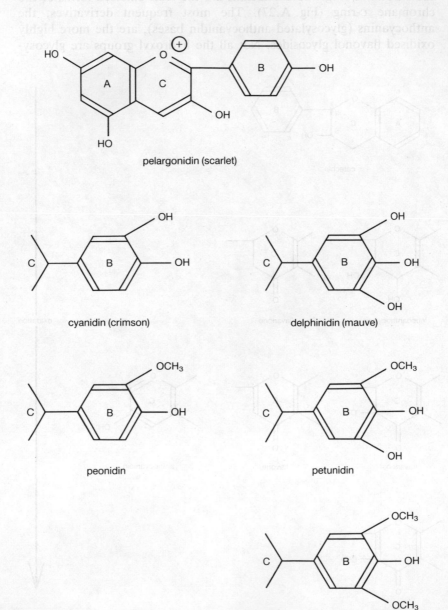

pelargonidin (scarlet)

cyanidin (crimson)

delphinidin (mauve)

peonidin

petunidin

malvidin

Fig. A.28 Hydroxylation and methylation of the B-rings of anthocyanins

ring. Thus these six types can give rise to a very large number of different anthocyanins. The methyl ethers of cyanidin and delphinidin are peonidin, petunidin and malvidin as shown in (Fig. A.28). As the pyrone ring in the flavylium cation is electron deficient, the anthocyanidins are highly reactive and rapidly decolorise in fresh homogenised fruits and during preservation.

The aglycones of the common flavonol glycosides are kaempferol, quercetin and myricetin (Fig. A.29) found mainly in flowers and leaves and are colourless at the pH of the cell sap. In the flavone glycosides, the hydroxyl group in position 3 is absent. The flavones occur mainly in herbaceous plants.

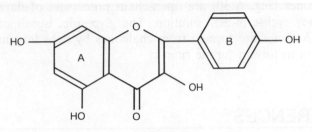

kaempferol

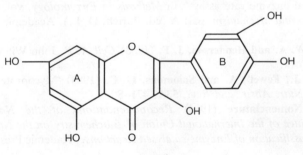

quercetin

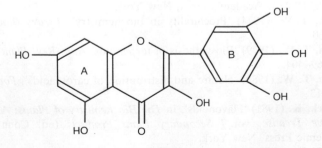

myricetin

Fig. A.29 The aglycones of flavonol glycosides

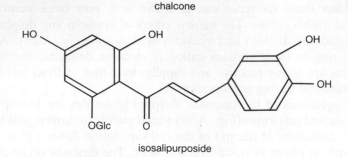

Fig. A.30   Chalcone

Chalcones (Fig. A.30) are open-chain precursors of flavanones to which they cyclise in acid solution. The glycoside, isosalipurposide is yellow. Aurones are formed from chalcones by dehydrogenation and cyclisation to form a furone ring.

REFERENCES

Allison, R. D. and Purich, D. L. (1979) 'Practical considerations in the design of initial enzyme rate assays', in *Methods in Enzymology*, vol. 63 *Enzyme Kinetics and Mechanism*, part A (ed. Purich, D. L.). Academic Press, New York.

Bridger, W. A. and Henderson, J. F. (1983) *Cell ATP*. John Wiley and Sons, New York.

Edelman, J., Fewell, A. and Solomons, G. C. (1983) 'Mycoprotein – a new food', *Nutr. Abstr. and Rev.*, **53A**, 471–80.

Enzyme Nomenclature (1984) *Recommendations of the Nomenclature Committee of the International Union of Biochemistry on the Nomenclature and Classification of Enzyme-catalysed Reactions*. Academic Press, Orlando, Florida.

Fromm, H. J. (1979) 'Summary of kinetic reaction mechanisms', in *Methods in Enzymology*, vol. 63 *Enzyme Kinetics and Mechanism*, part A (ed. Purich, D. L.). Academic Press, New York.

Goodwin, T. W. (1974) 'Prochirality in biochemistry', *Essays Biochem.*, **9**, 103–60.

Goodwin, T. W. (1979) 'Biosynthesis of terpenoids' *Ann. Rev. Plant Physiol.*, **30**, 369–404.

Goodwin, T. W. (1980) 'Nature and distribution of carotenoids', *Food Chem.* **5**, 3–13.

Hahlbrock, K. (1981) 'Flavonoids', in *The Biochemistry of Plants: A Comprehensive Treatise*, vol. 7 *Secondary Plant Products* (ed. Conn, E. E.). Academic Press, New York.

Holme, D. J. and Peck, H. (1983) *Analytical Biochemistry*. Longman, London.

JECFA (1978) Joint FAO/WHO Expert Committee on Food Additives. WHO Technical Report, series No. 617.

JECFA (1981) Food and Nutrition Paper no. 19, 25th session of the Joint Expert Committee on Food Additives. FAO/WHO, Rome.

MAFF (1982) Food Additives and Contaminants Committee, Report on the review of enzyme preparation FAC/REP 35 (includes the report of the committee on toxicity of chemicals in food, consumer products and the environment). HMSO, London.

NAS/NRC (1981a) The 1978 enzyme survey, National Academy of Sciences/National Research Council, Food and Nutrition Board, Committee on GRAS List Survey. National Academy Press, Washington DC.

NAS/NRC (1981b) *Food Chemicals Codex* (3rd edn.). National Academy of Sciences/National Research Council, Food and Nutrition Board, Committee on Codex Specifications. National Academy Press, Washington DC.

Rouseff, R. L. (1980) 'Flavonoids and citrus quality', in *Citrus Nutrition and Quality* (Eds. Nagy, S. and Attaway, J. A.). ACS Symposium Series 143, American Chemical Society, Washington DC.

Stryer, L. (1981) *Biochemistry* (2nd edn.). Freeman and Co., San Francisco, California

Thompson, J. (1978) '*In vivo* regulation of glycolysis and characterisation of sugar : phosphotransferase systems in *Streptococcus lactis*', *J. Bacteriol.*, **136**, 465–75.

Zioudrou, D., Streaty, R. A. and Klee, W. A. (1979) 'Opioid peptides derived from food proteins', *J. Biol. Chem.*, **254**, 2446–9.

Index

Note: illustrations (Figures) are indicated by *italic page numbers*, major sections by **bold page numbers**.